PRINCIPLES OF
MAGNETIC RESONANCE IMAGING

PRINCIPLES OF MAGNETIC RESONANCE IMAGING

A Signal Processing Perspective

Zhi-Pei Liang
Department of Electrical and Computer Engineering
University of Illinois at Urbana-Champaign
Urbana, Illinois

Paul C. Lauterbur
Department of Medical Information Sciences
University of Illinois at Urbana-Champaign
Urbana, Illinois

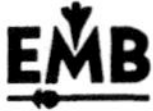

IEEE Engineering in Medicine and Biology Society, *Sponsor*

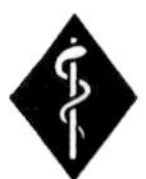

IEEE Press Series on Biomedical Engineering
Metin Akay, *Series Editor*

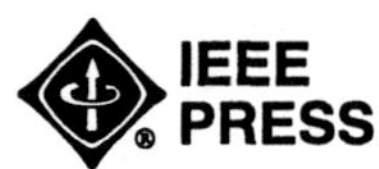

The Institute of Electrical and Electronics Engineers, Inc., New York

© 2000 by the Institute of Electrical and Electronics Engineers, Inc.
3 Park Avenue, 17th Floor, New York, NY 10016-5997

Printed in the United States of America

10   9   8   7   6   5   4   3   2   1

ISBN 0-7803-4723-4
IEEE Order Number: PC5769

SPIE ISBN 0-8194-3516-3

Library of Congress Cataloging-in-Publication Data

Liang, Zhi-Pei, 1961–
    Principles of magnetic resonance imaging : a signal processing
  perspective / Zhi-Pei Liang, Paul C. Lauterbur : IEEE Engineering in
  Medicine and Biology Society, sponsor.
        p.   cm. -- (IEEE Press series in biomedical engineering)
    Includes bibliographical references and index.
    ISBN 0-7803-4723-4
    1. Magnetic resonance imaging Congresses. 2. Nuclear magnetic
  resonance Congresses. 3. Signal processing Congresses.
    I. Lauterbur, Paul C., 1929–   . II. IEEE Engineering in Medicine
  and Biology Society.   III. Title.   IV. Series.
  RC78.7.N83L36   1999
    616.07'548--dc21   99-27706
                                                                 CIP

Books in the IEEE Press Series in Biomedical Engineering

Time Frequency and Wavelets in Biomedical Signal Processing
Edited by Metin Akay
1998   Hardcover   768 pp   IEEE Order No. PC5619   ISBN 0-7803-1147-7

Physiological Control Systems
Michael C.K. Khoo
2000   Hardcover   344 pp   IEEE Order No. PC5680   ISBN 0-7803-3408-6

Neural Networks and Artificial Intelligence for Biomedical Engineering
Donna L. Hudson and Maurice E. Cohen
2000   Hardcover   324 pp   IEEE Order No. PC5675   ISBN 0-7803-3404-3

Contents

Preface

The story is told that young King Solomon was given the choice between wealth and wisdom. When he chose wisdom, God was so pleased that he gave Solomon not only wisdom but wealth also. So it is with science.

Arthur Holly Compton

Because of the unique function of our visual system for information gathering and processing, images or pictures play a central role in our daily lives. In fact, much of what we know about ourselves and the world around us has been derived from images produced by various imaging devices. Magnetic resonance imaging (MRI), in particular, can produce images from human or any biological system noninvasively that reveal the structure, metabolism, and function of internal tissues or organs, greatly extending the range of human vision into realms that would otherwise be inaccessible. The impact of this imaging technique on diagnostic radiology has been revolutionary in the last two decades because of its capability to produce anatomical images with unprecedented quality and safety to the patient. With the ever-improving technology to produce images at higher speed (ultra-fast imaging), higher resolution (microimaging), and higher information content (combined anatomical, metabolic, and functional imaging), MRI will likely have similar impact in biology and neuroscience in the years to come.

Functionally, MRI can be regarded as one of the tomographic imaging techniques that produce images of the interior of an object from data collected outside. What really makes it more fascinating and attractive scientifically than many other techniques are its versatility and flexibility. To quote a popular saying of Erwin Hahn, "there is nothing that nuclear spins will not do for you, as long as you treat them as human beings."

This book is about MRI. Although its working principles are not the easiest to understand for beginning students, they are certainly fun to learn. This book is our attempt to help your endeavor. In contrast to many existing books on this subject, our discussions will be based on a signal processing approach in which the descriptions of the fundamental concepts and principles center around a signal. This approach is motivated largely by the consideration that understanding how MR signals are generated, detected, manipulated, and processed into an image is essential. The book has ten chapters covering five major topics of MRI: (1) signal generation, detection, and characteristics, (2) spatial localization principles, (3) image reconstruction, (4) image resolution, contrast, noise, and artifacts, and (5) advanced concepts on data acquisition (fast-scan imaging) and processing (constrained reconstruction). The style of presentation is aimed at upper-level undergraduate and graduate engineering students for use as a textbook on this subject. Toward this end, we have included homework problems in each chapter to assist the instructors in teaching and the students in learning the material. In addition, we hope that the materials are covered at an appropriate level to be useful as a reference for medical imaging scientists in this field.

Zhi-Pei Liang
Paul C. Lauterbur
University of Illinois at Urbana-Champaign

Acknowledgments

This book is based on the lecture notes developed for a senior to graduate-level course on magnetic resonance imaging in the Department of Electrical and Computer Engineering at the University of Illinois at Urbana-Champaign (UIUC). Many of my friends, colleagues, and students deserve much credit for helping bring this book to fruition. In particular, I wish to thank Professors Paul C. Lauterbur, E. Mark Haacke, Joan Dawson, Richard Magin, Jianming Jin, Steve Wright, Xiaohong Zhou, Fernando Boada, and Andrew Webb for discussions that were of great assistance to me in writing the book. These and many other researchers whom I may or may not have the opportunity of meeting personally have laid the foundation of this exciting field and helped make this book directly or indirectly. I would also like to thank Jill Hanson, Chris Hess, K.-T. Yang, Andrew Harris, Brian Stewart, Marc Kowalski, Jeffrey Tsao, and Weng Chew for their helpful comments and suggestions about the manuscript. I appreciate the efforts of Jamie Hutchinson and Betty C. Pessagno in copyediting the entire manuscript. I am grateful for the errors they caught but any remaining ones are mine alone. A special thanks goes to Fang-Pei Liang for his encouragement and moral support, to Metin Akay (the Series Editor) for his tremendous help and understanding during the preparation of the manuscript, and to Cherik Bulkes, Jingfei Ma, Qing-San Xiang, and Fernando Boada for providing some valuable MR images. I gratefully acknowledge Hong Xie, Jill Hanson, Nina Parsons, Chris Hess, Jim Ji, Song Wang, Hong Jiang, Mark Skouson, and Hao Pan for their help in preparing some of the figures. This project benefited considerably from research support from the National Science Foundation, National Institutes of Health, the UIUC Beckman Institute for Advanced Science and Technology, and the UIUC Center for Advanced Study.

Finally, and most important of all, I am greatly indebted to my wife, Bo, and my daughter, Annie, for their constant encouragement, understanding, support, and love, without which this book would not have been possible. This book is dedicated to them and to the memory of my younger brother Liang, Sheng-Pei, who selflessly devoted his short life to medicine.

Zhi-Pei Liang
University of Illinois at Urbana-Champaign

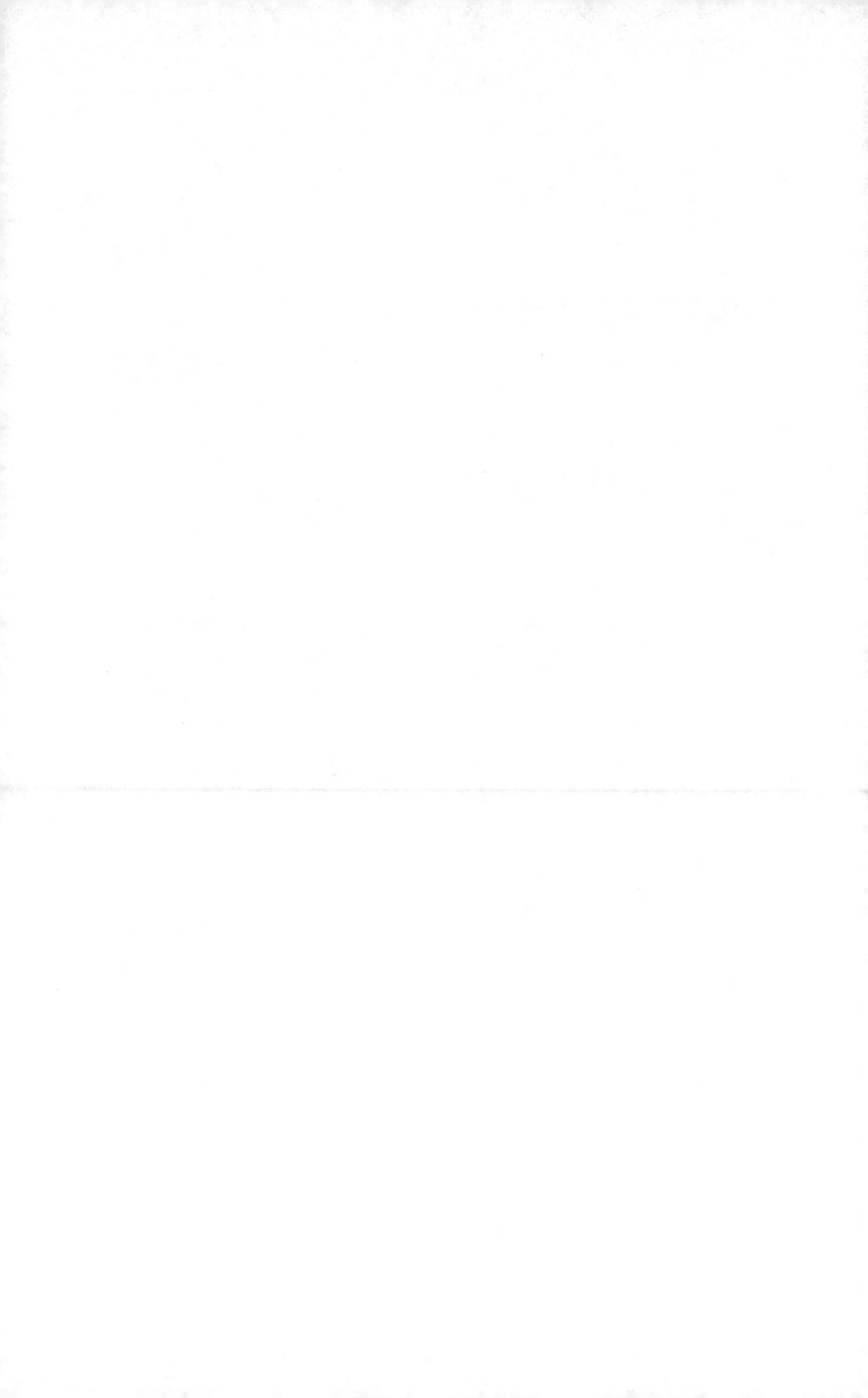

Chapter 1

Introduction

> *A journey of a thousand miles must begin with a single step.*
>
> *Lao Zi*

Tomography is an important area in the ever-growing field of imaging science. The term *tomos* ($\tau o\mu o\varsigma$) means "cut" in Greek, but tomography is concerned with creating images of the internal (anatomical or functional) organization of an object without physically cutting it open. To a beginner, it might seem inconceivable, but as your reading of this book progresses, you will appreciate not only the feasibility but also the inherent beauty and simplicity of tomography.

Tomographic imaging principles are rooted in physics, mathematics, computer science, and engineering. However, development of these principles is traditionally tied to solving application problems—particularly biomedical problems. Therefore, their theoretical significance has not been well appreciated by researchers outside this field. Like any other scientific discipline, tomography has a unique history. Radon was perhaps the first to address the tomographic imaging issue, albeit from a purely mathematical standpoint. Unfortunately, his seminal work published in 1917 went unnoticed for half a century. The sixties and the seventies were the formative years of tomography when ground-breaking work was done for both X-ray tomography and magnetic resonance imaging (MRI) . Now, a number of tomographic imaging modalities are available for medical and nonmedical uses. A partial list includes X-ray CT (computer tomography), MRI, PET (positron emission tomography), SPECT (single photon emission computed tomography), MEG (magnetoencephalography), SAR (synthetic aperture radar), and various acoustic imaging systems. Although these systems use different physical principles for signal generation and detection, the underlying signal processing principles for image formation are, to a large extent, the same. Therefore, it is fair to say that understanding how one imaging modality works will provide a significant insight into the working principles of other imaging modalities as well.

This book is about MRI. Its emphasis is on the principles of image formation rather than the hardware to build an MRI system or the applications of such a system. The reader is referred to the book by Chen and Hoult [13] on MRI technology or to the two volumes edited by Stark and Bradley [62] on MRI applications.

1.1   What Is MRI?

Simply put, MRI is a tomographic imaging technique that produces images of internal physical and chemical characteristics of an object from externally measured nuclear magnetic resonance (NMR) signals. Physically, MRI is based on the well-known NMR phenomenon observed in bulk matter independently by Felix Bloch at Stanford and Edward Purcell at Harvard in 1946. Image formation using NMR signals is made possible by the spatial information encoding principles, originally coined *zeugmatography* [182], developed by Paul Lauterbur in 1972. These principles enable one to uniquely encode spatial information into the activated MR signals detected outside an object. To help answer the question "What is MRI?" some notable features of MRI are listed below.

First, like any other tomographic imaging device, an MRI scanner outputs a multidimensional data array (or image) representing the spatial distribution of some measured physical quantity. But unlike many of them, MRI can generate two-dimensional sectional images at any orientation, three-dimensional volumetric images, or even four-dimensional images representing spatial-spectral distributions. In addition, no mechanical adjustments to the imaging machinery are involved in generating these images.

Second, MR signals used for image formation come directly from the object itself. In this sense, MRI is a form of *emission* tomography similar to PET and SPECT. But unlike PET or SPECT, no injection of radioactive isotopes into the object is needed for signal generation in MRI. There are other forms of tomography in use, including *transmission* tomography and *diffraction* tomography. X-ray CT belongs to the first category, while most acoustic tomography is of the diffraction type. In both cases, an external signal source is used to "probe" the object being imaged.

Third, MRI operates in the radio-frequency (RF) range, as shown in Fig. 1.1. Therefore, the imaging process does not involve the use of ionizing radiation and does not have the associated potential harmful effects. However, because of the unique imaging scheme used, the resulting spatial resolution of MRI is *not* limited by the "probing" (or working) frequency range as in other remote-sensing technologies.

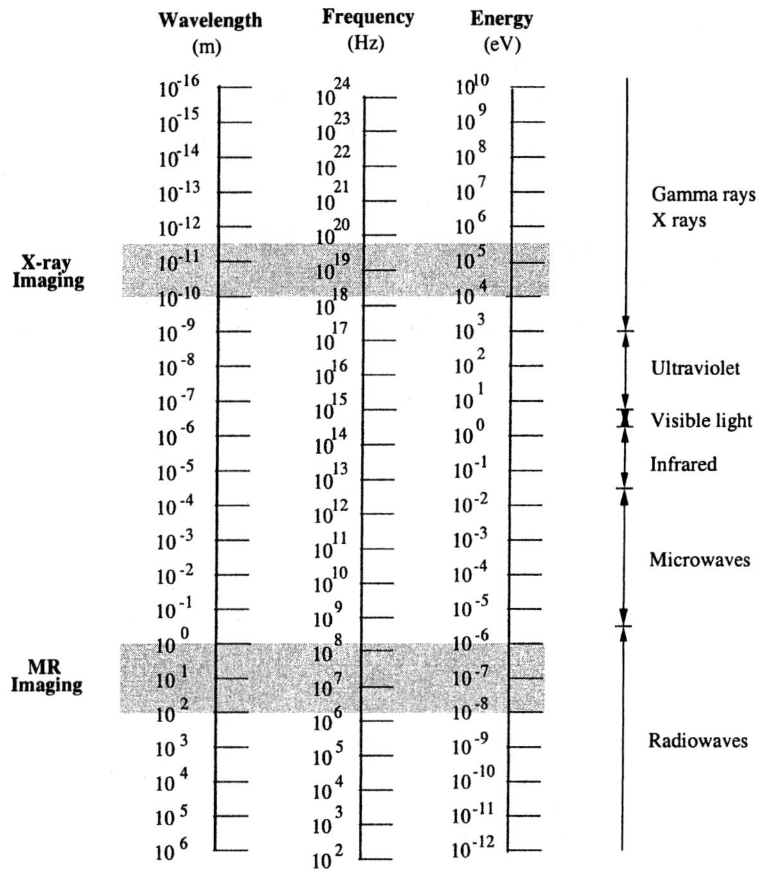

Figure 1.1 Electromagnetic spectrum.

Finally, and perhaps most importantly to an MRI user, MR images are extremely rich in information content. The image pixel value is in general dependent on a host of intrinsic parameters, including the nuclear spin density ρ, the spin-lattice relaxation time T_1, the spin-spin relaxation time T_2, molecular motions (such as diffusion and perfusion), susceptibility effects, and chemical shift differences. The imaging effects of these parameters can be suppressed or enhanced in a specific experiment by another set of operator-selectable parameters, such as repetition time (T_R), echo time (T_E), and flip angle (α). Therefore, an MR image obtained from the same anatomical site can look drastically different with different data acquisition protocols. An example is given in Fig. 1.2, in which the three images shown were obtained from the same cross section of a human head using a so-called spin-echo imaging sequence (discussed in Section 7.4). As can

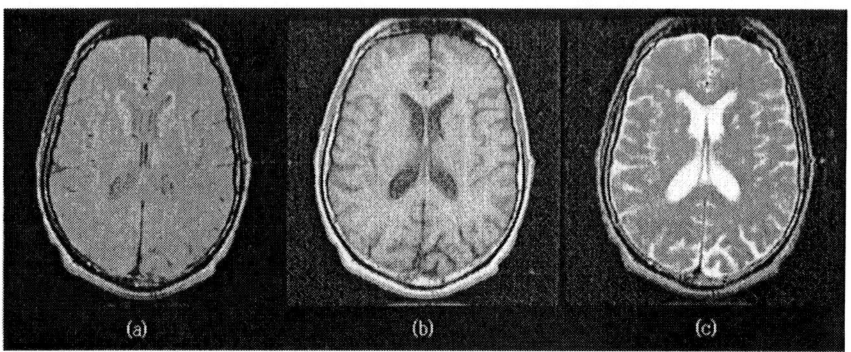

Figure 1.2 Cross-sectional head image obtained using a spin-echo excitation sequence with (a) spin density-weighted contrast ($T_E = 17$ ms, $T_R = 2000$ ms); (b) T_1-weighted contrast ($T_E = 18$ ms, $T_R = 400$ ms); and (c) T_2-weighted contrast ($T_E = 80$ ms, $T_R = 2500$ ms).

be seen, the image contrast corresponding to different T_R and T_E values is quite different. Another example is shown in Fig. 1.3, in which signals from stationary spins were suppressed so that only the flowing blood was imaged. In general, an MRI image can be made to be a spatial map of the density of stationary spins or moving spins, or of relaxation times, or of the water diffusion coefficients. These are the subjects of study for subareas known as spectroscopic imaging, diffusion-weighted imaging, angiographic imaging, and functional imaging. Arguably, it is the flexibility in data acquisition and the rich contrast mechanisms of MRI that endow the technique with superior scientific and diagnostic values.

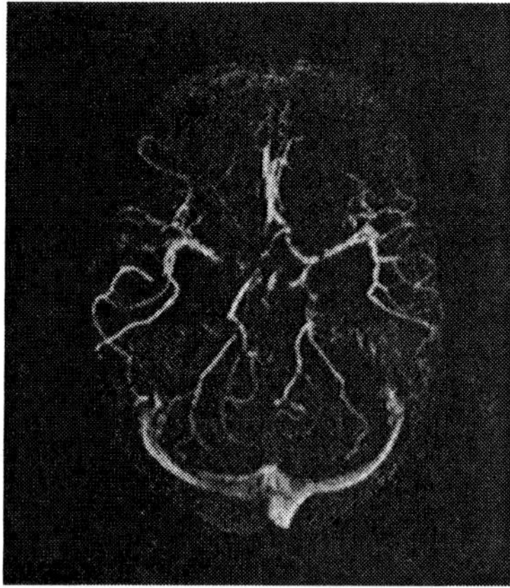

Figure 1.3 An example of angiographic imaging.

1.2   A System Perspective

An MR imager is shown in Fig. 1.4, which resembles an X-ray CT scanner. However, beyond the system appearance, an MR scanner and a CT scanner have little in common in terms of hardware components. An MR scanner consists of three main hardware components: a main magnet, a magnetic field gradient system, and an RF system. This section briefly describes their functional characteristics. For a more in-depth discussion, the reader is referred to the literature [8, 64].

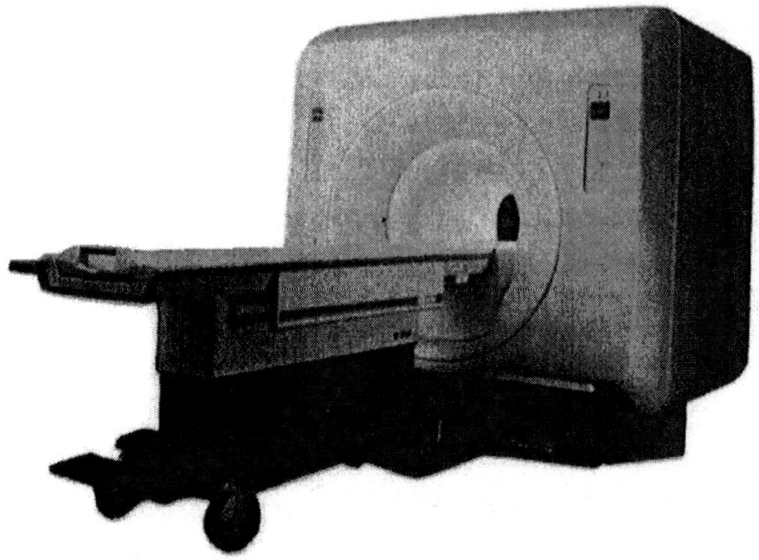

Figure 1.4 A typical clinical MRI scanner. (Images courtesy of GE Medical Systems.)

1.2.1   The Main Magnet

The main magnet is either a resistive, a permanent, or a superconducting magnet. Its primary function is to generate a strong uniform static field, referred to as the B_0 field,[1] for polarization of nuclear spins in an object. Resistive magnets are generally used at low field (< 0.15 T); permanent magnets can operate at field strengths up to 0.3 T; superconducting magnets are normally used for generating

---

[1] A magnetic field is a vector quantity, but we will use the conventional scalar notation for a magnetic field when only its magnitude is concerned and its direction need not be made explicit. Following convention, the B_0 field is assumed to point along the z-direction.

higher field strengths.[2]   The optimal field strength for imaging is application-dependent. Advantages of high fields are better signal-to-noise ratio and spectral resolution. Disadvantages include RF penetration problems and higher costs. The field strength commonly encountered in a clinical whole-body system ranges from 0.5 to 2 T.

The spatial homogeneity of the main magnetic field is defined as the maximum deviation of the field over a given volume within the region of interest:[3]

$$\text{Homogeneity} = \frac{B_{0,\max} - B_{0,\min}}{B_{0,\text{mean}}} \tag{1.1}$$

An imaging magnet requires moderate homogeneity over a large volume to provide good image quality. A typical requirement for a human system would be 10 to 50 parts per million (ppm) over a 30 to 50 cm diameter spherical volume. For spectroscopic imaging, the requirement for field homogeneity is much more stringent. In practice, the main magnet alone is not capable of generating such a highly homogeneous field. The common approach to overcoming this problem is to use a secondary compensating magnetic field generated by a set of so-called shim coils to bring the overall field to the level of desired homogeneity.

1.2.2   The Gradient System

The magnetic field gradient system normally consists of three orthogonal gradient coils, an example of which is shown in Fig. 1.5. Gradient coils are designed to produce time-varying magnetic fields of controlled spatial nonuniformity, whose formal definition is given in Section 4.4.1. The gradient system is a crucial component of an MRI scanner because gradient fields are essential for signal localization, as will become evident in Chapter 5.

Important specifications for a gradient system include maximum gradient strength and the rate at which this maximum gradient strength can be obtained. Gradient strength is normally measured in units of millitesla per meter (mT/m), and the higher it is the better. Most clinical imaging systems can provide a maximum gradient strength of approximately 10 mT/m. The lower limit of the gradient strength required is determined by the criterion that the gradient field must be stronger than the main field inhomogeneity.

The time interval for a gradient to ramp up to its full strength is called the *rise time*; the shorter the rise time, the better the gradient system. For conventional imaging methods, rise times of approximately 1.0 ms from 0 to 10 mT/m are considered to be good. For some fast imaging methods (especially echo-planar imaging methods to be discussed in Chapter 9), a shorter rise time is needed.

---

[2]The strength of a magnetic field is measured in the units of gauss (G) or tesla (T) with 1 T = 10^4 G. The earth's magnetic field is approximately equal to 0.5 G.

[3]Outside the region of interest, the B_0 field is highly inhomogeneous. Therefore, various expressions in the book are valid only within the region of interest and should be used as such.

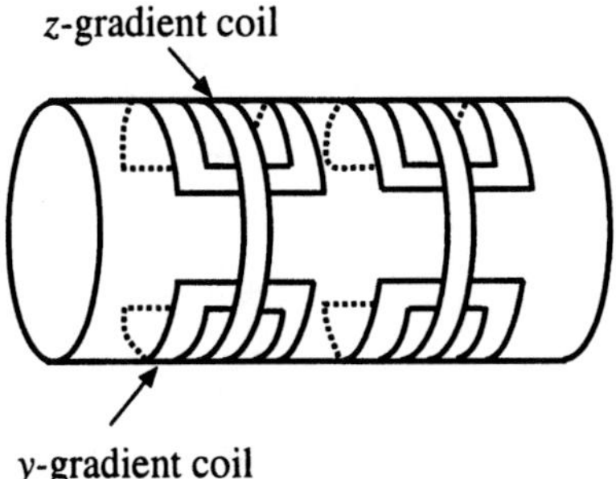

Figure 1.5   Schematic representation of the Maxwell coil pair (z-coil segment indicated) and the y-saddle coil set used to establish the z- and y-gradient, respectively.

1.2.3   The RF System

The RF system consists of a transmitter coil that is capable of generating a rotating magnetic field, often referred to as the B_1 field, for excitation of a spin system, and a receiver coil that converts a precessing magnetization into an electrical signal. Sometimes, a single coil can be used as both a transmitter and receiver coil, thus the name *transceiver* coil. Both the transmitter and receiver coils are usually called *RF coils* because they resonate at a radio frequency, as required by spin excitation and signal detection.

A desirable feature of the RF component is to provide a uniform B_1 field and high detection sensitivity. To do so, an MR system is often equipped with RF coils of different shapes and sizes for different applications. Some common examples are solenoidal coils, saddle coils, birdcage coils, and surface coils, as shown in Fig. 1.6. A long solenoidal coil consists of many closely spaced turns on a cylindrical form with a diameter much less than its length. It can produce a uniform B_1 field in its interior. A saddle coil has a pair of coils wound on a cylindrical surface and is able to generate a relatively homogeneous field near its center. A birdcage coil consists of a series of identical loops connected together and located on the surface of a cylinder giving the appearance of a birdcage. It provides the best RF field homogeneity of all the RF coils currently in use. Surface coils come in different forms and sizes. The simplest is a loop of wire that is useful for imaging of a limited region.

1.3   A Signal Processing Perspective

While an MRI system is rather complex, the imaging principles that such a system implements are much less intimidating. Especially when viewed from a signal processing standpoint, the imaging process essentially involves a pair of trans-

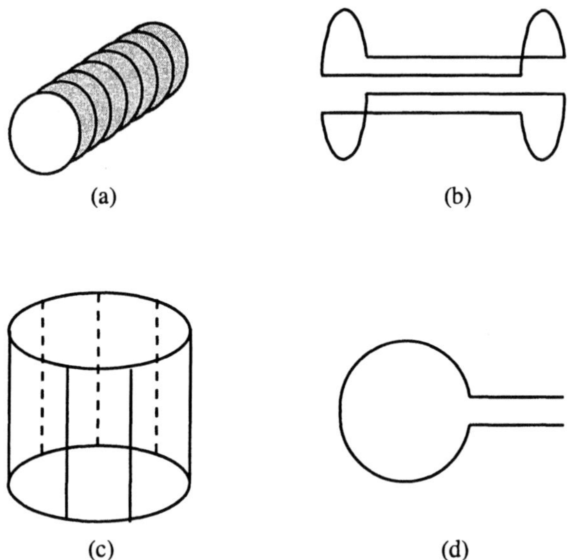

Figure 1.6 Some examples of RF coils: (a) solenoidal coil, (b) saddle coil, (c) birdcage coil, and (d) surface coil.

formations as shown in Fig. 1.7. The first transformation, often referred to as the *imaging equation*, governs how the experimental data are collected, and the second, often referred to as the *image reconstruction equation*, determines how the measured data are processed for image formation. In engineering, the first step is known as the *forward* problem and the second step is the so-called *inverse* problem. This book will adopt this transform-based approach to describe the principle of MR image formation. Specifically, we will focus on how MR signals are generated, detected, manipulated, and processed into an image. In doing so, we start with the microscopic magnetic moments $\vec{\mu}$ in an object and then trace step-by-step how they are subsequently converted to a bulk magnetization $\vec{M}$, a transverse magnetization $\vec{M}_{xy}$, an electrical signal $S(t)$, a k-space signal $S(\vec{k})$, and finally the desired image $I(\vec{x})$. Therefore, the main thread that links the book's materials together is

$$\vec{\mu} \longrightarrow \vec{M} \longrightarrow \vec{M}_{xy} \longrightarrow S(t) \longrightarrow S(\vec{k}) \longrightarrow I(\vec{x})$$

As will become evident later in this book, $\vec{\mu} \longrightarrow \vec{M}$ is accomplished by exposing the object to the B_0 field; $\vec{M} \longrightarrow \vec{M}_{xy}$ is done with RF excitations; $\vec{M}_{xy} \longrightarrow S(t)$, known as signal detection, is based on Faraday's law of induction; $S(t) \longrightarrow S(\vec{k})$ is the core of MRI, which involves the use of magnetic field gradients to encode spatial information into the transient responses of a spin system upon RF excitations; and finally, $S(\vec{k}) \longrightarrow I(\vec{x})$ is the well-known image reconstruction problem common to many tomographic imaging modalities. This book will focus on elucidating the underlying principles of each of these steps.

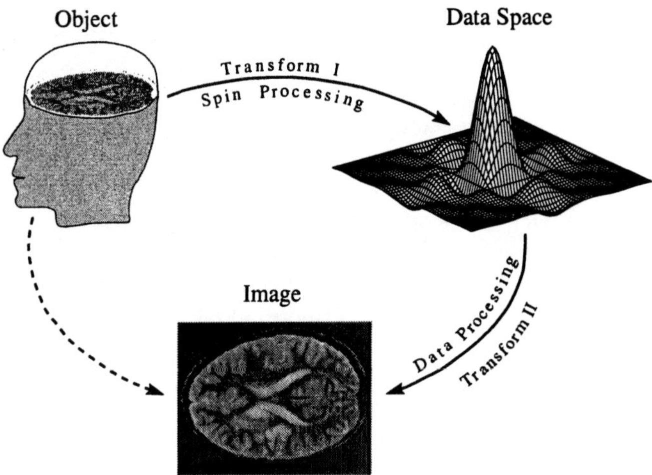

Figure 1.7   The MR imaging process viewed as two mathematical transformations.

1.4   Organization of the Book

This book is intended to be useful to upper-level undergraduate and graduate students in engineering or physical sciences as a textbook for a course on this subject, as well as to practicing MRI scientists as a reference. It emphasizes the fundamental principles and concepts underlying signal generation and detection, spatial information encoding, and image reconstruction. The remainder of the book is organized as follows.

Chapter 2 reviews some of the fundamental mathematical concepts that are key to understanding MRI principles. A primary objective is to make this book self-contained so that the reader will not require many reference books to review these materials.

Chapter 3 covers the basic physical principles for signal generation and detection.

Chapter 4 discusses the excitation requirements and general characteristics of transient signals of various types generated from a spin system after pulse excitations.

Chapter 5 discusses physical and mathematical principles for spatial localization of activated MR signals.

Chapter 6 discusses signal processing principles and techniques for image reconstruction from spatially encoded signals.

Chapter 7 describes the rich mechanisms unique to MRI for manipulating image contrast.

Chapter 8 deals with practical imaging issues such as limited resolution, signal-to-noise ratios, and image artifacts.

Chapter 9 discusses the principles and techniques of fast-scan imaging.

Chapter 10 introduces the concept of constrained image reconstruction.

Appendix A provides a summary of some commonly used mathematical formulas.

Appendix B contains a glossary of technical terms that frequently appear in the MR literature.

Appendix C presents a partial list of mathematical symbols used in the book.

Appendix D presents a partial list of abbreviations used in the book.

Appendix E contains the definitions of several physical constants.

The bibliography provides a list of relevant references. Although MRI has a relatively brief history, the number of publications on this subject is overwhelming. The bibliography included is by no means comprehensive. However, it should provide the reader with some useful guidance in searching for further details on the main ideas discussed in this book.

Exercises

1.1   What is the radio-frequency range?

1.2   What is roughly the strength of the earth's magnetic field? What is the strength of the main magnet of a clinical MR imager?

1.3   What are the main differences between emission, transmission, and diffraction tomography?

1.4   In what sense can MRI be viewed as a form of emission tomography?

1.5   MR imaging requires the use of three types of magnet fields: a strong uniform static field, an oscillating field, and three gradient fields.

   (a)   Identify the hardware components in an MRI system that produce these magnetic fields.

   (b)   Describe briefly the primary roles of these magnetic fields.

Chapter 2

Mathematical Fundamentals

If the only tool you have is a hammer, you tend to treat everything as if it were a nail.

Abraham Maslow

This chapter reviews some mathematical concepts essential for understanding MRI principles. We will begin with a brief description of vector quantities and then review the definitions of some commonly used mathematical functions and two integral transforms: the Fourier transform and the Radon transform.

Before we proceed, a word on the notation is in order. Throughout this text, we will use $f(x), g(x), h(x)$, and so on, to represent continuous-variable functions, and $f[n], g[n], h[n]$, or f_n, g_n, h_n, and the like to represent discrete-variable functions (or sequences) with the understanding that n is an integer variable. In many situations when there is no confusion, we will also use $f[n]$ or f_n to represent data samples from $f(x)$ such that $f_n = f[n] = f(n\Delta x)$ for some Δx. Multivariable functions are sometimes expressed in vector notation such that $f(r)$ may refer to $f(x, y)$ or $f(x, y, z)$, depending on the context.

2.1   Vectors

Many physical quantities, such as velocity, magnetic field, and angular momentum, have both magnitude and direction. These quantities, called *vectors*, are represented in this book by two types of symbols: symbols with an overhead arrow such as $\vec{A}$ (called *explicit vector notations*) and boldface symbols such as A (called *implicit vector notations*). To understand the subtle difference between these two notations, consider a three-dimensional vector $\vec{A}$ shown in Fig. 2.1. In explicit form,

$$\vec{A} = A_x\vec{i} + A_y\vec{j} + A_z\vec{k} \tag{2.1}$$

and in implicit form

$$\boldsymbol{A} = (A_x, A_y, A_z) \tag{2.2}$$

where A_x, A_y, and A_z are the x-, y-, and z-components of $\vec{A}$, and $\vec{i}$, $\vec{j}$, and $\vec{k}$ are the unit directional vectors along the x-, y-, and z-axes, respectively. By definition,

$$\begin{cases} \vec{i} \sim (1,0,0) \\ \vec{j} \sim (0,1,0) \\ \vec{k} \sim (0,0,1) \end{cases} \tag{2.3}$$

Within a single reference frame, both types of notations uniquely specify a vector, and we will use them interchangeably when there is no confusion. However, when multiple reference frames are used, as is often the case in describing MRI techniques, it is important to know which reference frame is used for vectors in the implicit notation.

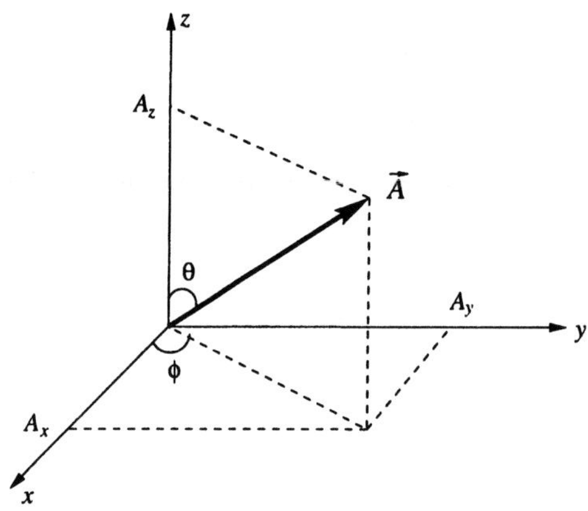

Figure 2.1   Graphical representation of a vector.

The magnitude and direction of $\boldsymbol{A}$ are represented by $|\boldsymbol{A}|$ and $\boldsymbol{\mu}_A$, respectively, such that

$$\boldsymbol{A} = |\boldsymbol{A}|\boldsymbol{\mu}_A \tag{2.4}$$

where $\boldsymbol{\mu}_A$ is the unit directional vector of $\boldsymbol{A}$. $|\boldsymbol{A}|$ and $\boldsymbol{\mu}_A$ can be determined from the components of $\boldsymbol{A}$ using the following formulas:

$$|\boldsymbol{A}| = \sqrt{A_x^2 + A_y^2 + A_z^2} \tag{2.5}$$

and

$$\mu_A = \frac{1}{\sqrt{A_x^2 + A_y^2 + A_z^2}} (A_x, A_y, A_z) \tag{2.6}$$

Alternatively, μ_A can be expressed in terms of the polar and azimuthal angles as follows:

$$\mu_A = (\sin\theta\cos\phi, \sin\theta\sin\phi, \cos\theta) \tag{2.7}$$

where

$$\theta = \tan^{-1}\left(\frac{\sqrt{A_x^2 + A_y^2}}{A_z}\right) \tag{2.8}$$

and

$$\phi = \arctan\left(\frac{A_y}{A_x}\right) \tag{2.9}$$

For planar vectors, a complex notation is often used in the MR literature. Specifically, let $A = (A_x, A_y)$. We regard A as equivalent to A if A is constructed as

$$A \triangleq A_x + iA_y \tag{2.10}$$

where $i \triangleq \sqrt{-1}$. In the polar (or exponential) form, A can be expressed as

$$A = |A|e^{i\phi} = |A|(\cos\phi + i\sin\phi) \tag{2.11}$$

where $|A| = \sqrt{A_x^2 + A_y^2}$, and ϕ is given in Eq. (2.9). Geometrically, ϕ is the smaller angle between A and the x-axis (real axis).

The exponential form in Eq. (2.11) is used frequently at various places in this book. A special example is

$$A(t) = A_0 e^{i\omega_0 t} \tag{2.12}$$

which represents a vector of length A_0 rotating counterclockwise at an angular speed ω_0.

Vector quantities can be used in various operations. The simplest one is vector addition, which is defined as follows:

$$\vec{A} + \vec{B} \triangleq (A_x + B_x, A_y + B_y, A_z + B_z) \tag{2.13}$$

Vector addition can be performed graphically using the so-called *parallelogram rule* shown in Fig. 2.2. It is obvious that vector addition obeys the commutative and associative laws:

$$\text{Commutative law:} \quad \vec{A} + \vec{B} = \vec{B} + \vec{A} \tag{2.14a}$$

$$\text{Associative law:} \quad \vec{A} + (\vec{B} + \vec{C}) = (\vec{A} + \vec{B}) + \vec{C} \tag{2.14b}$$

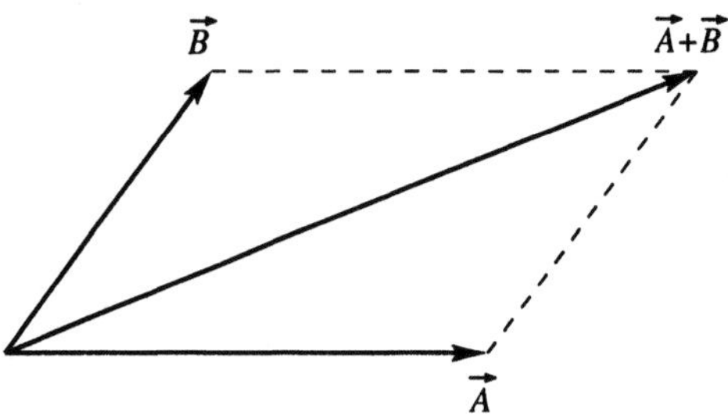

Figure 2.2 Parallelogram rule for vector addition.

Vector multiplication exists in two forms: scalar (or dot) product and vector (or cross) product.[1] The dot product of two vectors $\vec{A}$ and $\vec{B}$, denoted by $\vec{A} \cdot \vec{B}$, is a scalar that is equal to the product of the magnitudes of $\vec{A}$ and $\vec{B}$ and the cosine of the (smaller) angle between them. Let ϕ_{AB} be the smaller angle between $\vec{A}$ and $\vec{B}$. Then,

$$\vec{A} \cdot \vec{B} \triangleq |\vec{A}||\vec{B}| \cos \phi_{AB} \tag{2.15}$$

It is easy to see that the dot product is commutative and distributive:

$$\text{Commutative law:} \quad \vec{A} \cdot \vec{B} = \vec{B} \cdot \vec{A} \tag{2.16a}$$
$$\text{Distributive law:} \quad \vec{A} \cdot (\vec{B} + \vec{C}) = \vec{A} \cdot \vec{B} + \vec{A} \cdot \vec{C} \tag{2.16b}$$

The associative law, however, does not apply to the dot product. Using the distributive property, one can show that

$$\vec{A} \cdot \vec{B} = A_x B_x + A_y B_y + A_z B_z \tag{2.17}$$

The cross product of two vectors, $\vec{A}$ and $\vec{B}$, is defined by

$$\vec{A} \times \vec{B} \triangleq |\vec{A}||\vec{B}||\sin \phi_{AB}|\vec{\mu}_{AB} \tag{2.18}$$

where $\vec{\mu}_{AB}$ is determined according to the *right-hand rule*. That is, $\vec{\mu}_{AB}$ takes the direction of the thumb of the right hand when the fingers rotate from $\vec{A}$ to $\vec{B}$ through the angle ϕ_{AB}, as shown in Fig. 2.3.

The cross product obeys the distributive law:

$$\vec{A} \times (\vec{B} + \vec{C}) = \vec{A} \times \vec{B} + \vec{A} \times \vec{C} \tag{2.19}$$

However,

$$\vec{A} \times \vec{B} = -\vec{B} \times \vec{A} \tag{2.20}$$

---

[1] It is important to note that while addition of planar vectors is equivalent to addition of the corresponding complex numbers, vector multiplication (dot or cross product) does not correspond to complex multiplication. Therefore, the complex notation of planar vectors should be used with caution.

and

$$\vec{A} \times (\vec{B} \times \vec{C}) \neq (\vec{A} \times \vec{B}) \times \vec{C} \tag{2.21}$$

Therefore, the cross product is neither commutative nor associative.

Based on the distributive property, one can show that

$$\vec{A} \times \vec{B} = (A_y B_z - A_z B_y)\vec{i} + (A_z B_x - A_x B_z)\vec{j} + (A_x B_y - A_y B_x)\vec{k} \tag{2.22}$$

or in determinant form

$$\vec{A} \times \vec{B} = \begin{vmatrix} \vec{i} & \vec{j} & \vec{k} \\ A_x & A_y & A_z \\ B_x & B_y & B_z \end{vmatrix} \tag{2.23}$$

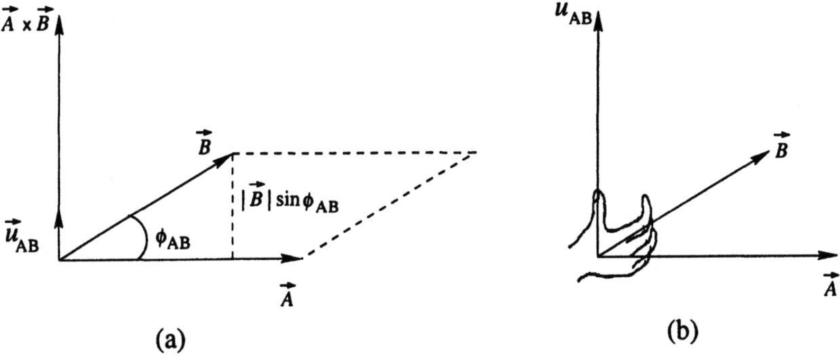

Figure 2.3   (a) $\vec{A} \times \vec{B}$, and (b) the right-hand rule. Note that μ_{AB} is orthogonal to the plane containing $\vec{A}$ and $\vec{B}$.

The following identities for the unit directional vectors of the x-, y- and z-axes directly follow from the definition of dot and cross products:

$$\vec{i} \cdot \vec{i} = \vec{j} \cdot \vec{j} = \vec{k} \cdot \vec{k} = 1 \tag{2.24a}$$

$$\vec{i} \times \vec{i} = \vec{j} \times \vec{j} = \vec{k} \times \vec{k} = 0 \tag{2.24b}$$

$$\vec{i} \times \vec{j} = \vec{k}; \quad \vec{j} \times \vec{k} = \vec{i}; \quad \vec{k} \times \vec{i} = \vec{j} \tag{2.24c}$$

2.2   Basic Concepts of Matrix Algebra

The (implicit) vector notation is often used to represent one-dimensional data sequences. Specifically, a column vector containing N elements is denoted as

$$v \triangleq \begin{bmatrix} v_1 \\ v_2 \\ \vdots \\ v_N \end{bmatrix} \tag{2.25}$$

Similarly, a row vector of size N is denoted as

$$v \triangleq [v_1, v_2, \cdots, v_N] \tag{2.26}$$

A column vector of size N is also called an $N \times 1$ vector and is written as

$$v = \{v_n\}_{N \times 1} \tag{2.27}$$

Likewise, a row vector of size N is called a $1 \times N$ vector and written as

$$v = \{v_n\}_{1 \times N} \tag{2.28}$$

Two-dimensional data sequences can be represented by matrices, which are represented by boldface Roman symbols. A matrix of size $M \times N$ has M rows and N columns and is written as

$$\mathbf{W} = \{w_{mn}\}_{M \times N} = \begin{bmatrix} w_{11} & w_{12} & \cdots & w_{1N} \\ w_{21} & w_{22} & \cdots & w_{2N} \\ \vdots & \vdots & \vdots & \vdots \\ w_{M1} & w_{M2} & \cdots & w_{MN} \end{bmatrix} \tag{2.29}$$

Some basic matrix definitions are summarized as follows:

- Identity matrix: $\mathbf{I} = \{\delta(m - n)\}_{M \times M}$

- Determinant: $|\mathbf{W}| = |\{w_{mn}\}_{M \times M}|$

- Inverse, $\mathbf{W}^{-1}$: $\mathbf{W}^{-1}\mathbf{W} = \mathbf{W}\mathbf{W}^{-1} = \mathbf{I}$

- Transpose: $\mathbf{W} = \{w_{mn}\}_{M \times N} \longrightarrow \mathbf{W}^T = \{w_{nm}\}_{N \times M}$

- Complex conjugate: $\mathbf{W} = \{w_{mn}\}_{M \times N} \longrightarrow \mathbf{W}^* = \{w_{mn}^*\}_{M \times N}$

- Hermitian: $\mathbf{W} = \{w_{mn}\}_{M \times N} \longrightarrow \mathbf{W}^H = \{w_{nm}^*\}_{N \times M}$

- Matrix addition: $\mathbf{A} + \mathbf{B} \triangleq \{a_{mn} + b_{mn}\}_{M \times N}$

- Scalar multiplication: $c\mathbf{W} = \{cw_{mn}\}_{M \times N}$

- Matrix multiplication: $\mathbf{C}_{M \times N} \triangleq \mathbf{A}_{M \times L}\mathbf{B}_{L \times N} \longrightarrow c_{mn} = \sum_{\ell=1}^{L} a_{m\ell}b_{\ell n}$

- Eigenvalues, λ: Roots of $|\mathbf{W} - \lambda\mathbf{I}|$

- Eigenvectors, v: Nonzero solutions of $\mathbf{W}v = \lambda v$

- Orthogonal matrix: $\mathbf{W}^{-1} = \mathbf{W}^T$ or $\mathbf{W}\mathbf{W}^T = \mathbf{W}^T\mathbf{W} = \mathbf{I}$

- Unitary matrix: $\mathbf{W}^{-1} = \mathbf{W}^H$ or $\mathbf{W}\mathbf{W}^H = \mathbf{W}^H\mathbf{W} = \mathbf{I}$

2.3 Some Commonly Used Functions

This section reviews the definitions of several commonly used functions.

2.3.1 Unit Step Function

The unit step function, denoted by $u(\cdot)$, is defined by

$$u(x) \triangleq \begin{cases} 1 & x > 0 \\ 0 & x < 0 \end{cases} \tag{2.30}$$

2.3.2 Signum Function

The signum function, denoted by $\mathrm{sgn}(\cdot)$, is defined by

$$\mathrm{sgn}(x) \triangleq \begin{cases} 1 & x > 0 \\ -1 & x < 0 \end{cases} \tag{2.31}$$

It can be expressed in terms of the unit step function as

$$\mathrm{sgn}(x) = 2u(x) - 1 \tag{2.32}$$

2.3.3 Rectangular Window Function

The unit-width rectangular window function, denoted as $\Pi(\cdot)$, is defined by

$$\Pi(x) \triangleq \begin{cases} 1 & |x| < 1/2 \\ 0 & \text{otherwise} \end{cases} \tag{2.33}$$

Clearly,

$$\Pi(x) = u\left(x + \tfrac{1}{2}\right) - u\left(x - \tfrac{1}{2}\right) \tag{2.34}$$

2.3.4 Triangle Window Function

The unit triangle window function, denoted by $\Lambda(\cdot)$, is defined by

$$\Lambda(x) \triangleq \begin{cases} 1 - |x| & |x| \leq 1 \\ 0 & \text{otherwise} \end{cases} \tag{2.35}$$

2.3.5 Hamming Window Function

The Hamming window function is a raised cosine function defined by

$$H(x) \triangleq \begin{cases} 0.54 + 0.46\cos(2\pi x) & |x| \leq 1/2 \\ 0 & \text{otherwise} \end{cases} \tag{2.36}$$

2.3.6   Gaussian Function

The Gaussian window function is defined as

$$G(\mu, \sigma, x) \triangleq \frac{1}{\sqrt{2\pi}\sigma} e^{-\frac{(x-\mu)^2}{2\sigma^2}} \tag{2.37}$$

where μ and σ are the mean and standard deviation of the Gaussian distribution because of the following properties:

$$\mu = \int_{-\infty}^{\infty} x G(\mu, \sigma, x) dx \tag{2.38}$$

and

$$\sigma^2 = \int_{-\infty}^{\infty} (x - \mu)^2 G(\mu, \sigma, x) dx \tag{2.39}$$

2.3.7   Dirac Delta Function

The Dirac delta function or impulse function, denoted by $\delta(x)$, is a mathematical abstraction for pulses that are so brief and intense that making them any briefer and more intense does not matter as long as their integral stays the same. Mathematically, $\delta(x)$ is a generalized function because we cannot define its value point by point as with ordinary functions. A formal definition of $\delta(x)$ is based on the distribution theory. In this definition, $\delta(x)$ is a functional such that

$$\int_{-\infty}^{\infty} \varphi(x)\delta(x) dx = \varphi(0) \tag{2.40}$$

for any $\varphi(x)$ that is continuous at the origin. The definition above implies the following properties:

(a) $\delta(x) = 0$ for $x \neq 0$

(b) $\delta(x)$ is unbounded at $x = 0$

(c) $\int_{-\infty}^{\infty} \delta(x) dx = 1$

Pictorially, $\delta(x)$ is represented by an upward arrow at the origin, as shown in Fig. 2.4, which signifies a pulse at the origin with an unbounded amplitude and zero duration.

In practice, $\delta(x)$ is taken to be the limit of a function sequence $g_n(x)$:

$$\delta(x) = \lim_{n \to \infty} g_n(x) \tag{2.41}$$

provided that

$$\lim_{n \to \infty} \int_{-\infty}^{\infty} \varphi(x) g_n(x) dx = \varphi(0) \tag{2.42}$$

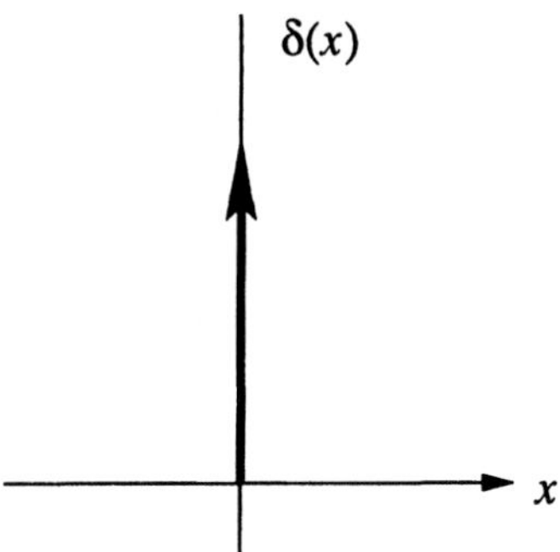

Figure 2.4   Pictorial representation of the delta function.

Many sequences with this property are available. Four well-known examples are as follows:

$$\delta(x) \;=\; \lim_{\Delta x \to 0} \frac{1}{\Delta x}\Pi\left(\frac{x}{\Delta x}\right) \tag{2.43a}$$

$$\delta(x) \;=\; \lim_{\Delta x \to 0} \frac{1}{\Delta x}\,\text{sinc}\left(\frac{\pi x}{\Delta x}\right) \tag{2.43b}$$

$$\delta(x) \;=\; \lim_{\Delta x \to 0} \frac{1}{\Delta x}\Lambda\left(\frac{x}{\Delta x}\right) \tag{2.43c}$$

$$\delta(x) \;=\; \lim_{\Delta x \to 0} \frac{1}{\Delta x}e^{-\frac{\pi x^2}{\Delta x^2}} \tag{2.43d}$$

The impulse function $\delta(x)$ and the unit step function $u(x)$ are closely related to each other by

$$\frac{du(x)}{dx} = \delta(x) \tag{2.44}$$

This relationship can be proved from the distribution definition of $\delta(x)$ by noting that

$$\int_{-\infty}^{\infty} \frac{du(x)}{dx}\varphi(x)\,dx = u(x)\varphi(x)\Big|_{-\infty}^{\infty} - \int_{-\infty}^{\infty} u(x)\frac{d\varphi(x)}{dx}\,dx$$

$$= \varphi(\infty) - [\varphi(\infty) - \varphi(0)] = \varphi(0)$$

The following properties of the impulse function $\delta(x)$ immediately follow from the defining integral:

(a) *Scaling property*:

$$\delta(ax) = \frac{1}{|a|}\delta(x) \qquad a \neq 0 \tag{2.45}$$

(b) *Sampling property*:

$$\varphi(x)\delta(x - x_0) = \varphi(x_0)\delta(x - x_0) \qquad (2.46a)$$

$$\int_{-\infty}^{\infty} \varphi(x)\delta(x - x_0)dx = \varphi(x_0) \qquad (2.46b)$$

(c) *Derivative property*:

$$\int_{-\infty}^{\infty} \varphi(x)\delta^{(n)}(x - x_0)dx = (-1)^n \varphi^{(n)}(x_0) \qquad (2.47)$$

2.3.8   Kronecker Delta Function

The discrete counterpart of the Dirac delta function is the Kronecker delta function, written as $\delta[n]$ or simply δ_n. Mathematically, it is defined as

$$\delta[n] = \begin{cases} 1 & n = 0 \\ 0 & \text{otherwise} \end{cases} \qquad (2.48)$$

Note that $\delta[n]$ is not a generalized function, but it has similar effects on discrete functions as $\delta(x)$ does on continuous functions. For example, similarly to Eqs. (2.44) and (2.46), we have

$$\delta[n] = u[n] - u[n - 1] \qquad (2.49)$$

and

$$\sum_{n=-\infty}^{\infty} \varphi[n]\delta[n - n_0] = \varphi[n_0] \qquad (2.50)$$

2.3.9   Comb Function

The comb function is a periodic function consisting of a sequence of equally spaced Dirac delta functions. A formal definition of $\text{comb}(x)$ is

$$\text{comb}(x) = \sum_{n=-\infty}^{\infty} \delta(x - n) \qquad (2.51)$$

It is easy to show that

$$\sum_{n=-\infty}^{\infty} \delta(x - n\Delta x) = \frac{1}{\Delta x}\text{comb}\left(\frac{x}{\Delta x}\right) \qquad (2.52)$$

2.3.10   Sinc Function

The sinc function is defined by

$$\mathrm{sinc}(x) = \frac{\sin(x)}{x} \tag{2.53}$$

This function is rather popular in the imaging literature because it is directly tied to the Fourier transform of a rectangular window function, as discussed in Section 2.5. Inspection of both Eq. (2.53) and the plot in Fig. 2.5 reveals the following properties of the sinc function:

(a) It is an even function.

(b) It has a peak value 1 at $x = 0$ by the L'Hôpital rule.

(c) Its zero crossings are located at $\pm n\pi$. The region between $x = -\pi$ and $x = \pi$ is called the *main lobe*, and the regions between $x = -(n+1)\pi$ and $x = -n\pi$ or between $x = n\pi$ and $x = (n+1)\pi$ for $n > 1$ are called the *side lobes*.

(d) Since $\mathrm{sinc}(x)$ is the product of an oscillating $\sin(x)$ and a monotonically decreasing function $1/x$, $\mathrm{sinc}(x)$ exhibits sinusoidal oscillations of period 2π, with amplitude decreasing continuously as $1/x$.

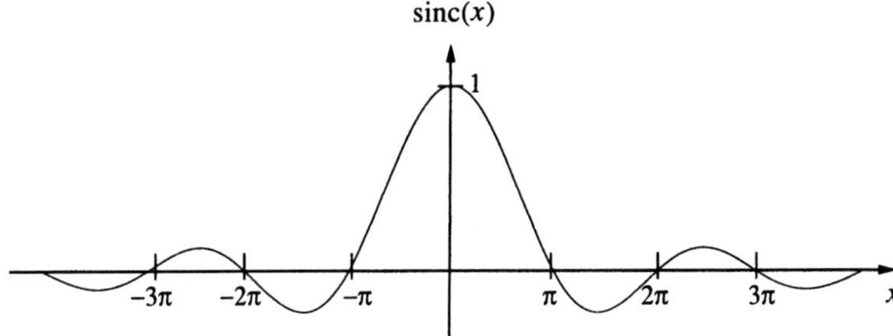

Figure 2.5   Pictorial representation of the sinc function.

2.3.11   Dirichlet Function

The Dirichlet function is defined as

$$\mathrm{Dir}(N, x) = \frac{\sin(Nx)}{\sin(x)} \tag{2.54}$$

It is easy to show that $\mathrm{Dir}(N, x)$ is a periodic function of period π for N odd but 2π for N even. Within the region $-\pi/2 < x < \pi/2$, $\mathrm{Dir}(N, x)$ looks like a sinc function in the sense that it has a main lobe spanning over the region between $x = -\pi/N$ and $x = \pi/N$ and a sequence of side lobes spanning over the regions between $x = -(n+1)\pi/N$ and $x = -n\pi/N$ or between $x = n\pi/N$ and $x = (n+1)\pi/N$. Two examples of $\mathrm{Dir}(N, x)$ are shown in Fig. 2.6.

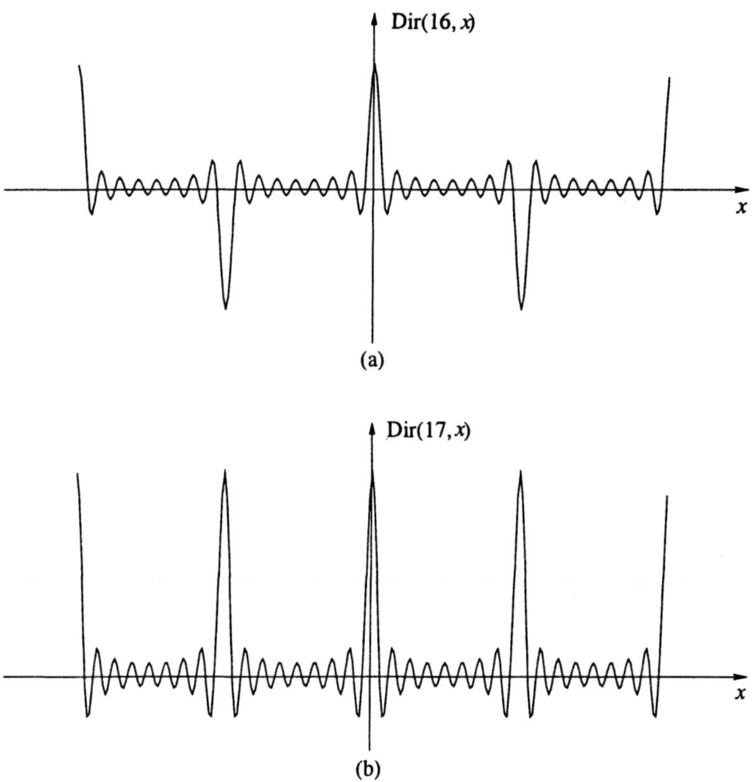

Figure 2.6 Plots of $\mathrm{Dir}(N, x)$ for (a) $N = 16$ and (b) $N = 17$, respectively.

2.3.12 Bessel Functions

Bessel functions of the first kind of integer order n, denoted by $J_n(x)$, are useful for describing some imaging effects. One definition of $J_n(x)$ is given in terms of the following integral:

$$J_n(x) = \frac{1}{2\pi} \int_{-\pi}^{\pi} e^{i(n\theta - x\sin\theta)}\,d\theta \qquad (2.55)$$

A special case is the zero-order Bessel function of the first kind, which, according to Eq. (2.55), is defined by

$$J_0(x) = \frac{1}{2\pi} \int_{-\pi}^{\pi} e^{ix \sin \theta} d\theta \tag{2.56}$$

Equivalently, we have

$$J_0(x) = \frac{1}{2\pi} \int_{-\pi}^{\pi} e^{-ix \sin \theta} d\theta = \frac{1}{2\pi} \int_{-\pi}^{\pi} e^{ix \cos \theta} d\theta = \frac{1}{2\pi} \int_{-\pi}^{\pi} e^{-ix \cos \theta} d\theta \tag{2.57}$$

Some useful relations of $J_n(x)$ are summarized below.

$$J_n(-x) = (-1)^n J_n(x) \tag{2.58a}$$

$$J_{-n}(x) = (-1)^n J_n(x) \tag{2.58b}$$

$$e^{ix \sin \theta} = \sum_{n=-\infty}^{\infty} J_n(x) e^{in\theta} \tag{2.58c}$$

$$e^{ix \cos \theta} = \sum_{n=-\infty}^{\infty} i^n J_n(x) e^{in\theta} \tag{2.58d}$$

$$\cos(x \sin \theta) = J_0(x) + 2 \sum_{n=1}^{\infty} J_{2n}(x) \cos 2n\theta \tag{2.58e}$$

$$\sin(x \sin \theta) = 2 \sum_{n=1}^{\infty} J_{2n+1}(x) \sin(2n + 1)\theta \tag{2.58f}$$

Plots of $J_0(x)$, $J_1(x)$, and $J_2(x)$ are given in Fig. 2.7. As can be seen, the Bessel functions oscillate (but are not exactly periodic), and their amplitudes decay gradually (asymptotically as $1/\sqrt{x}$).

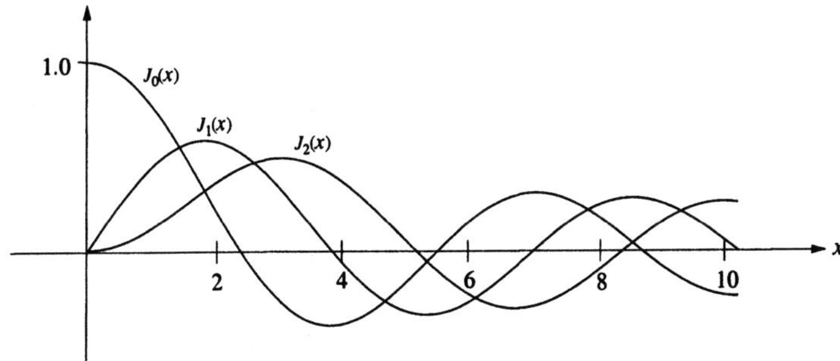

Figure 2.7   Plots of Bessel functions $J_0(x)$, $J_1(x)$, and $J_2(x)$.

2.4 Convolution

Convolution is an important mathematical operation between two functions. For two continuous-variable functions $g(x)$ and $h(x)$, their convolution is defined as

$$f(x) = \int_{-\infty}^{\infty} g(\tau)h(x-\tau)d\tau = \int_{-\infty}^{\infty} g(x-\tau)h(\tau)d\tau \qquad (2.59)$$

Symbolically, Eq. (2.59) is often written as

$$f(x) = g(x) * h(x) \qquad (2.60)$$

For discrete-variable functions (or data sequences), the integration in Eq. (2.59) is replaced by a summation such that

$$f[n] = g[n] * h[n] = \sum_{m=-\infty}^{\infty} g[m]h[n-m] \qquad (2.61)$$

The following is a summary of some useful properties of convolution:

(a) *Commutativity*:
$$g * h = h * g \qquad (2.62)$$

(b) *Associativity*:
$$f * (g * h) = (f * g) * h \qquad (2.63)$$

(c) *Distributivity*:
$$f * (g + h) = f * g + f * h \qquad (2.64)$$

(d) *Differentiation property*:
For continuous convolution, it is easy to show that

$$\frac{d}{dx}(g * h) = \frac{dg}{dx} * h = g * \frac{dh}{dx} \qquad (2.65)$$

(e) *Shifting property*:
If $g * h = f$, then

$$g(x - x_0) * h(x) = g(x) * h(x - x_0) = f(x - x_0) \qquad (2.66)$$

(f) *Width property*:
If $g(x)$ and $h(x)$ are functions of finite widths W_g and W_h, respectively, then $g(x) * h(x)$ is another finite duration function with width $W_g + W_h$.

The width property can be extended to discrete convolution, but it takes a slightly different form. Suppose that $g[n]$ and $h[n]$ are sequences of finite widths N_g and N_h, respectively; then $g[n] * h[n]$ is another finite duration sequence with width $N_g + N_h - 1$. This property can be understood by considering the simple example, where $g[n] = h[n] = \{1, 1, 1\}$ are sequences of width 3, while $g[n] * h[n] = \{1, 2, 3, 2, 1\}$ is a sequence of width 5.

Theorem 2.1 (Central Limit Theorem)   *When a function $h(x)$ is convolved with itself n times, in the limit $n \to \infty$, the convolution product is a Gaussian function with a variance that is n times the variance of $h(x)$, provided the area, mean, and variance of $h(x)$ are finite.*

One may have seen this theorem in the statistical literature. It can be interpreted here as saying that convolution is a smoothing process. Therefore, it is often appropriate to say that an image obtained from a practical imaging system is a smoothed version of the true image function.

■ **Example 2.1**

This example evaluates the convolution of two exponential functions from the definition.

$$ae^{-\alpha x}u(x) * be^{-\beta x}u(x) = \int_{-\infty}^{\infty} ae^{-\alpha \tau}u(\tau)be^{-\beta(x-\tau)}u(x-\tau)d\tau$$

$$= ab\left[\int_0^x e^{-(\alpha-\beta)\tau-\beta x}d\tau\right]u(x)$$

$$= \frac{ab}{\beta-\alpha}(e^{-\alpha x} - e^{-\beta x})u(x)$$

Note that both exponential functions have a step discontinuity at the origin, but their convolution is smooth throughout the entire x-axis, as shown in Fig. 2.8.

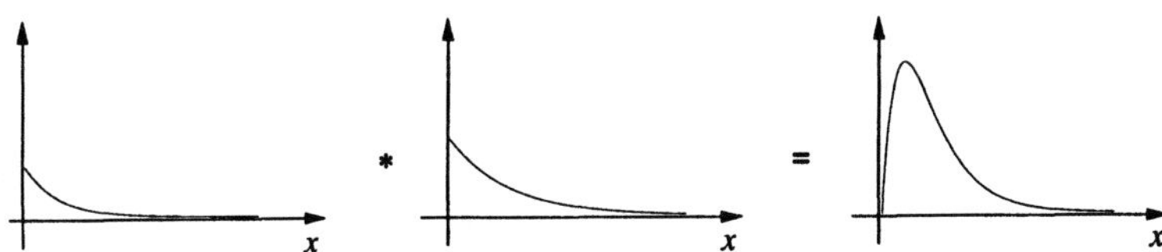

Figure 2.8   Convolution of two exponential functions.

■ Example 2.2

This example calculates $\Pi(x) * \Pi(x)$ using the derivative property.

First, the derivative property gives

$$\frac{d}{dx}\left[\Pi(x) * \Pi(x)\right] = \left[\frac{d}{dx}\Pi(x)\right] * \Pi(x)$$

$$= [\delta(x + \tfrac{1}{2}) - \delta(x - \tfrac{1}{2})] * \Pi(x)$$

$$= \Pi(x + \tfrac{1}{2}) - \Pi(x - \tfrac{1}{2})$$

Then,

$$\Pi(x) * \Pi(x) = \int_{-\infty}^{x} \left[\Pi(\tau + \tfrac{1}{2}) - \Pi(\tau - \tfrac{1}{2})\right] d\tau$$

$$= \begin{cases} 1 - |x| & |x| \leq 1 \\ 0 & \text{otherwise} \end{cases}$$

which is a triangular pulse, as shown in Fig. 2.9. Note that the resulting triangular pulse is wider and smoother than the rectangular pulse. This result is to be expected from the central limit theorem.

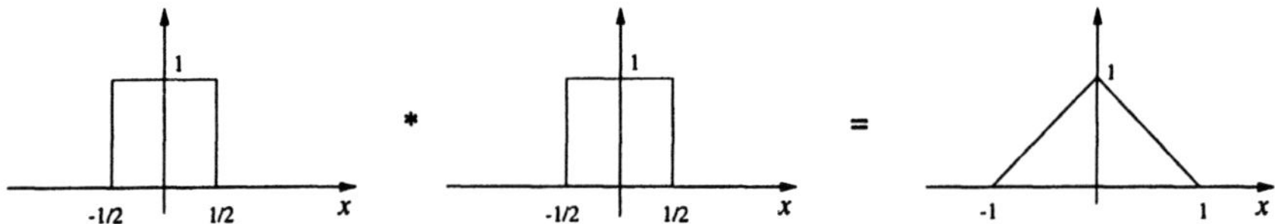

Figure 2.9   Convolution of two identical rectangular pulses yields a triangular pulse.

2.5   The Fourier Transform

The Fourier transform is of fundamental importance in MRI as will become evident in the subsequent chapters. This section reviews its definition and some of its properties relevant to MRI. A number of excellent books provide in-depth discussions of the theory and applications of the Fourier transform. For engineering students, Bracewell [6] and Papoulis [51] are especially suitable.

2.5.1 Definition

The Fourier transform of a spatial function $\rho(x)$, denoted by $\mathcal{F}\{\rho(x)\}$, or $\{\mathcal{F}\rho\}(k)$, or simply $S(k)$, is defined as

$$S(k) = \mathcal{F}\{\rho(x)\} = \mathcal{F}\rho = \int_{-\infty}^{\infty} \rho(x)e^{-i2\pi kx}\,dx \qquad (2.67)$$

where k is a spatial frequency variable having the unit of cycles per unit distance.

In signal processing, $S(k)$ is called the *frequency spectrum* of $\rho(x)$. In general, $S(k)$ is a complex-valued function of k and is often conveniently written as

$$S(k) = |S(k)|e^{i\varphi(k)} \qquad (2.68)$$

where $|S(k)|$ is the magnitude spectrum and $\varphi(k)$ is the phase spectrum. In MRI, $S(k)$ are the experimental data measured in the Fourier space (often called *k-space*), while $\rho(x)$ is the desired image function representing, for example, the spin density function. Variables x and k are termed *conjugate variables* of the Fourier transform. Another pair of conjugate variables frequently mentioned in the MRI literature consists of time t and spectral frequency f.

Given $S(k)$, we can recover $\rho(x)$ using the *inverse* Fourier transform:

$$\rho(x) = \mathcal{F}^{-1}\{S(k)\} = \int_{-\infty}^{\infty} S(k)e^{i2\pi kx}\,dk \qquad (2.69)$$

The functions $\rho(x)$ and $S(k)$ are said to constitute a Fourier transform pair. A shorthand notation "$\longleftrightarrow$" is often used to signify this pairing relationship such that

$$\rho(x) \overset{\mathcal{F}}{\longleftrightarrow} S(k) \quad \text{or simply} \quad \rho(x) \longleftrightarrow S(k) \qquad (2.70)$$

The definitions above can be extended to higher dimensions. In vector notation, the forward and inverse Fourier transforms can be written as

$$S(\boldsymbol{k}) = \int_{-\infty}^{\infty} \cdots \int_{-\infty}^{\infty} \rho(\boldsymbol{r})e^{-i2\pi \boldsymbol{k}\cdot\boldsymbol{r}}\,d\boldsymbol{r} \qquad (2.71)$$

and

$$\rho(\boldsymbol{r}) = \int_{-\infty}^{\infty} \cdots \int_{-\infty}^{\infty} S(\boldsymbol{k})e^{i2\pi \boldsymbol{k}\cdot\boldsymbol{r}}\,d\boldsymbol{k} \qquad (2.72)$$

These formulas apply to functions of any dimensionality if $\boldsymbol{k}$ and $\boldsymbol{r}$ are defined appropriately. For instance, in two dimensions, $\boldsymbol{k} = (k_x, k_y)$ and $\boldsymbol{r} = (x, y)$; then

$$S(k_x, k_y) = \int_{-\infty}^{\infty} \int_{-\infty}^{\infty} \rho(x, y)e^{-i2\pi(k_x x + k_y y)}\,dx\,dy \qquad (2.73)$$

and

$$\rho(x, y) = \int_{-\infty}^{\infty} \int_{-\infty}^{\infty} S(k_x, k_y)e^{i2\pi(k_x x + k_y y)}\,dk_x\,dk_y \qquad (2.74)$$

An important property of higher-dimensional Fourier transforms is that they can be expressed as sequential one-dimensional transforms along each dimension. For example, the two-dimensional forward Fourier transform can be written as

$$\{\mathcal{F}\rho\}(k_x, k_y) = \int_{-\infty}^{\infty} \left\{ \int_{-\infty}^{\infty} \rho(x, y) e^{-i2\pi k_x x} dx \right\} e^{-i2\pi k_y y} dy \qquad (2.75)$$

This property makes it possible to treat higher-dimensional Fourier transform imaging problems in the one-dimensional setting. In general, the following recursive relationship exists for expressing the n-dimensional Fourier transform in terms of lower-dimensional transforms:

$$\mathcal{F}_n = \mathcal{F}_m \mathcal{F}_{n-m} \qquad (2.76)$$

where $\mathcal{F}_n$ is the n-dimensional Fourier transform operator. As an example, we have $\mathcal{F}_4 = \mathcal{F}_3 \mathcal{F}_1 = \mathcal{F}_2 \mathcal{F}_2 = \mathcal{F}_1 \mathcal{F}_1 \mathcal{F}_1 \mathcal{F}_1$, which means that the four-dimensional Fourier transform can be decomposed into one three-dimensional transform cascaded with a one-dimensional transform, or into two cascaded two-dimensional transforms, or into four cascaded one-dimensional transforms.

2.5.2 Properties

Some properties of the Fourier transform relevant to MRI are summarized below for easy reference. For notational simplicity, we assume $\rho(x) \overset{\mathcal{F}}{\longleftrightarrow} S(k)$ whenever appropriate. All the formulas listed are based on the one-dimensional Fourier transform; extension to higher dimensions is in most cases straightforward and left to the reader.

(a) *Uniqueness*:
$$\rho_1(x) = \rho_2(x) \longrightarrow S_1(k) = S_2(k) \qquad (2.77)$$

(b) *Linearity*:
$$a\rho_1(x) + b\rho_2(x) \longleftrightarrow aS_1(k) + bS_2(k) \qquad (2.78)$$

(c) *Shifting theorem*:
$$\rho(x - x_0) \longleftrightarrow S(k) e^{-i2\pi k x_0} \qquad (2.79a)$$

$$e^{i2\pi k_0 x} \rho(x) \longleftrightarrow S(k - k_0) \qquad (2.79b)$$

(d) *Modulation*:
$$\rho(x) \cos(2\pi k_0 x) \longleftrightarrow \tfrac{1}{2}[S(k + k_0) + S(k - k_0)] \qquad (2.80a)$$

$$\rho(x) \sin(2\pi k_0 x) \longleftrightarrow \tfrac{1}{2}i[S(k + k_0) - S(k - k_0)] \qquad (2.80b)$$

(e) *Conjugate symmetry*:

$$\rho^*(x) \longleftrightarrow S^*(-k) \tag{2.81}$$

Specifically, if $\rho(x)$ is a real-valued function, that is, $\rho(x) = \rho^*(x)$, then $S(k) = S^*(-k)$.

(f) *Scaling property*:

$$\rho(ax) \longleftrightarrow \frac{1}{|a|} S\left(\frac{k}{a}\right) \tag{2.82}$$

(g) *Parseval's formula*:

$$\int_{-\infty}^{\infty} \rho_1(x)\rho_2^*(x)dx = \int_{-\infty}^{\infty} S_1(k)S_2^*(k)dk \tag{2.83}$$

Setting $\rho_1(x) = \rho_2(x) = \rho(x)$ yields

$$\int_{-\infty}^{\infty} |\rho(x)|^2 dx = \int_{-\infty}^{\infty} |S(k)|^2 dk \tag{2.84}$$

which states that energy is conserved in both the space and frequency domains.

(h) *Derivative property*:

$$(-i2\pi x)^n \rho(x) \longleftrightarrow \frac{d^n S(k)}{dk^n} \tag{2.85a}$$

$$\frac{d^n \rho(x)}{dx^n} \longleftrightarrow (i2\pi k)^n S(k) \tag{2.85b}$$

(i) *Convolution theorem*:

$$\rho_1(x) * \rho_2(x) \longleftrightarrow S_1(k)S_2(k) \tag{2.86}$$
$$\rho_1(x)\rho_2(x) \longleftrightarrow S_1(k) * S_2(k) \tag{2.87}$$

(j) *Analyticity*:
Functions that we deal with in imaging applications have nonzero values only in a finite spatial region. Functions of this type are called spatially *support-limited*, and their Fourier transform are analytic over the entire k-space. In the one-dimensional case, this property states that

$$\frac{d^n S(k)}{dk^n} \quad \text{exists for all } n \text{ and } k$$

(k) *Asymptotic property*:
If $\rho(x)$ and all of its derivatives up to order n exist and are bounded, then $S(k)$ decays as fast as $1/k^{n+1}$ as $|k| \to \infty$.

2.5.3 Examples

This section presents several examples of Fourier transform calculations based on the definition or properties.

■ **Example 2.3**

This example analyzes the Fourier transform of a rectangular pulse with unit width and amplitude. From the definition,

$$\int_{-\infty}^{\infty} \Pi(x)e^{-i2\pi kx}dx = \int_{-\frac{1}{2}}^{\frac{1}{2}} e^{-i2\pi kx}dx$$

$$= \frac{1}{-i2\pi k}e^{-i2\pi kx}\Big|_{x=-\frac{1}{2}}^{\frac{1}{2}}$$

$$= \text{sinc}(\pi k) \tag{2.88}$$

Several properties of the Fourier transform can be observed from the above result.

(a) *Analyticity*: $\mathcal{F}\{\Pi(x)\} = \text{sinc}(\pi k)$ is analytic along the entire k-axis because $\Pi(x)$ is support-limited.

(b) *Asymptotic property*: $\mathcal{F}\{\Pi(x)\}$ decays as fast as $1/k$ as $|k|$ approaches infinity because $\Pi(x)$ has zero-order discontinuities.

(c) By the *scaling property*,

$$a\Pi\left(\frac{x}{W_x}\right) \longleftrightarrow aW_x\Pi(\pi W_x k) \tag{2.89}$$

(d) Based on the *Parseval formula*,

$$\int_{-\infty}^{\infty} \text{sinc}^2(\pi k)dk = \int_{-\infty}^{\infty} \Pi^2(x)dx = 1 \tag{2.90}$$

Also of interest is that

$$\int_{-\infty}^{\infty} \text{sinc}(\pi k)dk = \lim_{x\to 0}\int_{-\infty}^{\infty} \text{sinc}(\pi k)e^{i2\pi kx}dk = \Pi(0) = 1 \tag{2.91}$$

■ **Example 2.4**

This example illustrates the use of the properties for simplifying Fourier transform calculations.

Consider the unit triangular pulse $\Lambda(x)$ defined in Section 2.3. Noting that

$$\frac{d\Lambda(x)}{dx} = \Pi\left(x + \tfrac{1}{2}\right) - \Pi\left(x - \tfrac{1}{2}\right)$$

and the derivative property, we have

$$\{\mathcal{F}\Lambda\}(k) = \frac{1}{i2\pi k}\mathcal{F}\left\{\frac{d\Lambda(x)}{dx}\right\}$$

$$= \frac{1}{i2\pi k}\left[\mathcal{F}\left\{\Pi\left(x + \tfrac{1}{2}\right)\right\} - \mathcal{F}\left\{\Pi\left(x - \tfrac{1}{2}\right)\right\}\right] \qquad (2.92)$$

$$= \frac{1}{i2\pi k}\left[\operatorname{sinc}(x)e^{i\pi k} - \operatorname{sinc}(x)e^{-i\pi k}\right]$$

$$= \operatorname{sinc}^2(\pi k) \qquad (2.93)$$

■ **Example 2.5**

The Gaussian function has an interesting Fourier transform relationship. For simplicity, consider the normalized Gaussian function ($\mu = 0$ and $\sigma = 1$). Its Fourier transform is given by

$$\mathcal{F}\left\{\frac{1}{\sqrt{2\pi}}e^{-x^2/2}\right\}(k) = \int_{-\infty}^{\infty}\frac{1}{\sqrt{2\pi}}e^{-x^2/2}e^{-i2\pi kx}dx$$

$$= \frac{1}{\sqrt{2\pi}}\int_{-\infty}^{\infty}e^{-(x/\sqrt{2}+i\pi\sqrt{2}k)^2-(\sqrt{2}\pi k)^2}dx$$

$$= \frac{1}{\sqrt{\pi}}e^{-(\sqrt{2}\pi k)^2}\int_{-\infty}^{\infty}e^{-y^2}dy$$

$$= e^{-(\sqrt{2}\pi k)^2} \qquad (2.94)$$

which is another Gaussian pulse of variances $1/(4\pi^2)$.

■ Example 2.6

In this example, we derive the following transform pairs:

$$\delta(x) \xleftrightarrow{\;\mathcal{F}\;} 1 \tag{2.95a}$$

$$\mathrm{sgn}(x) \xleftrightarrow{\;\mathcal{F}\;} \frac{1}{i\pi k} \tag{2.95b}$$

$$u(x) \xleftrightarrow{\;\mathcal{F}\;} \tfrac{1}{2}\delta(k) + \tfrac{1}{i2\pi k} \tag{2.95c}$$

First, Eq. (2.95a) can easily be obtained from the definition. That is,

$$\int_{-\infty}^{\infty} \delta(x)e^{-i2\pi kx}dx = 1$$

Second, Eq. (2.95b) can be derived as follows.

$$\mathcal{F}\{\mathrm{sgn}(x)\} = \lim_{a\to 0}\left[\int_{0}^{\infty} e^{-ax}e^{-i2\pi kx}dx - \int_{-\infty}^{0} e^{ax}e^{-i2\pi kx}dx\right]$$

$$= \lim_{a\to 0}\left[\frac{1}{a + i2\pi k} - \frac{1}{a - i2\pi k}\right]$$

$$= \frac{1}{i\pi k}$$

Incidentally, the preceding expression implies that $\mathrm{sgn}(x)$ has an unbounded dc term; in fact, $\mathcal{F}\{\mathrm{sgn}(x)\} = 0$ for $k = 0$ because $\mathrm{sgn}(x)$ is an odd function. However, this subtlety is widely ignored in the signal processing texts.

Finally, the Fourier transform of $u(x)$ can be derived from the forgoing results. Specifically, noting that

$$u(x) = \tfrac{1}{2} + \tfrac{1}{2}\mathrm{sgn}(x)$$

and

$$\mathcal{F}\{1\} = \delta(k)$$

we have

$$\mathcal{F}\{u(x)\} = \mathcal{F}\left\{\tfrac{1}{2} + \tfrac{1}{2}\mathrm{sgn}(x)\right\} = \tfrac{1}{2}\delta(k) + \tfrac{1}{i2\pi k}$$

■ Example 2.7

In this example, we derive the Fourier transform of the comb function defined in Section 2.3.

First, recognizing that $\mathrm{comb}(x)$ is a periodic function of period 1, we can express it in terms of a Fourier series as

$$\mathrm{comb}(x) = \sum_{n=-\infty}^{\infty} c_n e^{i2\pi nx} \tag{2.96}$$

where the coefficients c_n are determined by

$$c_n = \int_{-\frac{1}{2}}^{\frac{1}{2}} \mathrm{comb}(x) e^{-i2\pi nx} dx = \int_{-\frac{1}{2}}^{\frac{1}{2}} \delta(x) e^{-i2\pi nx} dx = 1$$

Second, applying the Fourier transform to both sides of Eq. (2.96) yields

$$\mathcal{F}\{\mathrm{comb}(x)\} = \sum_{n=-\infty}^{\infty} \mathcal{F}\left\{e^{i2\pi nx}\right\}$$

$$= \sum_{n=-\infty}^{\infty} \delta(k-n) = \mathrm{comb}(k) \tag{2.97}$$

Using the scaling property of the delta function and that of the Fourier transform, we have the following more general result (shown in Fig. 2.10):

$$\sum_{n=-\infty}^{\infty} \delta(x - n\Delta x) \xleftrightarrow{\mathcal{F}} \Delta k \sum_{n=-\infty}^{\infty} \delta(k - n\Delta k) \tag{2.98}$$

where $\Delta k = 1/\Delta x$.

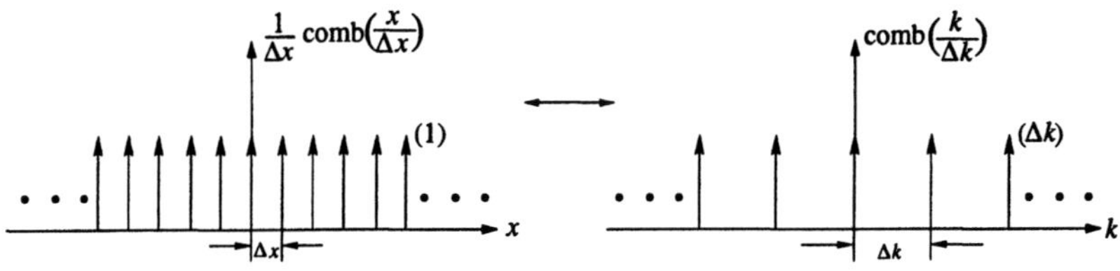

Figure 2.10   The Fourier transform of a delta function train.

2.6 The Radon Transform

The Radon transform is known as the mathematical basis for tomographic imaging from projection (line, plane, or hyperplane integral) data. Unlike the case of the Fourier transform, the popularity and growth of the Radon transform have been closely tied to tomographic imaging [16, 32]. In fact, the basic Radon transform theory was ignored for nearly half a century following its invention in 1917 until its first successful use for generating X-ray tomographic images in 1972. For this reason, this transform has been reinvented several times in different forms and in different areas. In this section, we first present its mathematical definition and then discuss some of its fundamental properties. To bring out the concept, we begin with the definition of the two-dimensional Radon transform. Then we will define higher-dimensional Radon transforms and partial Radon transforms. Finally, we describe the projection-slice theorem and other properties of the Radon transform. The inverse Radon transform is discussed in Chapter 6 in the context of image reconstruction from projection data.

2.6.1 Two-Dimensional Radon Transforms

The two-dimensional Radon transform is simply a line integral, as shown in Fig. 2.11. More specifically, for an arbitrary function $\rho(x, y)$, its Radon transform, denoted as $\mathcal{R}\{\rho(x, y)\}$, or $\{\mathcal{R}\rho\}(p, \phi)$, or simply $P(p, \phi)$, is the integration of $\rho(x, y)$ along a line (ray) L,

$$P(p, \theta) = \mathcal{R}\{\rho(x, y)\} = \int_L \rho(x, y) dl \qquad (2.99)$$

where the integral path L is defined by

$$x \cos \phi + y \sin \phi = p \qquad (2.100)$$

In some medical imaging literature, $\{\mathcal{R}\rho\}(p, \phi)$ is called a *raysum* since the line integral is accomplished physically by passing a ray through an object. For a fixed ϕ, $\{\mathcal{R}\rho\}(p, \phi)$, as a function of p, is a projection of $\rho(x, y)$ along L, and ϕ is referred to as the *projection angle*. It is important to note, however, that the projection angle is defined as the angle between the x-axis and the line normal to the ray path (not the orientation angle of the ray path itself).

Mathematically, $\mathcal{R}\{\rho(x, y)\}$ can be written in several equivalent forms. For example, the line integral in Eq. (2.99) can be converted to a one-dimensional integration as

$$\{\mathcal{R}\rho\}(p, \phi) = \int_{-\infty}^{\infty} \rho(p \cos \phi - q \sin \phi, p \sin \phi + q \cos \phi) dq \qquad (2.101)$$

Equation (2.101) is obtained by transforming the (x, y) coordinate system to the rotated coordinate system (p, q), shown in Fig. 2.12. The required transformation

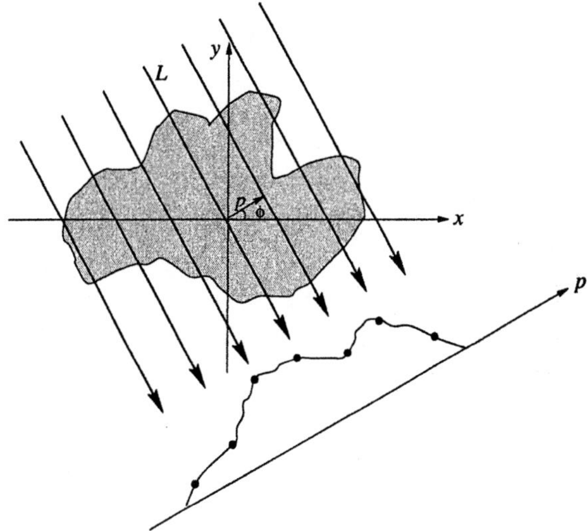

Figure 2.11   Two-dimensional Radon transform as line integrals.

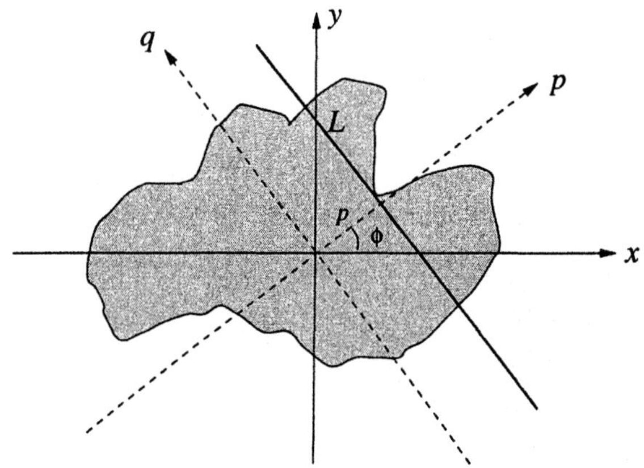

Figure 2.12   Ray path L relative to the original and rotated coordinates.

is given by

$$\begin{cases} p = x\cos\phi + y\sin\phi \\ q = -x\sin\phi + y\cos\phi \end{cases} \quad \text{or} \quad \begin{cases} x = p\cos\phi - q\sin\phi \\ y = p\sin\phi + q\cos\phi \end{cases} \qquad (2.102)$$

Another more convenient form of the two-dimensional Radon transform is

$$\{\mathcal{R}\rho\}(p,\phi) = \int_{-\infty}^{\infty}\int_{-\infty}^{\infty} \rho(x,y)\delta(x\cos\phi + y\sin\phi - p)\,dx\,dy \qquad (2.103)$$

The equivalence between Eqs. (2.101) and (2.103) can be justified using the coordinate transformation defined in Eq. (2.102). Specifically, upon performing the variable substitution

$$\begin{cases} x = \hat{p}\cos\phi - \hat{q}\sin\phi \\ y = \hat{p}\sin\phi + \hat{q}\cos\phi \end{cases} \tag{2.104}$$

Eq. (2.103) becomes

$$\{\mathcal{R}\rho\}(p,\phi) = \iint \rho(\hat{p}\cos\phi - \hat{q}\sin\phi, \hat{p}\sin\phi + \hat{q}\cos\phi)\delta(\hat{p}-p)|\mathbf{J}|d\hat{p}d\hat{q} \tag{2.105}$$

Equation (2.101) immediately follows by making use of the property of the delta function and noting that

$$|\mathbf{J}| = \begin{vmatrix} \dfrac{\partial x}{\partial \hat{p}} & \dfrac{\partial x}{\partial \hat{q}} \\[2mm] \dfrac{\partial y}{\partial \hat{p}} & \dfrac{\partial y}{\partial \hat{q}} \end{vmatrix} = \begin{vmatrix} \cos\phi & -\sin\phi \\ \sin\phi & \cos\phi \end{vmatrix} = 1 \tag{2.106}$$

■ **Example 2.8**

This examples calculates $\{\mathcal{R}\rho\}(p, 0°)$ for $\rho(x,y) = \Pi(\frac{x}{a})\Pi(\frac{y}{b})$. Based on the definition, we have

$$\{\mathcal{R}\rho\}(p, 0°) = \int_{-\infty}^{\infty} \int_{-\infty}^{\infty} \Pi\left(\frac{x}{a}\right) \Pi\left(\frac{y}{b}\right) \delta(x\cos 0° + y\sin 0° - p)dxdy$$

$$= \int_{-b/2}^{b/2} \int_{-a/2}^{a/2} \delta(x-p)dxdy$$

$$= b\int_{-a/2}^{a/2} \delta(x-p)dxdy$$

$$= \begin{cases} b & -a/2 \leq p \leq a/2 \\ 0 & \text{otherwise} \end{cases}$$

$$= b\,\Pi\left(\frac{p}{a}\right)$$

2.6.2   Higher-Dimensional Radon Transforms

The Radon transform of higher-dimensional functions can be defined by extending Eq. (2.103) to higher dimensions. First, we rewrite Eq. (2.103) in vector form with the dimension of the transform operator and the vector variables being made explicit:

$$\{\mathcal{R}_2\rho\}(p, \boldsymbol{\mu}_2) = \int_{\mathbb{R}^2} \rho(\boldsymbol{r}_2)\delta(p - \boldsymbol{\mu}_2 \cdot \boldsymbol{r}_2)d\boldsymbol{r}_2 \qquad (2.107)$$

where $\boldsymbol{\mu}_2 = (\cos\phi, \sin\phi)$, $\boldsymbol{r}_2 = (x, y)$, and $d\boldsymbol{r}_2 = dxdy$. Extending Eq. (2.107) to n dimensions gives

$$\{\mathcal{R}_n\rho\}(p, \boldsymbol{\mu}_n) = \int_{\mathbb{R}^n} \rho(\boldsymbol{r}_n)\delta(p - \boldsymbol{\mu}_n \cdot \boldsymbol{r}_n)d\boldsymbol{r}_n \qquad (2.108)$$

which is called the *nth-dimensional Radon transform* of $\rho(\boldsymbol{r}_n)$.

To gain a better understanding of Eq. (2.108), consider the three-dimensional case. In the spherical coordinate system,

$$\boldsymbol{\mu}_3 = (\sin\theta\cos\phi, \sin\theta\sin\phi, \cos\theta) \qquad (2.109)$$

and

$$\boldsymbol{\mu}_3 \cdot \boldsymbol{r}_3 = x\sin\theta\cos\phi + y\sin\theta\sin\phi + z\cos\theta \qquad (2.110)$$

where θ and ϕ are the polar and azimuthal angles, respectively. Substituting Eq. (2.110) into Eq. (2.108) yields

$$\{\mathcal{R}_3\rho\}(p, \boldsymbol{\mu}_3) = \iiint \rho(x, y, z)\delta(x\sin\theta\cos\phi + y\sin\theta\sin\phi + z\cos\theta - p)dxdydz$$
$$(2.111)$$

Noting that
$$x\sin\theta\cos\phi + y\sin\theta\sin\phi + z\cos\theta = p \qquad (2.112)$$

defines a plane as shown in Fig. 2.13, it is clear that Eq. (2.111) is a plane integral in contrast to the line integral given by Eq. (2.103) for the two-dimensional case.

For $n > 3$, it is convenient to employ the hyperspherical polar coordinates $(r, \theta_1, \cdots, \theta_{n-2}, \phi)$ with

$$\begin{cases} r_1 = r\cos\theta_1 \\ r_2 = r\sin\theta_1\cos\theta_2 \\ \quad\vdots \\ r_{n-2} = r\sin\theta_1\cdots\sin\theta_{n-3}\cos\theta_{n-2} \\ r_{n-1} = r\sin\theta_1\cdots\sin\theta_{n-2}\cos\phi \\ r_n = r\sin\theta_1\cdots\sin\theta_{n-2}\sin\phi \end{cases} \qquad (2.113)$$

for $0 \le \theta_\ell \le \pi$, $0 \le \phi \le 2\pi$, and $r \ge 0$. The unit vector in Eq. (2.108) is now given by

$$\boldsymbol{\mu}_n = (\cos\theta_1, \sin\theta_1\cos\theta_2, \cdots, \sin\theta_1\cdots\sin\theta_{n-2}\sin\phi) \qquad (2.114)$$

and the volume element is

$$d\boldsymbol{r} = r^{n-1}(\sin\theta_1)^{n-2}(\sin\theta_2)^{n-3}(\sin\theta_2)d\theta_1 d\theta_2 \cdots d\theta_{n-2}d\phi \qquad (2.115)$$

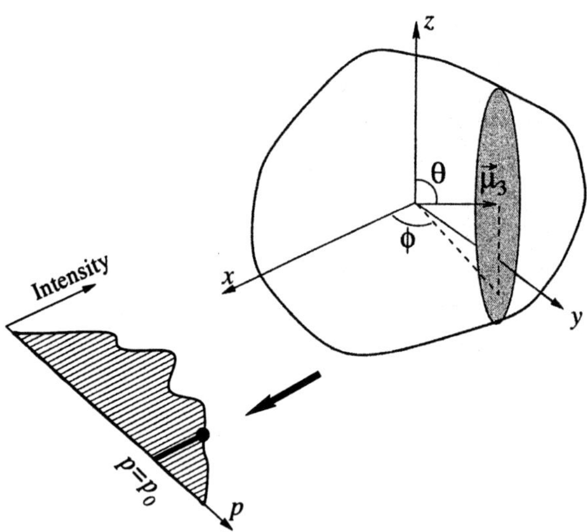

Figure 2.13   Three-dimensional Radon transform as plane integrals.

2.6.3   Partial Radon Transforms

For functions of more than two dimensions, it is sometimes useful to define a *partial Radon transform*, which is the mathematical foundation for the multistage projection reconstruction algorithm to be described in Chapter 6. Before introducing the general definition, let us first consider the three-dimensional Radon transform. From Eq. (2.111), we have

$$
\begin{aligned}
\mathcal{R}_3\rho &= \iiint \rho(x,y,z)\delta(x\cos\phi\sin\theta + y\sin\phi\sin\theta + z\cos\theta - p)\,dxdydz \\
&= \iiint \rho(x,y,z)\delta[(x\cos\phi + y\sin\phi)\sin\theta + z\cos\theta - p]\,dxdydz \\
&= \iiiint \rho(x,y,z)\delta(q\sin\theta + z\cos\theta - p) \\
&\qquad \delta(x\cos\phi + y\sin\phi - q)\,dqdxdydz \\
&= \iint \left[\iint \rho(x,y,z)\delta(x\cos\phi + y\sin\phi - q)\,dxdy \right] \\
&\qquad \delta(q\sin\theta + z\cos\theta - p)\,dqdz
\end{aligned}
\tag{2.116}
$$

The double integral inside the brackets is a line integral in the (x,y)-plane. Treating $\rho(x,y,z)$ as a function of x and y with z being a free parameter, the bracketed double integral can be viewed as a two-dimensional Radon transform and written as

$$\{\mathcal{R}_2\rho\}(q,\phi;z) = \iint \rho(x,y,z)\delta(x\cos\phi + y\sin\phi - q)dxdy \qquad (2.117)$$

where $\mu_2 = (\cos\phi, \sin\phi)$. Substituting Eq. (2.117) into Eq. (2.116) yields

$$\{\mathcal{R}_3\rho\}(p,\phi,\theta) = \iint \mathcal{R}_2\rho(q,\phi;z)\delta(q\sin\theta + z\cos\theta - p)dqdz \qquad (2.118)$$

We refer to $\{\mathcal{R}_2\rho\}(q,\phi;z)$ as a *partial* Radon transform of $\rho(x,y,z)$ because the function is only partially transformed (along the x- and y-directions). As with Eq. (2.117), we also have other partial transforms such as $\{\mathcal{R}_2\rho\}(q,\phi;x)$ and $\{\mathcal{R}_2\rho\}(q,\phi;y)$, as well as those not in the cardinal directions. In general, we define a partial Radon transform as a lower-dimensional transform of a higher-dimensional function. A more formal definition is as follows.

Definition 2.1 *For an n-dimensional function $\rho(r)$, its m-dimensional partial Radon transform along the first m cardinal directions $r_1, r_2, \ldots, r_m$ with $m \leq n$ is defined as*

$$\mathcal{R}_m\rho(p,\boldsymbol{\mu}_m; r_{m+1},\ldots,r_n) = \int_{\mathbb{R}^m} \rho(\boldsymbol{r}_m; r_{m+1},\ldots,r_n)\delta(p - \boldsymbol{\mu}_m \cdot \boldsymbol{r}_m)d\boldsymbol{r}_m$$

$$(2.119)$$

where $\boldsymbol{r}_m = (r_1, r_2, \ldots, r_m)$ and $\boldsymbol{\mu}_m$ is a unit directional vector in $\mathbb{R}^m$ defining the projection direction.

It is clear from this definition and from Fig. 2.14 that a notable distinction between partial and full Radon transforms is that, for a given projection angle, the Radon transform reduces a function $\rho(r)$ to a one-dimensional projection profile, while the partial Radon transforms are planar or hyperplanar projections of $\rho(r)$. Specifically, for an n-dimensional function, its m-dimensional partial Radon transform has $(n-m)$ untransformed spatial dimensions which, combined with distributions along the p-axis, form an $(n - m + 1)$-dimensional projection of the function for $2 \leq m \leq n$. For the special case $m = n$, the partial Radon transform becomes the (full) Radon transform.

Similarly to the Fourier transform, a higher-dimensional Radon transform can be expressed as cascaded lower-dimensional (partial) Radon transforms. This is demonstrated by Eq. (2.118), in which the three-dimensional Radon transform is equivalent to two cascaded two-dimensional Radon transforms. It is also easy to visualize that a four-dimensional Radon transform can be expressed as three cascaded two-dimensional Radon transforms, or as one two-dimensional Radon transform followed by a three-dimensional Radon transform, or vice versa. In general, the following recursive relationship exists for the partial Radon transform operator:

$$\mathcal{R}_n = \mathcal{R}_{n-m+1}\mathcal{R}_m \qquad 2 \leq m \leq n - 1 \text{ and } n > 2 \qquad (2.120)$$

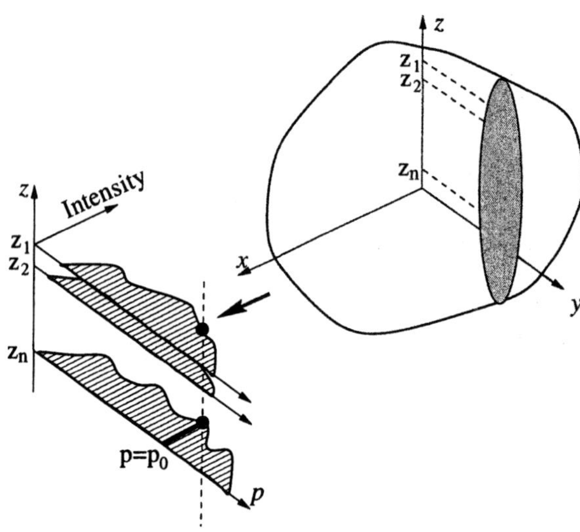

Figure 2.14 Graphical representation of two-dimensional partial Radon transforms of a three-dimensional object.

where $\mathcal{R}_n$ represents the n-dimensional (partial) Radon transform operator. To prove the decomposition in Eq. (2.120), we rewrite Eq. (2.108) as

$$\{\mathcal{R}_n\rho\}(p,\boldsymbol{\mu}_n) = \int_{\mathbb{R}^n} \rho(\boldsymbol{r}_n)\delta(p - \boldsymbol{\mu}'_m\cdot\boldsymbol{r}_m - \boldsymbol{\mu}'_{n-m}\cdot\boldsymbol{r}_{n-m})d\boldsymbol{r}_m d\tilde{\boldsymbol{r}}_{n-m} \quad (2.121)$$

where it is assumed that

$$\boldsymbol{\mu}'_m = (\mu_1, \mu_2, \ldots, \mu_m) \tag{2.122a}$$

$$\boldsymbol{r}_m = (r_1, r_2, \ldots, r_m) \tag{2.122b}$$

$$\tilde{\boldsymbol{\mu}}'_{n-m} = (\mu_{m+1}, \mu_{m+2}, \ldots, \mu_n) \tag{2.122c}$$

$$\tilde{\boldsymbol{r}}_{n-m} = (r_{m+1}, r_{m+2}, \ldots, r_n) \tag{2.122d}$$

such that

$$\boldsymbol{\mu}_n = (\boldsymbol{\mu}'_m, \tilde{\boldsymbol{\mu}}'_{n-m}) \tag{2.123a}$$

$$\boldsymbol{r}_n = (\boldsymbol{r}'_m \tilde{\boldsymbol{r}}_{n-m}) \tag{2.123b}$$

The prime superscripts on $\boldsymbol{\mu}'_m$ and $\tilde{\boldsymbol{\mu}}'_{n-m}$ are used to indicate that they are not unit vectors. Let $q = \frac{\boldsymbol{\mu}'_m}{|\boldsymbol{\mu}'_m|}\cdot\boldsymbol{r}_m$. Then

$$\{\mathcal{R}_n\rho\}(p,\boldsymbol{\mu}_n) = \int_{\mathbb{R}^{n-m+1}}\left[\int_{\mathbb{R}^m}\rho(\boldsymbol{r}_m,\tilde{\boldsymbol{r}}_{n-m})\delta\left(q - \frac{\boldsymbol{\mu}'_m}{|\boldsymbol{\mu}'_m|}\cdot\boldsymbol{r}_m\right)d\boldsymbol{r}_m\right]$$

$$\delta(p - |\boldsymbol{\mu}'_m|q - \tilde{\boldsymbol{\mu}}'_{n-m}\cdot\tilde{\boldsymbol{r}}_{n-m})dq d\tilde{\boldsymbol{r}}_{n-m} \tag{2.124}$$

Equation (2.120) immediately follows from Eq. (2.124) by noting that $\frac{\mu'_m}{|\mu'_m|}$ is a unit directional vector in $\mathbb{R}^m$ and $(|\mu'_m|, \mu'_{n-m})$ forms a unit directional vector in $\mathbb{R}^{n-m+1}$.

2.6.4 Basic Properties

The Radon transform possesses many useful properties. Some of the straightforward ones for the two-dimensional case are listed below; others are discussed subsequently in detail. Most of them can be extended to higher dimensions. For notational simplicity, we assume that $\rho(x,y) \overset{\mathcal{R}}{\longleftrightarrow} P(p,\phi)$.

(a) *Linearity*:

$$a\rho_1(x,y) + b\rho_2(x,y) \longleftrightarrow aP_1(p,\phi) + bP_2(p,\phi) \tag{2.125}$$

(b) *Symmetry*:

$$P(p,\phi) = P(-p, \phi \pm \pi) \tag{2.126}$$

(c) *Periodicity*:

$$P(p,\phi) = P(p, \phi + 2n\pi) \qquad \text{for integer } n \tag{2.127}$$

(d) *Shifting property*:

$$\rho(x - x_0, y - y_0) \longleftrightarrow P(p - x_0 \cos\phi - y_0 \sin\phi, \phi) \tag{2.128}$$

(e) *Rotation by ϕ_0*:

$$\rho(x \cos\phi_0 - y \sin\phi_0, x \sin\phi_0 + y \cos\phi_0) \longleftrightarrow P(p, \phi + \phi_0) \tag{2.129}$$

(f) *Scaling property*:

$$\rho(ax, ay) \longleftrightarrow \frac{1}{|a|} P(ap, \phi) \tag{2.130}$$

(g) *Energy conservation*

$$\int_{-\infty}^{\infty} \int_{-\infty}^{\infty} \rho(x,y)\,dx\,dy = \int_{-\infty}^{\infty} P(p,\phi)\,dp \tag{2.131}$$

2.6.5 Sinogram

The two-dimensional Radon transform maps the spatial domain (x,y) to the Radon domain (p,ϕ). This mapping exhibits some interesting properties. For example, each point in the Radon space corresponds to a straight line in the spatial domain; in other words, the data value at a particular point in the Radon space receives contributions from data points along a line in the spatial domain. On the other hand, a point in the spatial domain is mapped to a sinusoid in the Radon space. The first point is clear from the definition of the Radon transform. The latter point can be understood by considering a point source located at $r_0 = (x_0, y_0)$ with intensity A. Its Radon transform is

$$\mathcal{R}\{A\delta(r - r_0)\} = \int_{-\infty}^{\infty} \int_{-\infty}^{\infty} A\delta(r - r_0)\delta(p - \mu \cdot r)dr$$

$$= A\delta(p - \mu \cdot r_0)$$

$$= A\delta(x_0 \cos \phi + y_0 \sin \phi - p) \tag{2.132}$$

which is a sheet of impulses supported on a sinusoidal curve in the (p, ϕ)-plane, as shown in Fig. 2.15, defined by

$$p = x_0 \cos \phi + y_0 \sin \phi = r_0 \cos(\phi - \phi_0) \tag{2.133}$$

where $r_0 = \sqrt{x_0^2 + y_0^2}$ and $\phi_0 = \arctan(y_0/x_0)$. For this reason, the two-dimensional function formed by stacking up all the projections taken sequentially along the angular direction is called a *sinogram*.

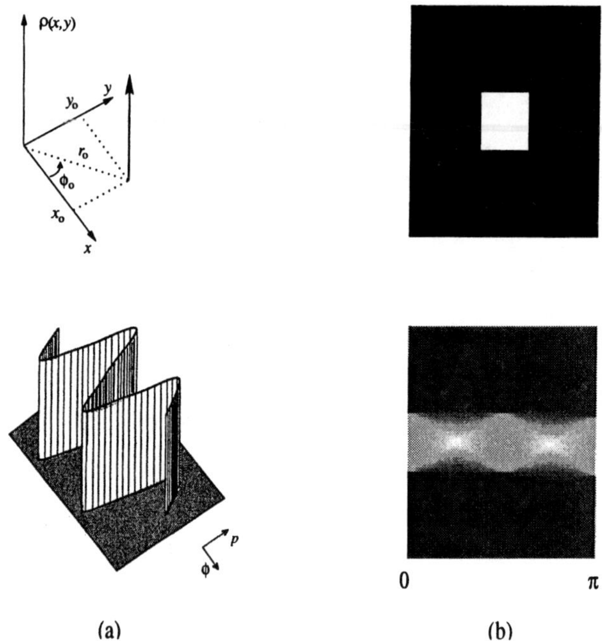

Figure 2.15 Sinograms of (a) a point source and (b) a rectangular function.

For an arbitrary function $\rho(x, y)$, the sinogram may be more complicated. Based on the sampling property of the delta function, we can rewrite $\rho(x, y)$ as

$$\rho(x, y) = \int_{-\infty}^{\infty} \int_{-\infty}^{\infty} \rho(x_0, y_0)\delta(x - x_0, y - y_0)dx_0 dy_0 \qquad (2.134)$$

Since the Radon transform operation is linear, by superposition the sinogram for $\rho(x, y)$ is a continuous sum of sinusoidal sheets with intensity $\rho(x_0, y_0)$, amplitude $r_0 = \sqrt{x_0^2 + y_0^2}$, and initial phase $\phi_0 = \arctan(y_0/x_0)$.

2.6.6   The Projection-Slice Theorem

The Radon transform is closely related to the Fourier transform by the famous projection-slice theorem, which is the theoretical basis for several image reconstruction algorithms. This theorem actually exists in two forms, although only the first form is popularly known. We will describe them both here. The first form of this theorem is for the (full) Radon transform, which relates a one-dimensional projection to a line of data in k-space, while the second form is for the partial Radon transform, which connects planar or hyperplanar projections to the k-space data.

Theorem 2.2 (Projection-Slice Theorem)   *For an n-dimensional function $\rho(r)$, the one-dimensional Fourier transform of $\{\mathcal{R}\rho\}(p, \mu)$ along the p-axis for a fixed projection angle μ is identical to the n-dimensional Fourier transform of $\rho(r)$ evaluated along a line passing through the origin with the same orientation angle in the Fourier space. Mathematically, this theorem can expressed as*

$$\mathcal{F}_p\{\{\mathcal{R}\rho\}(p, \mu)\} = \{\mathcal{F}\rho\}(k\mu) \qquad (2.135)$$

where $\mathcal{F}_p$ represents one-dimensional Fourier transform along the p-axis.

This theorem can be proven easily from the definition as follows:

$$\mathcal{F}_p\{\{\mathcal{R}\rho\}(p, \mu)\} = \int_{-\infty}^{\infty} \{\mathcal{R}\rho\}(p, \mu)e^{-i2\pi kp}dp$$

$$= \int_{-\infty}^{\infty} \left[\int_{r \in R^n} \rho(r)\delta(p - \mu \cdot r)dr \right] e^{-i2\pi kp}dp$$

$$= \int_{r \in R^n} \rho(r) \left[\int_{-\infty}^{\infty} \delta(p - \mu \cdot r)e^{-i2\pi kp}dp \right] dr$$

$$= \int_{r \in R^n} \rho(r)e^{-i2\pi k\mu \cdot r}dr$$

$$= \{\mathcal{F}\rho\}(k\mu)$$

For a better appreciation of the theorem, we take a closer look at it for the two- and three-dimensional cases. In two dimensions, we have $\mu = (\cos\phi, \sin\phi)$ and, consequently,

$$\mathcal{F}_p\{\{\mathcal{R}\rho\}(p, \phi)\} = \{\mathcal{F}\rho\}(k\cos\phi, k\sin\phi) \tag{2.136}$$

which is depicted in Fig. 2.16. It is clear from this example that projections of $\rho(x, y)$ correspond to slices of its Fourier transform $\{\mathcal{F}\rho\}(k_x, k_y)$, thus the name *projection-slice theorem*.

In three dimensions, $\mu = (\sin\theta\cos\phi, \sin\theta\sin\phi, \cos\theta)$ and the projection-slice theorem states that

$$\mathcal{F}_1\{\{\mathcal{R}\rho\}(p, \phi, \theta)\} = \{\mathcal{F}\rho\}(k\sin\theta\cos\phi, k\sin\theta\sin\phi, k\cos\theta) \tag{2.137}$$

Note that

$$\begin{cases} k_x = k\sin\theta\cos\phi \\ k_y = k\sin\theta\sin\phi \\ k_z = k\cos\theta \end{cases} \tag{2.138}$$

or equivalently,

$$\frac{k_x}{\sin\theta\cos\phi} = \frac{k_y}{\sin\theta\sin\phi} = \frac{k_z}{\cos\theta} \tag{2.139}$$

defines a line along the direction of μ in the three-dimensional k-space.

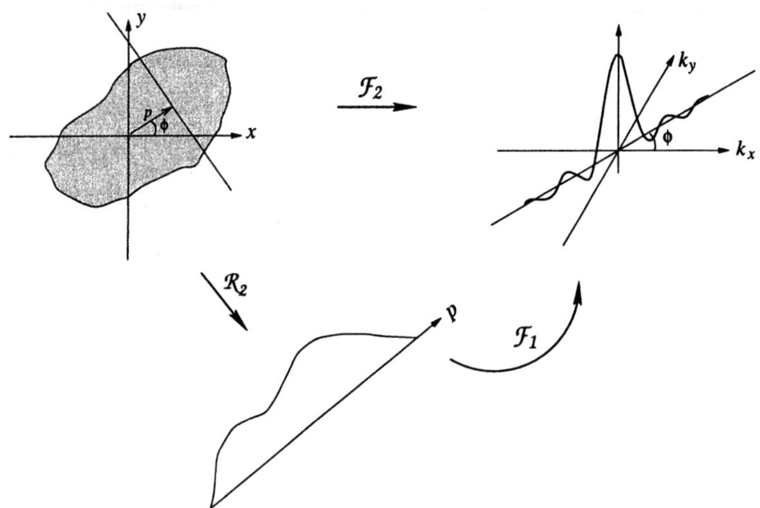

Figure 2.16 Pictorial representation of the projection-slice theorem in two dimensions.

■ Example 2.9

This example calculates the Radon transform of the object shown in Fig. 2.17.

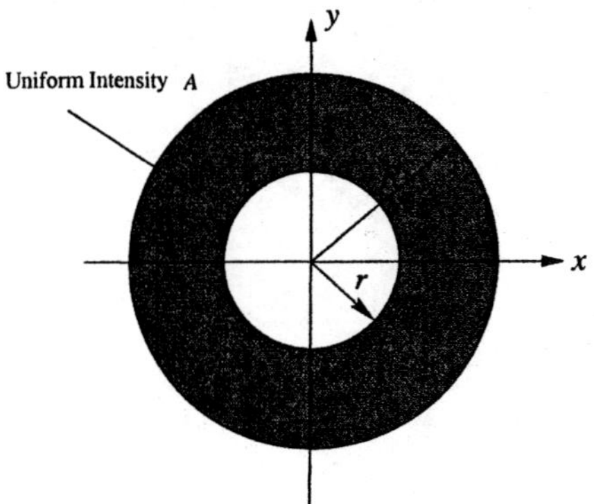

Figure 2.17   Graphical representation of $\rho(x, y)$.

First, we express the object function as

$$\rho(x, y) = \begin{cases} A & r^2 \le x^2 + y^2 \le R^2 \\ 0 & \text{otherwise} \end{cases}$$

Second, noting the object has a circular symmetry, it suffices to calculate $\{\rho\}(p, \phi)$ for only one projection angle, say $\phi = 0°$.

Third, let $\rho(x, y) = \rho_1(x, y) - \rho_2(x, y)$, where

$$\rho_1(x, y) = \begin{cases} A & x^2 + y^2 \le R^2 \\ 0 & \text{otherwise} \end{cases} \qquad \rho_2(x, y) = \begin{cases} A & x^2 + y^2 \le r^2 \\ 0 & \text{otherwise} \end{cases}$$

By definition,

$$\{\mathcal{R}\rho_1\}(p, \phi = 0°) = \int_{-\infty}^{\infty} \int_{-\infty}^{\infty} \rho_1(x, y)\delta(p - x)dx\,dy$$

$$= \int_{-R}^{R} \int_{-\sqrt{R^2 - x^2}}^{\sqrt{R^2 - x^2}} A\delta(p - x)dy\,dx$$

$$= \int_{-R}^{R} 2A\sqrt{R^2 - x^2}\delta(p - x)dx$$

$$= \begin{cases} 2A\sqrt{R^2 - p^2} & -R \le p \le R \\ 0 & \text{otherwise} \end{cases}$$

Similarly, we have

$$\{\mathcal{R}\rho_2\}(p, \phi = 0°) = \begin{cases} 2A\sqrt{r^2 - p^2} & -r \le p \le r \\ 0 & \text{otherwise} \end{cases}$$

Finally, based on the linearity of the Radon transform, we have

$$\mathcal{R}\{\rho(x,y)\} = \{\mathcal{R}\rho_1\}(p, \phi = 0°) - \{\mathcal{R}\rho_2\}(p, \phi = 0°)$$

$$= \begin{cases} 2A\sqrt{R^2 - p^2} & -R \le p \le -r, r \le p \le R \\ 2A\left[\sqrt{R^2 - p^2} - \sqrt{r^2 - p^2}\right] & -r \le p \le r \\ 0 & \text{otherwise} \end{cases}$$

■ Example 2.10

This example calculates the Fourier transform of $\mathcal{R}\{\rho\}(p, 45°)$ for a square object defined by $\rho(x, y) = \Pi(x/2)\Pi(y/2)$. We will do so directly and by the projection-slice theorem.

First, we evaluate $\{\mathcal{R}\rho\}(p, 45°)$ for the given object. It is clear from Fig. 2.18 that the projection is taken along the diagonal of the square. Simple geometric analysis shows that the result is a triangular pulse. Namely,

$$\{\mathcal{R}\rho\}(p, 45°) = 2\sqrt{2}\Lambda\left(\frac{p}{\sqrt{2}}\right)$$

Based on the result in Example 2.4 and the scaling property of the Fourier transform, we have

$$\mathcal{F}\{\{\mathcal{R}\rho\}(p, 45°)\} = \mathcal{F}\left\{2\sqrt{2}\Lambda\left(\frac{p}{\sqrt{2}}\right)\right\} = 4\operatorname{sinc}^2(\sqrt{2}\pi k)$$

We next derive the result by using the projection-slice theorem. We first find the two-dimensional Fourier transform of $\rho(x, y)$, which is

$$\{\mathcal{F}\rho\}(k_x, k_y) = 4\operatorname{sinc}(2\pi k_x)\operatorname{sinc}(2\pi k_y)$$

Then, from the projection-slice theorem, we immediately get the following result.

$$\mathcal{F}\{\{\mathcal{R}\rho\}(p, 45°)\} = \{\mathcal{R}\rho\}(k\cos 45°, k\sin 45°)$$
$$= 4\,\text{sinc}(\sqrt{2}\pi k)\text{sinc}(\sqrt{2}\pi k)$$
$$= 4\,\text{sinc}^2(\sqrt{2}\pi k)$$

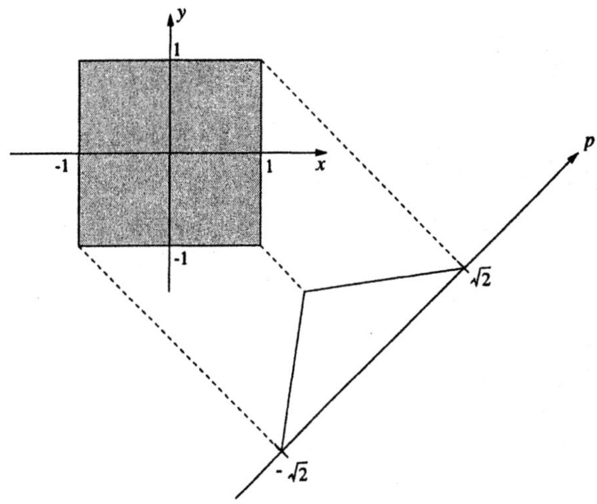

Figure 2.18 Projection of a square object.

Theorem 2.3 (Generalized Projection-Slice Theorem) *For an n-dimensional function $\rho(\mathbf{r})$, the Fourier transform of its partial Radon transform $\mathcal{R}_m\rho$ is related to its Fourier transform $\mathcal{F}\rho$ by the following relationship:*

$$\{\mathcal{F}_{n-m+1}\mathcal{R}_m\rho\}(k, k_{m+1}, \ldots, k_n) = \{\mathcal{F}\rho\}(k\mu_m, k_{m+1}, \ldots, k_n) \quad (2.140)$$

where it is understood that $\mathcal{R}_m\rho$ is a function of $(p, \mu_m; x_{m+1}, \ldots, x_n)$ such that p and k, and $(x_{m+1}, \ldots, x_n)$ and $(k_{m+1}, \ldots, k_n)$ are conjugate variable pairs of $\mathcal{F}_{n-m+1}$. The function on the right-hand side of Eq. (2.140) should be interpreted as $\{\mathcal{F}_n\rho\}(k_1, k_2, \ldots, k_n)$ evaluated at $(k_1, k_2, \ldots, k_m) = k\mu_m$.

We call Eq. (2.140) the *generalized projection-slice theorem* because it includes the basic projection-slice theorem as a special case with $m = n$. This theorem can be proven following the same procedure used to prove the basic projection-slice theorem as follows.

$$\{\mathcal{F}_{n-m+1}\mathcal{R}_m\rho\}(k, k_{m+1}, \ldots, k_n)$$

$$= \int_{R^{n-m}} \int_{-\infty}^{\infty} \left[\int_{R^m} \rho(\boldsymbol{r}_m; x_{m+1}, \ldots, x_n)\delta(p - \boldsymbol{\mu}_m \cdot \boldsymbol{r}_m)d\boldsymbol{r}_m \right]$$

$$e^{-i2\pi kp}e^{-i2\pi(k_{m+1}x_{m+1}+\cdots+k_n x_n)}dp\,dx_{m+1}\cdots dx_n$$

$$= \int_{R^n} \rho(\boldsymbol{r}_m; x_{m+1}, \ldots, x_n)e^{-i2\pi(k\boldsymbol{\mu}_m \cdot \boldsymbol{r}_m + k_{m+1}x_{m+1}+\cdots+k_n x_n)}$$

$$dr_m\,dx_{m+1}\cdots dx_n$$

$$= \{\mathcal{F}\rho\}(k\boldsymbol{\mu}_m, k_{m+1}, \ldots, k_n)$$

■ **Example 2.11**

In this example, we take a look at the generalized projection-slice theorem for a special case with $n = 3$ and $m = 2$. Specifically, if we choose the projection direction such that $\boldsymbol{\mu}_2 = (\cos 90°, \sin 90°) = (0, 1)$, we have

$$\{\mathcal{R}_2\rho\}(p = y, z) = \int_{-\infty}^{\infty} \int_{-\infty}^{\infty} \rho(x, y, z)\delta(p - y)dx\,dy$$

$$= \int_{-\infty}^{\infty} \rho(x, y, z)dx$$

which is a two-dimensional projection of the object along the x-axis. Based on the foregoing result, we easily get

$$\{\mathcal{F}_2\mathcal{R}_2\rho\}(k_y, k_z) = \int_{-\infty}^{\infty} \int_{-\infty}^{\infty} \int_{-\infty}^{\infty} \rho(x, y, z)e^{-i2\pi(k_y y + k_z z)}dx\,dy\,dz$$

$$= \mathcal{F}\rho(0, k_y, k_z)$$

which is exactly what the generalized projection-slice theorem predicts noting that $k\boldsymbol{\mu}_2 = (0, k) = (0, k_y)$.

2.6.7　Convolution Theorem

Another useful relationship associated with the Radon transform is the convolution theorem, which states that the Radon transform of the convolution of two functions $\rho_1(\boldsymbol{r})$ and $\rho_2(\boldsymbol{r})$ is equal to the one-dimensional convolution of their Radon transforms. That is,

$$\mathcal{R}\left\{ \int \rho_1(\hat{\boldsymbol{r}})\rho_2(\boldsymbol{r} - \hat{\boldsymbol{r}})d\hat{\boldsymbol{r}} \right\} = \int_{-\infty}^{\infty} \{\mathcal{R}\rho_1\}(q, \boldsymbol{\mu})\{\mathcal{R}\rho_2\}(p - q, \boldsymbol{\mu})dq \quad (2.141)$$

Equation (2.141) can be obtained directly from the definition of convolution and the Radon transform. Specifically,

$$
\begin{aligned}
\mathcal{R}\{\rho_1 * \rho_2\}(p, \boldsymbol{\mu}) &= \int_{\mathbb{R}^n} \left[\int_{\mathbb{R}^n} \rho_1(\hat{\boldsymbol{r}})\rho_2(\boldsymbol{r} - \hat{\boldsymbol{r}})d\hat{\boldsymbol{r}} \right] \delta(p - \boldsymbol{\mu} \cdot \boldsymbol{r})d\boldsymbol{r} \\
&= \int_{\mathbb{R}^n} \rho_1(\hat{\boldsymbol{r}}) \left[\int_{\mathbb{R}^n} \rho_2(\boldsymbol{r} - \hat{\boldsymbol{r}})\delta(p - \boldsymbol{\mu} \cdot \boldsymbol{r})d\boldsymbol{r} \right] d\hat{\boldsymbol{r}} \\
&= \int_{\mathbb{R}^n} \rho_1(\hat{\boldsymbol{r}}) \left[\int_{\mathbb{R}^n} \rho_2(\hat{\boldsymbol{r}}_1)\delta[(p - \boldsymbol{\mu} \cdot \hat{\boldsymbol{r}}) - \boldsymbol{\mu} \cdot \hat{\boldsymbol{r}}_1]d\hat{\boldsymbol{r}}_1 \right] d\hat{\boldsymbol{r}} \\
&= \int_{\mathbb{R}^n} \rho_1(\hat{\boldsymbol{r}})\{\mathcal{R}\rho_2\}(p - \boldsymbol{\mu} \cdot \hat{\boldsymbol{r}}, \boldsymbol{\mu})d\hat{\boldsymbol{r}} \\
&= \int_{\mathbb{R}^n} \rho_1(\hat{\boldsymbol{r}}) \left[\int_{\infty}^{\infty} \{\mathcal{R}\rho_2\}(p - q, \boldsymbol{\mu})\delta(q - \boldsymbol{\mu} \cdot \hat{\boldsymbol{r}})dq \right] d\hat{\boldsymbol{r}} \\
&= \int_{\infty}^{\infty} \{\mathcal{R}\rho_2\}(p - q, \boldsymbol{\mu}) \left[\int_{\mathbb{R}^n} \rho_1(\hat{\boldsymbol{r}})\delta(q - \boldsymbol{\mu} \cdot \hat{\boldsymbol{r}})d\hat{\boldsymbol{r}} \right] dq \\
&= \int_{\infty}^{\infty} \{\mathcal{R}\rho_1\}(q, \boldsymbol{\mu})\{\mathcal{R}\rho_2\}(p - q, \boldsymbol{\mu})dq
\end{aligned}
$$

Exercises

2.1   Let $v = (1, -2, 3)$. Determine $|v|$ and μ_v, and graph v.

2.2   Let $A = (1, 1, 0)$ and $B = (1, 2, -2)$.

   (a)   Graph A and B.

   (b)   Evaluate and graph $A + B$, $A \cdot B$, and $A \times B$.

   (c)   Determine the angle between A and B.

2.3   Derive Eq. (2.17) from Eq. (2.15).

2.4   Derive Eq. (2.22) from Eq. (2.18).

2.5   Consider the following two matrices:

$$\mathbf{W}_1 = \frac{1}{\sqrt{2}} \begin{bmatrix} 1 & 1 \\ 1 & -1 \end{bmatrix} \quad \text{and} \quad \mathbf{W}_2 = \begin{bmatrix} \sqrt{2} & i \\ -i & \sqrt{2} \end{bmatrix}$$

   (a)   Determine if they are orthogonal or unitary matrices.

   (b)   Evaluate $\mathbf{W}_1 \mathbf{W}_2$.

   (c)   Determine $\mathbf{W}_1^{-1}$ and $\mathbf{W}_2^{-1}$.

2.6   Sketch the following functions:

   (a) $\Pi(\frac{x}{2})$

   (b) $\Pi(2x - 10)$

   (c) $\Lambda(2x + 5)$

   (d) $\Lambda(-2x + 5)$

   (e) $\text{sinc}(\frac{x-3}{2})$

   (f) $\text{sinc}(\frac{x}{5})\Pi(\frac{x}{10\pi})$

   (g) $n^2\{u[n] - u[n - 4]\}$

   (h) $u[n + 3] - u[n - 5]$

   (i) $u[-n + 5]u[n + 3]$

   (j) $u[-n]u[n - 1]$

2.7 For the Gaussian function defined in Eq. (2.37), show that

$$\mu = \int_{-\infty}^{\infty} xG(\mu, \sigma, x)dx$$

and

$$\sigma^2 = \int_{-\infty}^{\infty} (x - \mu)^2 G(\mu, \sigma, x)dx$$

Hint:

$$\int_{-\infty}^{\infty} e^{-(x-\mu)^2/(2\sigma^2)}dx = \sqrt{2\pi}\sigma$$

2.8 Prove the following properties of the Dirichlet function $\mathrm{Dir}(N, x)$ defined in Eq. (2.54):

(a) $\mathrm{Dir}(N, x)$ is a periodic function of period π for N odd but 2π for N even.

(b)

$$\sum_{n=0}^{N-1} e^{i2nx} = \mathrm{Dir}(N, x)e^{i(N-1)x}$$

(c)

$$\int_{-\pi}^{\pi} \mathrm{Dir}(N, x)dx = \begin{cases} 2\pi & N \text{ odd} \\ 0 & N \text{ even} \end{cases}$$

2.9 Use the distribution definition to show that

$$\int_{-\infty}^{\infty} \varphi(x)\delta'(x)dx = -\varphi'(0)$$

2.10 Justify the formula given in Eq. (2.43a).

2.11 Show that

$$\int_{0}^{\pi} \delta(x \cos\phi + y \sin\phi)d\phi = \frac{1}{\sqrt{x^2 + y^2}}$$

Hint: $x \cos\phi + y \sin\phi = \sqrt{x^2 + y^2}\cos(\phi - \phi_0)$ where $\phi_0 = \arctan(y/x)$.

2.12 Based on Eq. (2.55), show that

$$J_n(x) = \frac{1}{\pi}\int_{0}^{\pi} \cos(n\theta - x \sin\theta)d\theta$$

2.13   Show that

$$J_0(x) = \frac{1}{2\pi} \int_{-\pi}^{\pi} e^{-ix\sin\theta}\, d\theta = \frac{1}{2\pi} \int_{-\pi}^{\pi} e^{ix\cos\theta}\, d\theta = \frac{1}{2\pi} \int_{-\pi}^{\pi} e^{-ix\cos\theta}\, d\theta$$

2.14   Show that

$$e^{ix\sin\theta} = J_0(x) + 2\sum_{n=1}^{\infty} J_{2n}(x)\cos(2n\theta) + i2\sum_{n=1}^{\infty} J_{2n-1}(x)\sin[(2n-1)\theta]$$

2.15   Show that $\frac{1}{\Delta x}\mathrm{comb}(x/\Delta x)$ is a comb function of periodicity Δx, namely,

$$\frac{1}{\Delta x}\mathrm{comb}(x/\Delta x) = \sum_{n=-\infty}^{\infty} \delta(x - n\Delta x)$$

2.16   Calculate the following convolutions and sketch the resulting functions:

(a) $\Pi(x/a) * \Pi(x/b)$

(b) $\Pi(x/a) * \Lambda(x/b)$

(c) $\frac{1}{x} * \frac{1}{x}$

(d) $G(\mu_1, \sigma_1, x) * G(\mu_2, \sigma_2, x)$

(e) $\{\cdots, 0, 0.5, 0, 1, 0, 0.5, 0, \cdots\} * \{\frac{1}{3}, \frac{1}{3}, \frac{1}{3}\}$

2.17   Show that

$$f_1(t)e^{-i2\pi f_0 t} * f_2(t)e^{-i2\pi f_0 t} = [f_1(t) * f_2(t)]e^{-i2\pi f_0 t}$$

2.18   Let $S(k) = \mathcal{F}\{\rho(x)\}$. Prove the following properties:

(a)   *Hermitian symmetry*:
    If $\rho(x)$ is a real function, then $S(k) = S^*(-k)$

(b)   *Modulation property*:

$$\mathcal{F}\{\rho(x)\cos(2\pi k_0 x)\} = \frac{1}{2}[S(k + k_0) + S(k - k_0)]$$

2.19   Prove the convolution theorem, namely,

$$\rho_1(x)\rho_2(x) \longleftrightarrow \{\mathcal{F}\rho_1\}(k) * \{\mathcal{F}\rho_2\}(k)$$

2.20   Calculate $\mathcal{F}\{\mathrm{sinc}^2(\pi a x)\}$ based on the convolution theorem.

2.21   Calculate the Fourier transform of the trapezoidal pulse in the following figure using the derivative and shift theorems.

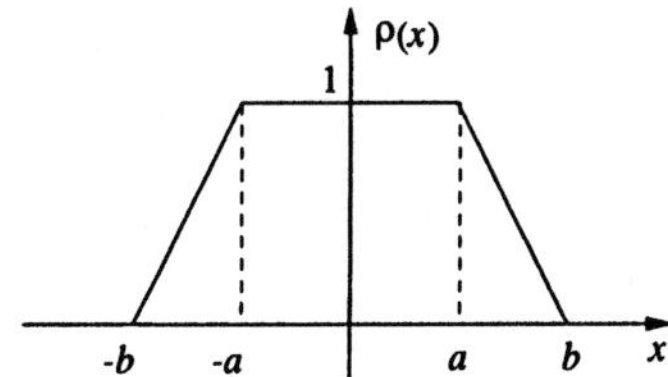

2.22   Calculate the Fourier transform of the following functions using the properties:

(a) $\Pi(\frac{t-t_0/2}{t_0})e^{-i2\pi f_0 t}$

(b) $\Pi(\frac{t-t_0/2}{t_0})e^{-i2\pi f_0(t-t_0/2)}$

(c) $\text{sinc}[\pi f_w(t-t_0)]e^{-i2\pi f_0 t}$

(d) $\text{sinc}[\pi f_w(t-t_0)]e^{-i2\pi f_0(t-t_0)}$

2.23   Show that any periodic function $f(t)$ of period T can be written as

$$f(t) = f_T(t) * \frac{1}{T}\text{comb}\left(\frac{t}{T}\right)$$

where $f_T(t)$ is a period of $f(t)$.

2.24   Show the following Fourier transform relationship:

$$\mathcal{F}\left\{\frac{1}{\sqrt{x^2+y^2}}\right\} = \frac{1}{\sqrt{k_x^2+k_y^2}}$$

2.25   Calculate the following convolution:

$$\text{sinc}(\pi a_1 x) * \text{sinc}(\pi a_2 x) * \cdots * \text{sinc}(\pi a_n x)$$

where it is assumed that $0 < a_1 < a_2 < \cdots < a_n$.

2.26   A function $\rho(x)$ can be expressed as a sum of its even and odd components as $\rho(x) = \rho_e(x) + \rho_o(x)$.

(a)   If $\rho(x)$ is a real function, show that

$$\rho_e(x) \longleftrightarrow \Re\{\mathcal{F}\rho(k)\}$$
$$\rho_o(x) \longleftrightarrow i\Im\{\mathcal{F}\rho(k)\}$$

(b)   Verify the result in (a) with $\rho(x) = e^{-x}u(x)$.

2.27   Let $S(k)$ be the Fourier transform of a real function $\rho(x)$ with S_{r} and S_{i} being the real and imaginary parts of S, respectively. Find $\mathcal{F}^{-1}\{S_{\mathrm{r}}(k)\}$ and $\mathcal{F}^{-1}\{S_{\mathrm{i}}(k)\}$ and express the results in terms of $\rho(x)$.

2.28   Let $\rho(x, y)$ be a circularly symmetric function and let $S(k_x, k_y)$ be its Fourier transform. Show that

$$S(k\cos\phi, k\sin\phi) = 2\pi \int_0^{\infty} \rho(r\cos\phi, r\sin\phi) J_0(2\pi kr)\, r\, dr$$

2.29   Given that

$$\int_{\infty}^{-\infty} e^{-x^2}\, dx = \sqrt{\pi}$$

find the Radon transform of $e^{-\pi(x^2+y^2)}$.

2.30   Calculate the partial Radon transform $\{\mathcal{R}_2\rho\}(p, \phi; z)$ for the following function:

$$\rho(x, y, z) = \begin{cases} z & x^2 + y^2 \le 1 \text{ and } |z| \le 1 \\ 0 & \text{otherwise} \end{cases}$$

2.31   Prove the properties of the Radon transform listed in Section 2.6.4.

2.32   Let $S(k_x, k_y)$ be the two-dimensional Fourier transform of $\rho(x, y)$ and $\tilde{S}(k)$ be a one-dimensional obtained from it by setting $k_x = k\cos\phi_0$ and $k_y = k\sin\phi_0 + k_0$. Namely, $\tilde{S}(k)$ is the value of $S(k_x, k_y)$ evaluated along the line $k_y = \tan\phi_0 k_x + k_0$ in the two-dimensional k-space, as shown in the following figure. Find $\mathcal{F}^{-1}\{\tilde{S}(k)\}$ and express the result in terms of $\rho(x, y)$.

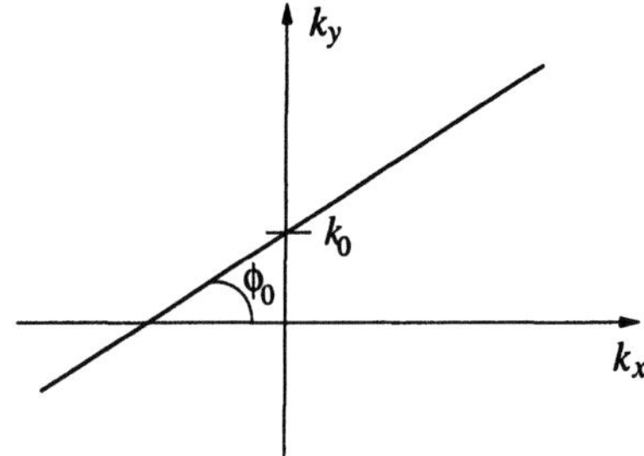

Chapter 3

Signal Generation and Detection

The magnetic moments of nuclei in normal matter will result in a nuclear paramagnetic polarization upon establishment of equilibrium in a constant magnetic field. It is shown that a radio-frequency field at right angles to the constant field causes a forced precession of the total polarization around the constant field with decreasing latitude as the Larmor frequency approaches adiabatically the frequency of the r-f field. Thus there results a component of the nuclear polarization in right angles to both the constant and the r-f field and it is shown that under normal laboratory conditions this component can induce observable voltages.

Felix Bloch

Having reviewed the mathematical fundamentals, we now begin to discuss the image formation principles of MRI. This chapter focuses on the signals: what they are, and how they are generated and detected from an object. To gain some fundamental understanding, we will start with a description of the nuclear magnetic resonance (NMR) phenomenon and then gradually arrive at various signal expressions.

As its name implies, NMR involves nuclei (of an object to be imaged), magnetic fields (generated by an imager), and the resonance phenomenon (arising from the interactions of the nuclei with the magnetic fields). Therefore, to master the mechanism underlying signal generation and detection in MRI and to understand the characteristics of the signals measured, we need, in principle, to start from the nuclear level. As we know, subatomic particles behave quantum-mechanically, but, fortunately, MRI principles can often be accurately described using classical vector models because MRI deals with the collective behavior of an ensemble of a huge number of nuclei present in a macroscopic object. Specifically, we will adopt a system approach for our discussions. In this approach, the object being imaged is viewed as a linear system[1] (magnetized nuclear spin system), and the signal detected is a response activated from the system by an input radio-frequency (RF) excitation that drives the system to a state of resonance. In the rest of the chapter, we will first describe what a magnetized spin system is, then discuss the effects of RF excitations on a spin system, and finally characterize the observed signals.

3.1   Magnetized Nuclear Spin Systems

To understand the NMR phenomenon, we begin with the object to be imaged. We know from basic chemistry that a biological sample or any physical object can be broken down successively into its constituent molecules, then to atoms, and then to nuclei and their orbiting electrons. Nuclei have a finite radius ($\sim 10^{-14}$ m), a finite mass ($\sim 10^{-27}$ kg), and a net electric charge ($\sim 10^{-19}$ coulomb). A fundamental property of nuclei is that those with odd atomic weights and/or odd atomic numbers, such as the nucleus of the hydrogen atom (which has one proton), possess an angular momentum $\vec{J}$, often called *spin*. Although nuclear spin is a property characterized by quantum mechanics, in the classical vector model, spin is visualized as a physical rotation similar to the rotation of a top about its axis. In MRI, an ensemble of nuclei of the same type present in an object being imaged is referred to as a (nuclear) spin system. For example, all the protons (attached either to water or fat) form one spin system while the nuclei of ^{31}P form another spin system. One important property of a nuclear spin system is the so-called *nuclear magnetism* created by placing it in an external magnetic field. This magnetism is the physical basis of MRI. In the rest of this section we will discuss its origin and characteristics.

3.1.1   Nuclear Magnetic Moments

Nuclear magnetism of a nuclear spin system originates from the microscopic magnetic field associated with a nuclear spin. A classical argument for the existence of this magnetic field is twofold: (1) a nucleus such as a proton has electrical charges, and (2) it rotates around its own axis if it has a nonzero spin. Like any spinning charged object, a nucleus with a nonzero spin creates a magnetic field around it, which is analogous to that surrounding a microscopic bar magnet, as shown in Fig. 3.1. Physically, it is represented by a vector quantity $\vec{\mu}$, which

---

[1] While imaging can be treated as a linear process, a spin system behaves nonlinearly during excitation, as described later in this chapter.

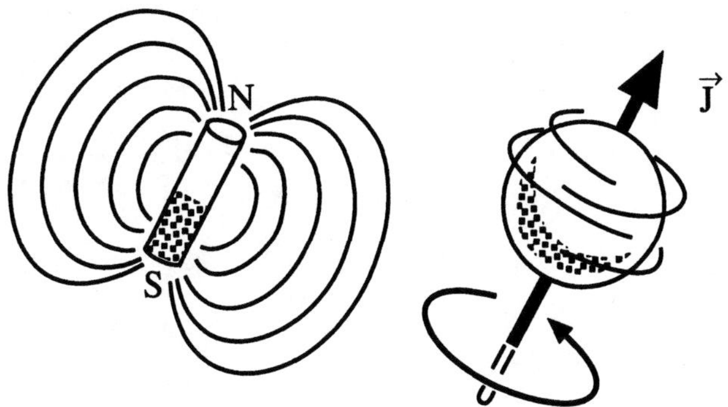

Figure 3.1 Nuclei with nonzero $\vec{\mu}$ are regarded as microscopic magnets.

is called the *nuclear magnetic dipole moment* or *magnetic moment*. One fundamental relationship of particle physics is that the spin angular momentum and
magnetic moment vectors are related to each other by

$$\vec{\mu} = \gamma \vec{J} \tag{3.1}$$

where γ is a physical constant known as the *gyromagnetic ratio*. A related constant $\boldsymbol{\gamma}$ is also widely used, which is defined as

$$\boldsymbol{\gamma} = \frac{\gamma}{2\pi} \tag{3.2}$$

Note that the value of γ or $\boldsymbol{\gamma}$ is nucleus-dependent. For instance, $\gamma = 2.675 \times$
10^8 rad/s/T ($\boldsymbol{\gamma} = 42.58$ MHz/T) for ^{1}H while $\gamma = 7.075 \times 10^7$ rad/s/T ($\boldsymbol{\gamma} =$
11.26 MHz/T) for ^{31}P. The $\boldsymbol{\gamma}$ values of some diagnostically relevant nuclei are
listed in Table 3.1.

Table 3.1 Properties of Some NMR-Active Nuclei

Nucleus	Spin	Relative Sensitivity[a]	Gyromagnetic Ratio $\boldsymbol{\gamma}$ (MHz/T)
^{1}H	1/2	1.000	42.58
^{13}C	1/2	0.016	10.71
^{19}F	1/2	0.870	40.05
^{31}P	1/2	0.093	11.26

[a] Calculated at constant field for an equal number of
nuclei.

Since magnetic moment is a vector quantity, we need to know both its magnitude and its orientation to define it uniquely. Based on the theories of quantum

mechanics, the magnitude of $\vec{\mu}$, often denoted as $|\vec{\mu}|$ or simply μ when there is no confusion, is

$$\mu = \gamma \hbar \sqrt{I(I+1)} \tag{3.3}$$

where $\hbar$ is Planck's constant h (6.6×10^{-34} J-s) divided by 2π and I is the nuclear *spin quantum number*. The spin quantum number takes integer or half-integer or zero values such that

$$I = 0, \frac{1}{2}, 1, \frac{3}{2}, 2, \frac{5}{2}, \cdots \tag{3.4}$$

The value that I assumes for a particular nucleus is governed by the following three simple rules:

(a)   Nuclei with an odd mass number have half-integral spin.

(b)   Nuclei with an even mass number and an even charge number have zero spin.

(c)   Nuclei with an even mass number but an odd charge number have integral spin.

For ^{1}H, ^{13}C, ^{19}F, and ^{31}P nuclei, $I = \frac{1}{2}$, and such a spin system is called a spin-$\frac{1}{2}$ system. A nucleus is NMR-active only if $I \neq 0$.

Although the magnitude of $\vec{\mu}$ is certain under any conditions (with or without an external magnetic field), its direction is completely random in the absence of an external magnetic field due to thermal random motion. This is somewhat analogous to the situation with a collection of compass needles (analogous to the magnetic moments) sitting on a vibrating table (analogous to thermal motion). Therefore, at thermal equilibrium, no *net* magnetic field exists around a macroscopic object.

To activate macroscopic magnetism from an object, it is necessary to line up the spin vectors. This is accomplished by exposing the object to a strong external magnetic field. Following convention, we assume that an external magnetic field of strength B_0 is applied in the z-direction of the laboratory frame such that

$$\vec{B}_0 = B_0 \vec{k} \tag{3.5}$$

Unlike a compass needle which lines up exactly with an external magnetic field, a magnetic moment vector can assume one of a discrete set of orientations, an essential characteristic of the quantum model. In this model, the z-component of $\vec{\mu}$ becomes certain due to the B_0 field and is given by

$$\mu_z = \gamma m_I \hbar \tag{3.6}$$

where m_I is called the *magnetic quantum number*. For any nucleus with nonzero spin, m_I takes the following set of $(2I+1)$ values:

$$m_I = -I, -I+1, \ldots, I \tag{3.7}$$

which corresponds to $(2I + 1)$ possible orientations for $\vec{\mu}$ with respect to the direction of the external field. The angle θ between $\vec{\mu}$ and $\vec{B}_0$ can be calculated using the following formula:

$$\cos\theta = \frac{\mu_z}{\mu} = \frac{m_I}{\sqrt{I(I+1)}} \tag{3.8}$$

While the orientation of $\vec{\mu}$ is quantized along the direction of the external field, the direction of its transverse component $\vec{\mu}_{xy}$ remains random. Specifically, let

$$\vec{\mu}_{xy} = \mu_x \vec{i} + \mu_y \vec{j} \tag{3.9}$$

Then, μ_x and μ_y can be expressed as

$$\begin{cases} \mu_x = |\vec{\mu}_{xy}| \cos\xi \\ \mu_y = |\vec{\mu}_{xy}| \sin\xi \end{cases} \tag{3.10}$$

where ξ is a random variable uniformly distributed over $[0, 2\pi)$ and $|\vec{\mu}_{xy}|$ is given by

$$|\vec{\mu}_{xy}| = \sqrt{\mu^2 - \mu_z^2} = \gamma\hbar\sqrt{I(I+1) - m_I^2} \tag{3.11}$$

For a spin-$\frac{1}{2}$ system, $I = \frac{1}{2}$ and $m_I = \pm\frac{1}{2}$. It is easy to show, based on Eqs. (3.8) and (3.11), that

$$\theta = \pm 54°44' \tag{3.12}$$

and

$$|\vec{\mu}_{xy}| = \frac{\gamma\hbar}{\sqrt{2}} \tag{3.13}$$

Equation (3.12) implies that in a spin-$\frac{1}{2}$ system, any magnetic moment vector takes one of two possible orientations: pointing up (parallel) and pointing down (antiparallel), as shown in Fig. 3.2.

We next describe the motion of $\vec{\mu}$ when placed in an external magnetic field. We will use a classical treatment by assuming that $\vec{\mu}$ is a classical magnetic moment vector without mutual interactions. According to classical mechanics, the torque that $\vec{\mu}$ experiences from the external magnetic field is given by $\vec{\mu} \times B_0\vec{k}$, which is equal to the rate of change of its angular momentum. That is,

$$\frac{d\vec{J}}{dt} = \vec{\mu} \times B_0\vec{k} \tag{3.14}$$

Since $\vec{\mu} = \gamma\vec{J}$, we have

$$\frac{d\vec{\mu}}{dt} = \gamma\vec{\mu} \times B_0\vec{k} \tag{3.15}$$

which is the equation of motion for isolated spins in the classical treatment. The solution to Eq. (3.15) can be expressed by (see derivation in Example 3.1)

$$\begin{cases} \mu_{xy}(t) = \mu_{xy}(0)e^{-i\gamma B_0 t} \\ \mu_z(t) = \mu_z(0) \end{cases} \tag{3.16}$$

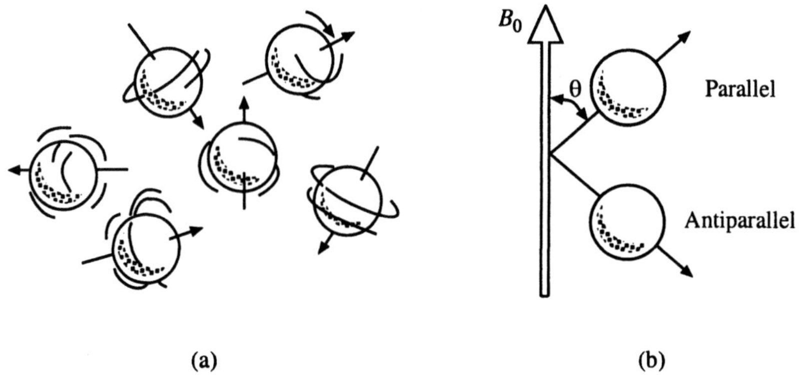

Figure 3.2 Nuclear magnetic moment vectors (a) pointing in random directions and (b) aligned in the direction of an external magnetic field.

where $\mu_{xy}(0)$ and $\mu_z(0)$ are the initial values and it is understood that

$$\mu_{xy} = \mu_x + i\mu_y \sim \vec{\mu}_{xy} = \mu_x \vec{i} + \mu_y \vec{j} \tag{3.17}$$

Equation (3.16) describes a precession of $\vec{\mu}$ about the z-axis (or the B_0 field), which is called *nuclear precession*. In the classical vector model, nuclear precession is similar to the wobbling of a spinning top about the gravitational axis, as illustrated in Fig. 3.3.

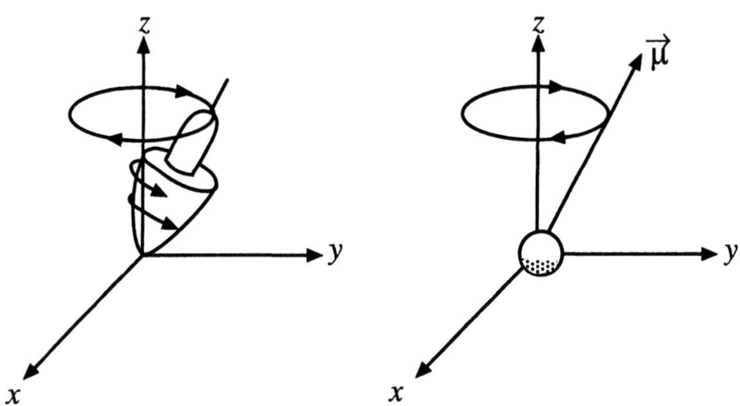

Figure 3.3 Precession of a nuclear spin about an external magnetic field is similar to the wobbling of a spinning top in a gravitational field.

Two important points about nuclear precession are evident from Eq. (3.16). First, the angular frequency of nuclear precession is

$$\omega_0 = \gamma B_0 \tag{3.18}$$

which is known as the Larmor frequency. Second, precession of $\vec{\mu}$ about $\vec{B}_0$ is clockwise if observed against the direction of the magnetic field. In practice, it is easy to determine the precession direction using the *left-hand rule*. That is, if the left thumb points in the direction of $\vec{B}_0$, nuclear precession follows the direction of other fingers.

In addition to Eq. (3.16), nuclear precession can be described by an angular velocity vector defined as

$$\vec{\omega} = -\gamma \vec{B}_0 = -\omega_0 \vec{k} \tag{3.19}$$

Another common way to describe the nuclear precession is through the use of a rotation matrix. Specifically, let

$$\mathbf{R}_z(\alpha) = \begin{bmatrix} \cos\alpha & \sin\alpha & 0 \\ -\sin\alpha & \cos\alpha & 0 \\ 0 & 0 & 1 \end{bmatrix} \tag{3.20}$$

Equation (3.25) can be expressed as

$$\boldsymbol{\mu}(t) = \mathbf{R}_z(\omega_0 t)\boldsymbol{\mu}(0) \tag{3.21}$$

where μ should be interpreted as a column vector $\mu = [\mu_x, \mu_y, \mu_z]^T$.

■ **Example 3.1**

This example derives the solution to Eq. (3.15). We first rewrite Eq. (3.15) in scalar form as

$$\begin{cases} \dfrac{d\mu_x}{dt} = \gamma B_0 \mu_y = \omega_0 \mu_y \\[2mm] \dfrac{d\mu_y}{dt} = -\gamma B_0 \mu_x = -\omega_0 \mu_x \\[2mm] \dfrac{d\mu_z}{dt} = 0 \end{cases} \tag{3.22}$$

The first two equations become decoupled after additional derivatives with respect to time. More specifically,

$$\frac{d^2 \mu_x}{dt^2} = -\omega_0^2 \mu_x \tag{3.23}$$

and

$$\frac{d^2\mu_y}{dt^2} = -\omega_0^2 \mu_y \tag{3.24}$$

These decoupled second-order differential equations have solutions of the general form $A\cos(\omega_0 t) + B\sin(\omega_0 t)$. Setting the initial conditions to $\mu_x(0)$, $\mu_y(0)$, and $\mu_z(0)$, we get

$$\begin{cases} \mu_x(t) = \mu_x(0)\cos(\omega_0 t) + \mu_y(0)\sin(\omega_0 t) \\ \mu_y(t) = -\mu_x(0)\sin(\omega_0 t) + \mu_y(0)\cos(\omega_0 t) \\ \mu_z(t) = \mu_z(0) \end{cases} \tag{3.25}$$

which yields the result in Eq. (3.16) immediately when put in complex notation.

3.1.2　Bulk Magnetization

To describe the collective behavior of a spin system, a macroscopic magnetization vector $\vec{M}$ is introduced, which is the vector sum of all the microscopic magnetic moments in the object. Specifically, let $\vec{\mu}_n$ represent the magnetic moment of the nth nuclear spin. Then,

$$\vec{M} = \sum_{n=1}^{N_s} \vec{\mu}_n \tag{3.26}$$

where N_s is the total number of spins in the object being imaged. This section analyzes $\vec{M}$ for a spin-$\frac{1}{2}$ system.

Recall that $\vec{M} = 0$ in the absence of an external magnetic field. We shall now focus on how $\vec{\mu}_n$ behaves collectively when the object is placed in $\vec{B}_0$. Based on the discussion in the previous section, $\vec{\mu}_n$ takes one of two possible orientations with respect to the z-axis at a given time. Spins in different orientations have different energy of interaction with the external magnetic field $\vec{B}_0$. Specifically, according to the quantum theory,

$$E = -\vec{\mu} \cdot \vec{B}_0 = -\mu_z B_0 = -\gamma \hbar m_I B_0 \tag{3.27}$$

Hence, for pointing-up spins ($m_I = \frac{1}{2}$),

$$E_\uparrow = -\tfrac{1}{2}\gamma \hbar B_0 \tag{3.28}$$

and for pointing-down spins ($m_I = -\frac{1}{2}$),

$$E_\downarrow = \tfrac{1}{2}\gamma \hbar B_0 \tag{3.29}$$

Equations (3.28) and (3.29) indicate that the spin-up state is the lower-energy state, while the spin-down state is the higher-energy state. The energy difference between the two spin states is given by

$$\Delta E = E_{\downarrow} - E_{\uparrow} = \gamma \hbar B_0 \qquad (3.30)$$

The nonzero difference in energy level between the two spin states is known as the *Zeeman splitting* phenomenon and is illustrated in Fig. 3.4.

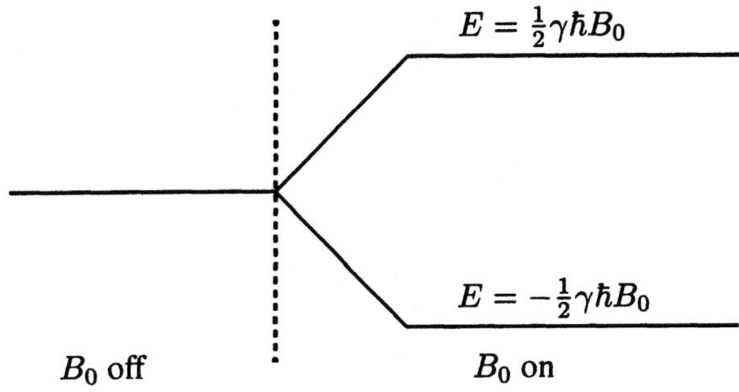

Figure 3.4   Zeeman splitting for a spin-$\frac{1}{2}$ system.

The spin population difference in the two spin states is related to their energy difference. According to the well-known Boltzmann relationship, we have

$$\frac{N_{\uparrow}}{N_{\downarrow}} = \exp\left(\frac{\Delta E}{KT_{\mathrm{s}}}\right) \qquad (3.31)$$

where

$N_{\uparrow}$:	number of pointing-up spins
$N_{\downarrow}$:	number of pointing-down spins
T_{s} :	absolute temperature of the spin system
K :	Boltzmann constant (1.38×10^{-23} J/K)

In practice,

$$\Delta E \ll KT_{\mathrm{s}} \qquad (3.32)$$

Consequently, by first-order approximation,

$$\exp\left(\frac{\Delta E}{KT_{\mathrm{s}}}\right) \approx 1 + \frac{\gamma \hbar B_0}{KT_{\mathrm{s}}} \qquad (3.33)$$

Therefore,

$$\frac{N_{\uparrow}}{N_{\downarrow}} \approx 1 + \frac{\gamma \hbar B_0}{KT_{\mathrm{s}}} \qquad (3.34)$$

and

$$N_\uparrow - N_\downarrow \approx N_\mathrm{s}\frac{\gamma\hbar B_0}{2KT_\mathrm{s}} \tag{3.35}$$

Equation (3.35) indicates that there is an excess of a very small fraction $\frac{\gamma\hbar B_0}{(2KT_\mathrm{s})}$ of spins in the lower-energy state. This uneven spin distribution between the two spin states occurs because a spin is more likely to take the lower-energy state (with higher stability) than the higher-energy state. Although it is very small, the population difference between the two spin states generates an observable macroscopic magnetization vector $\vec{M}$ from a spin system. Such a spin system is said to be *magnetized*. The resulting bulk magnetization, according to Eq. (3.26), is

$$\vec{M} = M_x\vec{i} + M_y\vec{j} + M_z\vec{k}$$
$$= \left(\sum_{n=1}^{N_\mathrm{s}}\mu_{x,n}\right)\vec{i} + \left(\sum_{n=1}^{N_\mathrm{s}}\mu_{y,n}\right)\vec{j} + \left(\sum_{n=1}^{N_\mathrm{s}}\mu_{z,n}\right)\vec{k} \tag{3.36}$$

where $\mu_{x,n}$, $\mu_{y,n}$ and $\mu_{z,n}$ are the projections of $\vec{\mu}_n$ along the x-, y-, and z-axes. The first two terms of Eq. (3.36) are zero because the projection of $\vec{\mu}_n$ onto the transverse plane has a random phase while it precesses about the z-axis,[2] as discussed in Section 3.1.1. The value of $\mu_{z,n}$ is given, according to Eq. (3.6), by

$$\mu_{z,n} = \begin{cases} +\frac{1}{2}\gamma\hbar & \text{if } \vec{\mu}_n \text{ is pointing up} \\ -\frac{1}{2}\gamma\hbar & \text{if } \vec{\mu}_n \text{ is pointing down} \end{cases} \tag{3.37}$$

Substituting Eq. (3.37) into Eq. (3.36) gives

$$\vec{M} = \left(\sum_{n=1}^{N_\uparrow}\tfrac{1}{2}\gamma\hbar - \sum_{n=1}^{N_\downarrow}\tfrac{1}{2}\gamma\hbar\right)\vec{k} = \tfrac{1}{2}(N_\uparrow - N_\downarrow)\gamma\hbar\vec{k} \tag{3.38}$$

Therefore, the bulk magnetization vector points exactly along the positive direction of the z-axis at equilibrium. Its magnitude is

$$M_z^0 = |\vec{M}| = \frac{\gamma^2\hbar^2 B_0 N_\mathrm{s}}{4KT_\mathrm{s}} \tag{3.39}$$

Equation (3.39) indicates that the magnitude of $\vec{M}$ is directly proportional to the external magnetic field strength B_0 and the total number of spins N_s. The value of N_s is characteristic of an object being imaged and cannot be changed in general; therefore, B_0 and T_s are the only controllable parameters. For a given spin system, one can increase the magnitude of $\vec{M}$ by increasing B_0 or decreasing

---

[2] According to Eq. (3.10), $\sum_{n=1}^{N_\mathrm{s}}\mu_{x,n} = \mu_{xy}\sum_{n=1}^{N_\mathrm{s}}\cos\xi_n = 0$ for a random variable ξ_n uniformly distributed over $[0, 2\pi]$.

T_s. Since MRI experiments are often carried out with the object being at room temperature, one is limited to increasing the magnitude of the applied magnetic field for an increase in the bulk magnetization. The optimal field strength for imaging is dependent on the application.[3] For most clinical MRI systems, B_0 ranges from 0.2 to 2 T.

Note that Eq. (3.39) is only valid for a spin-$\frac{1}{2}$ system. For a spin-I system, we have

$$M_z^0 = \frac{\gamma^2 \hbar^2 B_0 N_s I(I+1)}{3KT_s} \tag{3.40}$$

Detailed discussion of this formula can be found in [1].

■ **Example 3.2**

We calculate the spin population difference in the two energy states for a spin system consisting of protons.

According to Eq. (3.35), the fractional population difference is

$$\frac{N_\uparrow - N_\downarrow}{N_s} \approx \frac{\gamma \hbar B_0}{2KT_s} = \frac{\gamma h B_0}{2KT_s}$$

Substituting in the following values:

$$
\begin{aligned}
\gamma &= 42.58 \times 10^6 \text{ Hz/T} \\
h &= 6.6 \times 10^{-34} \text{ J-s} \\
T_s &= 300 \text{ K (room temperature)} \\
K &= 1.38 \times 10^{-23} \text{ J/K} \\
B_0 &= 1 \text{ T}
\end{aligned}
$$

we have

$$\frac{N_\uparrow - N_\downarrow}{N_s} \approx \frac{42.58 \times 10^6 \times 6.6 \times 10^{-34}}{2 \times 1.38 \times 10^{-23} \times 300} \approx 3 \times 10^{-6}$$

This means that, effectively, about three in a million protons in an object can be "activated" for generation of NMR signals. This is why NMR is known as a low-sensitive technique.

---

[3]The penetration depth of an RF field decreases with increasing frequency, but there is a dramatic increase in detection sensitivity with field strength, roughly proportional to $B_0^{7/4}$.

3.1.3   More on the Larmor Frequency

Let us restate that the precession frequency of $\vec{\mu}$ experiencing a B_0 field is given by

$$\omega_0 = \gamma B_0 \tag{3.41}$$

This relation, popularly known as the *Larmor equation*, is an important equation because the Larmor frequency is the natural resonance frequency of a spin system.

Equation (3.41) shows that the resonance frequency of a spin system is linearly dependent on both the strength of the external magnetic field B_0 and the value of the gyromagnetic ratio γ. This simple relationship is the physical basis for achieving nucleus specificity. As a case in point, nuclei of ^{1}H and ^{31}P in an object resonate at 42.58 MHz and 11.26 MHz, respectively, when the object is placed in $B_0 = 1$ T; this difference in resonance frequency enables us to selectively image one of them without "disturbing" the other.

In practice, a specific spin system (say, protons) may have a range of resonance frequencies. In this case, we call each group of nuclear spins that share the same resonance frequency an *isochromat*. There are two main reasons for a magnetized spin system to have multiple isochromats: (a) the existence of inhomogeneities in the B_0 field, and (b) the chemical shift effect.

It is obvious from Eq. (3.41) that when B_0 is not homogeneous, spins with the same γ value will have different Larmor frequencies at different spatial locations. It is easy to derive the frequency distribution of a spin system if the inhomogeneity of a given B_0 is known. The chemical shift effect is due to the fact that nuclei in a spin system are attached to different chemical environments (molecules) in a chemically heterogeneous object. Since each nucleus of a molecule is surrounded by orbiting electrons, these orbiting electrons produce their own weak magnetic fields, which "shield" the nucleus to varying degrees depending on the position of the nucleus in the molecule. As a result, the effective magnetic field that a nucleus "sees" is

$$\hat{B}_0 = B_0(1 - \delta) \tag{3.42}$$

where δ is a shielding constant taking on either positive or negative values. Based on the Larmor relationship, the resonance frequency for the nucleus is

$$\hat{\omega}_0 = \omega_0 - \Delta\omega = \omega_0(1 - \delta) \tag{3.43}$$

Equation (3.43) indicates that spins in different chemical environments will have relative shifts in their resonance frequency even when B_0 is perfectly homogeneous.

Clearly, the frequency shift $\Delta\omega$ is dependent on both the strength of the external field B_0 and the shielding constant δ. The value of δ is very small, usually on the order of a few parts per million (ppm) and is dependent on the local chemical environment in which the nucleus is situated. A well-known example is that "fat" (CH_2) protons in biological objects display about a 3.35 ppm shift in Larmor frequency from "water" (H_2O) protons.

For biological objects, a large range of δ values could exist, giving rise to many resonance frequencies. Assuming that the maximum chemical shift is $w_M/2$, the resonance frequency range of a spin system can be expressed as

$$|\omega - \omega_0| \leq \omega_M/2 \tag{3.44}$$

where ω_M is called the *(chemical shift) frequency bandwidth* of the spin system. Knowledge of these chemical shift frequencies and the corresponding spin densities is of great importance for determining the chemical structures of an object, which is the subject of NMR spectroscopy.

3.2   RF Excitations

We have thus far discussed two aspects of an NMR phenomenon: nuclei and a static magnetic field. The macroscopic effect of an external magnetic field $\vec{B}_0$ on an ensemble of nuclei with nonzero spins is the generation of an observable bulk magnetization vector $\vec{M}$ pointing along the direction of $\vec{B}_0$. Although there is a microscopic transverse component for each magnetic moment vector, the transverse component of $\vec{M}$ is zero at equilibrium because the precessing magnetic moments have random phases, as indicated by Eq. (3.16). A snapshot of an ensemble of a large number of spins ($I = \frac{1}{2}$) will be a set of vectors spreading out in the two precessing cones, as illustrated in Fig. 3.5. Establishment of a phase coherence among these "randomly" precessing spins in a magnetized spin system is referred to as *resonance*.

3.2.1   Resonance Condition

Before we state the resonance condition, let us look at the popular "swing" analogy. Suppose that a row of swings at a children's playground have the same length (thus, each swing-child complex has the same natural frequency). If the children do not begin swinging at the same time, a random phase relationship exists among the swings; that is, at a given time, the children are at different points of the swinging arc. For the swings to reach phase coherence, external forces must be applied at the natural frequency of the swings. For example, if all the swings are pushed in unison at the natural frequency of the swing by a parent placed behind each swing, the children will soon swing in phase, exerting a coherent force on the suspension bar.

For a magnetized spin system, the external force (energy) comes from an oscillating magnetic field denoted as $\vec{B}_1(t)$ in distinction from the static $\vec{B}_0$ field. The resonance condition based on classical physics is that $\vec{B}_1(t)$ rotates in the same manner as the precessing spins. A more rigorous argument is based on the quantum model. In this model, electromagnetic radiation of frequency ω_{rf} carries energy (Planck's law):

$$E_{\mathrm{rf}} = \hbar\omega_{\mathrm{rf}} \tag{3.45}$$

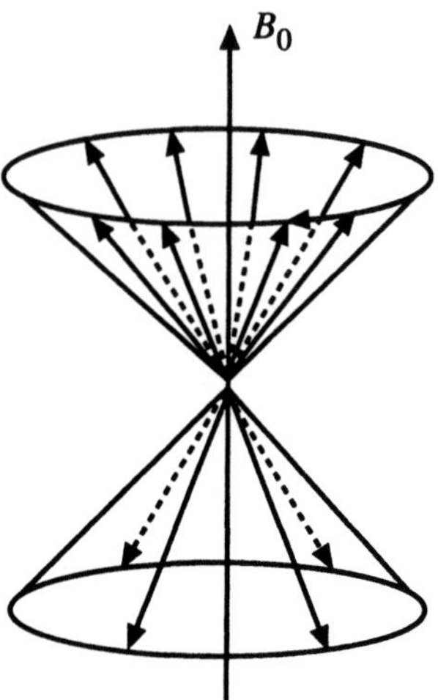

Figure 3.5 Distribution of nuclear magnetic moments observed at an arbitrary time instant. The excess of vectors pointing along the external field is greatly exaggerated.

To induce a coherent transition of spins from one energy state to another, the radiation energy must be equal to the energy difference ΔE between the adjacent spin states. That is,

$$\hbar\omega_{\text{rf}} = \Delta E = \gamma\hbar B_0 \tag{3.46}$$

or

$$\omega_{\text{rf}} = \omega_0 \tag{3.47}$$

Equation (3.47) is known as the *resonance condition*. In the following, we first describe what an RF pulse is and then discuss in detail the effect of RF excitations under on- and off-resonance conditions.

3.2.2   Characteristics of an RF Pulse

RF pulse is a synonym of the B_1 field, so called because the B_1 field is short-lived and oscillates in the radio-frequency range. Specifically, the B_1 field is normally turned on for a few microseconds or milliseconds Also, in contrast to the static magnetic field $\vec{B}_0$, the $\vec{B}_1$ field is much weaker (e.g., $B_1 = 50\,\text{mT}$ while $B_0 = 1.5\,\text{T}$).

A typical B_1 field takes the following form:

$$\vec{B}_1(t) = 2B_1^e(t)\cos(\omega_{rf}t + \varphi)\vec{i} \tag{3.48}$$

where

$$
\begin{array}{ll}
B_1^e(t): & \text{pulse envelope function} \\
\omega_{rf}: & \text{excitation carrier frequency} \\
\varphi: & \text{initial phase angle}
\end{array}
$$

This field is said to be *linearly polarized* because it oscillates linearly along the x-axis. Mathematically, it can be decomposed into two *circularly polarized* fields rotating in opposite directions, that is,

$$
\begin{aligned}
\vec{B}_1(t) = {} & B_1^e(t)[\cos(\omega_{rf}t + \varphi)\vec{i} - \sin(\omega_{rf}t + \varphi)\vec{j}] \\
& + B_1^e(t)[\cos(\omega_{rf}t + \varphi)\vec{i} + \sin(\omega_{rf}t + \varphi)\vec{j}]
\end{aligned} \tag{3.49}
$$

where the first bracketed term rotates clockwise and the second rotates counterclockwise, as illustrated in Fig. 3.6. Since the counterclockwise component rotates in the opposite direction of the precessing spins, it exerts negligible effects on a spin system if ω_{rf} is near the Larmor frequency.[4] Therefore, the effective $\vec{B}_1(t)$ field that needs to be considered here is

$$\vec{B}_1(t) = B_1^e(t)[\cos(\omega_{rf}t + \varphi)\vec{i} - \sin(\omega_{rf}t + \varphi)\vec{j}] \tag{3.50}$$

which has an x-component as

$$B_{1,x} = B_1^e(t)\cos(\omega_{rf}t + \varphi) \tag{3.51}$$

and a y-component as

$$B_{1,y} = -B_1^e(t)\sin(\omega_{rf}t + \varphi) \tag{3.52}$$

Many modern NMR systems use so-called quadrature RF transmitter coils to generate this circularly polarized field directly, with the advantage of reduced RF power deposition. Unless specified otherwise, the $\vec{B}_1(t)$ field used in the remainder of this book will be assumed to be in this form. For brevity, we will also adopt the following complex notation:

$$B_1(t) = B_{1,x}(t) + iB_{1,y}(t) = B_1^e(t)e^{-i(\omega_{rf}t + \varphi)} \tag{3.53}$$

In summary, an RF pulse generates an oscillating $\vec{B}_1(t)$ field perpendicular to the $\vec{B}_0$ field. The main parameters characterizing an RF pulse include (a) the envelope function $B_1^e(t)$, (b) the excitation carrier frequency ω_{rf}, and (c) the initial

---

[4]The main effect of this off-resonance component is a very slight shift of the observed resonance line, which is known as the *Bloch–Siegert shift*. This frequency shift disappears when the B_1 field is turned on.

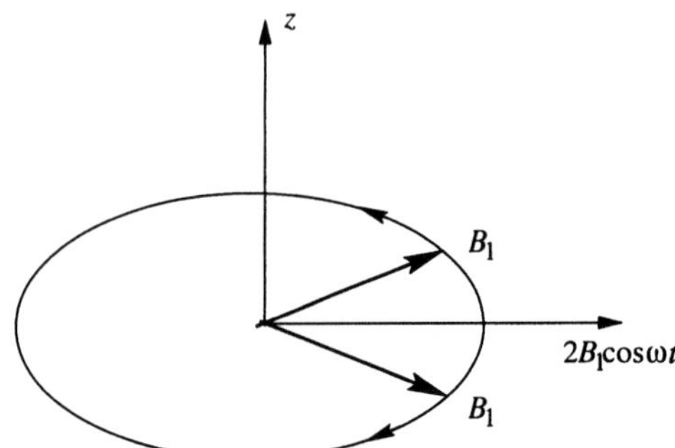

Figure 3.6   A linearly polarized field represented as two counter-rotating circularly polarized fields.

phase angle φ. The initial phase φ, if it is a constant, has no significant effect on the excitation result and is assumed to be zero for the present discussion. The excitation frequency ω_{rf} is a constant for most RF pulses[5] and is determined by the resonance condition. The envelope function $B_1^e(t)$ is the heart of an RF pulse. It uniquely specifies the shape and duration of an RF pulse, and thus its excitation property. In fact, many RF pulses are named based purely on the characteristics of this function. For example, the envelope function of the widely used *rectangular* pulse (shown in Fig. 3.7a), is defined as

$$B_1^e(t) = B_1\Pi\left(\frac{t - \tau_p/2}{\tau_p}\right) = \begin{cases} B_1 & 0 \le t \le \tau_p \\ 0 & \text{otherwise} \end{cases} \tag{3.54}$$

where τ_p is the pulse width. Another popular pulse, called the *sinc* pulse (Fig. 3.7b), uses the following envelope function:

$$B_1^e(t) = \begin{cases} B_1\mathrm{sinc}[\pi f_w(t - \tau_p/2)], & 0 \le t \le \tau_p \\ 0, & \text{otherwise} \end{cases} \tag{3.55}$$

Before describing the effect of such a pulse on a spin system, we next introduce two mathematical tools: the rotating reference frame and the Bloch equation.

3.2.3   Rotating Frame of Reference

A rotating frame is a coordinate system whose transverse plane is rotating clockwise at an angular frequency ω. To distinguish it from the conventional stationary frame, we use x', y', and z' to denote the three orthogonal axes of this frame, and correspondingly, $\vec{i}'$, $\vec{j}'$, and $\vec{k}'$ as their unit directional vectors. Mathematically, this frame is related to the stationary (laboratory) frame by the following

---

[5] For some special pulses, such as adiabatic pulses, ω_{rf} can be a function of time.

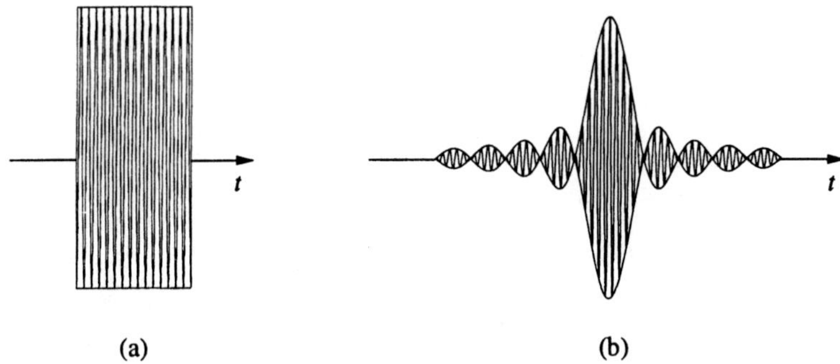

(a)   (b)

Figure 3.7 RF pulses with (a) a rectangular envelope function, and (b) a sinc envelope function.

transformation:

$$\begin{cases} \vec{i}\,' \triangleq \cos(\omega t)\vec{i} - \sin(\omega t)\vec{j} \\ \vec{j}\,' \triangleq \sin(\omega t)\vec{i} + \cos(\omega t)\vec{j} \\ \vec{k}\,' \triangleq \vec{k} \end{cases} \qquad (3.56)$$

Two special rotating frames are in use, which correspond to $\omega = \omega_0$ and $\omega = \omega_{\mathrm{rf}}$, respectively. In the first case, the (x', y')-plane precesses at the Larmor frequency of the spin system, and we call it the *Larmor-rotating frame*. In the second case, the (x', y')-plane rotates as the $\vec{B}_1(t)$ field, and we call it the *RF-rotating frame*. When $\omega_{\mathrm{rf}} = \gamma B_0$, both rotating frames are the same. Therefore, when there is no confusion, we use the generic term, rotating frame or ω-rotating frame, to refer to either, depending on the context.

The advantage of introducing the rotating frame lies in the conceptual simplicity it affords in describing the excitation effect of an RF pulse, as will become evident later in this chapter. In the sequel, we will present several useful relationships associated with this transformation.

First, the time derivatives of the unit directional vectors of the rotating frame are given by

$$\begin{cases} \dfrac{d\vec{i}\,'}{dt} = \vec{\omega} \times \vec{i}\,' \\[2mm] \dfrac{d\vec{j}\,'}{dt} = \vec{\omega} \times \vec{j}\,' \\[2mm] \dfrac{d\vec{k}\,'}{dt} = \vec{\omega} \times \vec{k}\,' \end{cases} \qquad (3.57)$$

where $\vec{\omega}$ can be arbitrary but is equal to $-\omega\vec{k}$ for the transformation specified by Eq. (3.56).

Second, let

$$\vec{M} \triangleq M_x\vec{i} + M_y\vec{j} + M_z\vec{k} \qquad (3.58)$$

and

$$\vec{M}_{\text{rot}} \triangleq M_{x'}\vec{i'} + M_{y'}\vec{j'} + M_{z'}\vec{k'} \tag{3.59}$$

Setting $\vec{M} = \vec{M}_{\text{rot}}$ yields

$$\begin{bmatrix} M_{x'} \\ M_{y'} \\ M_{z'} \end{bmatrix} = \begin{bmatrix} \cos\omega t & -\sin\omega t & 0 \\ \sin\omega t & \cos\omega t & 0 \\ 0 & 0 & 1 \end{bmatrix} \begin{bmatrix} M_x \\ M_y \\ M_z \end{bmatrix} \tag{3.60}$$

Similarly, let

$$\vec{B}_1 \triangleq B_{1,x}\vec{i} + B_{1,y}\vec{j} \tag{3.61}$$

and

$$\vec{B}_{1,\text{rot}} \triangleq B_{1,x'}\vec{i'} + B_{1,y'}\vec{j'} \tag{3.62}$$

We then have

$$\begin{bmatrix} B_{1,x'} \\ B_{1,y'} \end{bmatrix} = \begin{bmatrix} \cos\omega t & -\sin\omega t \\ \sin\omega t & \cos\omega t \end{bmatrix} \begin{bmatrix} B_{1,x} \\ B_{1,y} \end{bmatrix} \tag{3.63}$$

Equations (3.60) and (3.63) specify how to convert the magnetization vector and B_1 vector between the laboratory and rotating frames. The transformation rules can also be succinctly written in complex notation. Specifically,

$$M_{x'y'} = M_{xy}e^{i\omega t} \tag{3.64}$$

where $M_{xy} = M_x + iM_y$ and $M_{x'y'} = M_{x'} + iM_{y'}$. Similarly,

$$B_{1,\text{rot}}(t) = B_1(t)e^{i\omega t} \tag{3.65}$$

where $B_1 = B_{1,x} + iB_{1,y}$ and $B_{1,\text{rot}} = B_{1,x'} + iB_{1,y'}$.

Third, let

$$\frac{d\vec{M}}{dt} \triangleq \frac{dM_x}{dt}\vec{i} + \frac{dM_y}{dt}\vec{j} + \frac{dM_z}{dt}\vec{k} \tag{3.66a}$$

$$\frac{\partial\vec{M}_{\text{rot}}}{\partial t} \triangleq \frac{dM_{x'}}{dt}\vec{i'} + \frac{dM_{y'}}{dt}\vec{j'} + \frac{dM_{z'}}{dt}\vec{k'} \tag{3.66b}$$

Then,

$$\frac{d\vec{M}}{dt} = \frac{\partial\vec{M}_{\text{rot}}}{\partial t} + \vec{\omega} \times \vec{M}_{\text{rot}} \tag{3.67}$$

Clearly, based on the definitions in Eq. (3.66), $\frac{d\vec{M}}{dt}$ is the rate of change of $\vec{M}$ as observed in the laboratory frame, while $\frac{\partial\vec{M}_{\text{rot}}}{\partial t}$ is the rate of change of $\vec{M}$ as observed in the rotating frame. Therefore,

$$\frac{d\vec{M}}{dt} = \frac{d\vec{M}_{\text{rot}}}{dt} \neq \frac{\partial\vec{M}_{\text{rot}}}{\partial t} \tag{3.68}$$

■ Example 3.3

We prove the first relationship in Eq. (3.57) with respect to the transform in Eq. (3.56). Taking the time derivative of the first equation in Eq. (3.56) gives

$$\frac{d\vec{i}'}{dt} = -\omega \sin \omega t \vec{i} - \omega \cos \omega t \vec{j}$$

Replacing $\vec{i}$ and $\vec{j}$ with $\vec{i}'$ and $\vec{j}'$ according to the transformation rule in Eq. (3.56), we obtain

$$\frac{d\vec{i}'}{dt} = -\omega \sin \omega t (\cos \omega t \vec{i}' + \sin \omega t \vec{j}') - \omega \cos \omega t (-\sin \omega t \vec{i}' + \cos \omega t \vec{j}')$$

$$= -\omega(\cos^2 \omega t + \sin^2 \omega t)\vec{j}'$$

$$= -\omega \vec{j}'$$

Noting that $\vec{j}' = \vec{k}' \times \vec{i}'$ and $\vec{\omega} = -\omega \vec{k}'$, we immediately obtain

$$\frac{d\vec{i}'}{dt} = -\omega(\vec{k}' \times \vec{i}') = (-\omega \vec{k}') \times \vec{i}' = \vec{\omega} \times \vec{i}'$$

■ Example 3.4

We derive the result in Eq. (3.67). Taking the first-order derivative with respect to time on both sides of Eq. (3.59) yields

$$\frac{d\vec{M}}{dt} = \left(\frac{dM_{x'}}{dt}\vec{i}' + \frac{dM_{y'}}{dt}\vec{j}' + \frac{dM_{z'}}{dt}\vec{k}' \right) + \left(M_{x'}\frac{d\vec{i}'}{dt} + M_{y'}\frac{d\vec{j}'}{dt} + M_{z'}\frac{d\vec{k}'}{dt} \right)$$

$$= \frac{\partial \vec{M}_{\text{rot}}}{\partial t} + \left(M_{x'}\frac{d\vec{i}'}{dt} + M_{y'}\frac{d\vec{j}'}{dt} + M_{z'}\frac{d\vec{k}'}{dt} \right)$$

Making use of Eq. (3.57), we have

$$M_{x'}\frac{d\vec{i}'}{dt} + M_{y'}\frac{d\vec{j}'}{dt} + M_{z'}\frac{d\vec{k}'}{dt} = \vec{\omega} \times (M_{x'}\vec{i}' + M_{y'}\vec{j}' + M_{z'}\vec{k}') = \vec{\omega} \times \vec{M}_{\text{rot}}$$

Combining the two foregoing equations yields

$$\frac{d\vec{M}}{dt} = \frac{\partial \vec{M}_{\text{rot}}}{\partial t} + \vec{\omega} \times \vec{M}_{\text{rot}}$$

■ **Example 3.5**

Given that

$$\vec{B}_1(t) = B_1 \cos \omega_{\mathrm{rf}} t\, \vec{i} - B_1 \sin \omega_{\mathrm{rf}} t\, \vec{j}$$

we determine the RF field as observed in the ω_{rf}-rotating frame.

Since

$$\left[\begin{array}{c} B_{1,x} \\ B_{1,y} \end{array} \right] = \left[\begin{array}{c} B_1 \cos \omega_{\mathrm{rf}} t \\ -B_1 \sin \omega_{\mathrm{rf}} t \end{array} \right]$$

the B_1 field observed in the ω_{rf}-rotating frame, according to Eq. (3.63), is given by

$$\left[\begin{array}{c} B_{1,x'} \\ B_{1,y'} \end{array} \right] = \left[\begin{array}{cc} \cos \omega_{\mathrm{rf}} t & -\sin \omega_{\mathrm{rf}} t \\ \sin \omega_{\mathrm{rf}} t & \cos \omega_{\mathrm{rf}} t \end{array} \right] \left[\begin{array}{c} B_1 \cos \omega_{\mathrm{rf}} t \\ -B_1 \sin \omega_{\mathrm{rf}} t \end{array} \right]$$

$$= \left[\begin{array}{c} B_1 \\ 0 \end{array} \right]$$

In vector notation,

$$\vec{B}_{1,\mathrm{rot}}(t) = B_1 \vec{i}'$$

Therefore, the given RF field becomes a stationary field pointing along the x'-axis in the ω_{rf}-rotating frame.

3.2.4 The Bloch Equation

The time-dependent behavior of $\vec{M}$ in the presence of an applied magnetic field $\vec{B}_1(t)$ is described quantitatively by the *Bloch equation*. In the context of MRI, the Bloch equation takes the following general form:[6]

$$\frac{d\vec{M}}{dt} = \gamma \vec{M} \times \vec{B} - \frac{M_x \vec{i} + M_y \vec{j}}{T_2} - \frac{(M_z - M_z^0)\vec{k}}{T_1} \tag{3.69}$$

where M_z^0 is the thermal equilibrium value for $\vec{M}$ in the presence of $\vec{B}_0$ only, which can be calculated from Eq. (3.39) or (3.40); T_1 and T_2 are time constants characterizing the relaxation process of a spin system after it has been disturbed from its thermal equilibrium state, a topic to be further discussed in Section 3.3 and in Chapter 7. For the present discussion, we drop the last two terms in Eq. (3.69) because we are interested only in the behavior of $\vec{M}$ during the RF excitation period. This treatment is acceptable if the duration of an RF pulse is short compared to T_1 and T_2, as is often the case in practice.

---

[6] A more general form of the Bloch equation was given by Torrey [256].

Under this assumption, the Bloch equation takes a simpler form:

$$\frac{d\vec{M}}{dt} = \gamma \vec{M} \times \vec{B} \tag{3.70}$$

One may recognize that this Bloch equation is identical to the equation of motion for a free spin in Eq. (3.15) if $\vec{M}$ is replaced by $\vec{\mu}$. We next express the equation in the rotating frame. Substituting Eq. (3.67) into Eq. (3.70), we get

$$\frac{\partial \vec{M}_{\text{rot}}}{\partial t} = \gamma \vec{M}_{\text{rot}} \times \vec{B}_{\text{rot}} - \vec{\omega} \times \vec{M}_{\text{rot}}$$

$$= \gamma \vec{M}_{\text{rot}} \times \left(\vec{B}_{\text{rot}} + \frac{\vec{\omega}}{\gamma} \right) \tag{3.71}$$

We may rewrite Eq. (3.71) as

$$\frac{\partial \vec{M}_{\text{rot}}}{\partial t} = \gamma \vec{M}_{\text{rot}} \times \vec{B}_{\text{eff}} \tag{3.72}$$

where

$$\vec{B}_{\text{eff}} = \vec{B}_{\text{rot}} + \frac{\vec{\omega}}{\gamma} \tag{3.73}$$

is the effective magnetic field that the bulk magnetization vector "experiences" in the rotating frame. The second term in Eq. (3.73) represents a fictitious field component for simplified behavior of $\vec{M}_{\text{rot}}$. To see this more clearly, let $\vec{B} = B_0 \vec{k}$ and $\vec{\omega} = -\gamma B_0 \vec{k}$. Then,

$$\vec{B}_{\text{eff}} = \vec{B}_{\text{rot}} - \frac{\gamma B_0 \vec{k}}{\gamma} = B_0 \vec{k} - B_0 \vec{k} = 0 \tag{3.74}$$

Therefore, the apparent longitudinal field vanishes and $\vec{M}_{\text{rot}}$ appears to be stationary in the rotating frame.

Following the same analysis, the general Bloch equation in Eq. (3.69) can be expressed in the rotating frame as

$$\frac{\partial \vec{M}_{\text{rot}}}{\partial t} = \gamma \vec{M}_{\text{rot}} \times \vec{B}_{\text{eff}} - \frac{M_{x'}\vec{i'} + M_{y'}\vec{j'}}{T_2} - \frac{(M_{z'} - M_z^0)\vec{k'}}{T_1} \tag{3.75}$$

3.2.5 On-Resonance Excitations

We now look into the effects of an RF pulse on a spin system by examining the time-dependent behavior of $\vec{M}$ during the excitation period. We first consider the simple case in which a spin system has a single isochromat resonating at $\omega_0 = \gamma B_0$. For simplicity, we further assume that the initial phase angle φ is zero for the generic RF pulse defined in Eq. (3.50). Using the transformation rule specified by Eq. (3.63), we have

$$\vec{B}_{1,\text{rot}} = B_1^e(t)\vec{i'} \tag{3.76}$$

The effective field that the nuclear spins see in the rotating frame is

$$\vec{B}_{\text{eff}} = B_0\vec{k'} + B_1^e(t)\vec{i'} + \frac{\vec{\omega}_{\text{rf}}}{\gamma}$$

$$= \left(B_0 - \frac{\omega_{\text{rf}}}{\gamma}\right)\vec{k'} + B_1^e(t)\vec{i'} \tag{3.77}$$

Invoking the on-resonance excitation condition that

$$\omega_{\text{rf}} = \omega_0 = \gamma B_0 \tag{3.78}$$

we immediately get

$$\vec{B}_{\text{eff}} = B_1^e(t)\vec{i'} \tag{3.79}$$

Substituting the above result into the Bloch equation in Eq. (3.72) yields the following equation of motion for the bulk magnetization vector $\vec{M}$:

$$\frac{\partial \vec{M}_{\text{rot}}}{\partial t} = \gamma \vec{M}_{\text{rot}} \times B_1^e(t)\vec{i'} \tag{3.80}$$

In scalar form, we have

$$\begin{cases} \dfrac{dM_{x'}}{dt} = 0 \\[2mm] \dfrac{dM_{y'}}{dt} = \gamma B_1^e(t)M_{z'} \\[2mm] \dfrac{dM_{z'}}{dt} = -\gamma B_1^e(t)M_{y'} \end{cases} \tag{3.81}$$

A closed-form solution to Eq. (3.81) under the initial conditions $M_{x'}(0) = M_{y'}(0) = 0$ and $M_{z'}(0) = M_z^0$ is as follows:

$$\begin{cases} M_{x'}(t) = 0 \\[2mm] M_{y'}(t) = M_z^0 \sin\left(\displaystyle\int_0^t \gamma B_1^e(\hat{t})d\hat{t}\right) \\[2mm] M_{z'}(t) = M_z^0 \cos\left(\displaystyle\int_0^t \gamma B_1^e(\hat{t})d\hat{t}\right) \end{cases} \quad 0 \leq t \leq \tau_p \tag{3.82}$$

These equations indicate that the effect of the on-resonance excitation $\vec{B}_1$ field, as observed in the RF-rotating frame, is a precession of the bulk magnetization about the x'-axis. This is not surprising since the effective field $\vec{B}_{\text{eff}}$ points along the x'-axis. As an example, consider the case where

$$B_1^e(t) = B_1 \Pi \left(\frac{t - \tau_p/2}{\tau_p} \right) \tag{3.83}$$

Then, Eq. (3.82) becomes

$$\begin{cases} M_{x'}(t) = 0 \\ M_{y'}(t) = M_z^0 \sin(\omega_1 t) \qquad 0 \le t \le \tau_p \\ M_{z'}(t) = M_z^0 \cos(\omega_1 t) \end{cases} \tag{3.84}$$

where $\omega_1 = \gamma B_1$. It is now apparent that the bulk magnetization vector precesses about the x'-axis with angular velocity

$$\vec{\omega}_1 = -\gamma \vec{B}_1 \tag{3.85}$$

as shown in Fig. 3.8. The precession of $\vec{M}$ about the B_1 field is called *forced precession*. Equation (3.85) can be derived directly from the Larmor relationship, since the effective field that the spins see in the rotating frame is $B_1 \vec{i'}$.

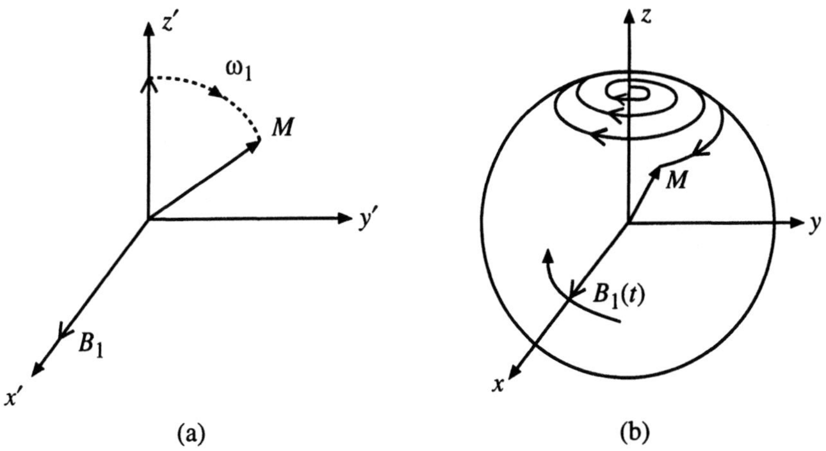

Figure 3.8   Motion of the bulk magnetization vector in the presence of a rotating RF field as observed in (a) the RF-rotating frame, and (b) the laboratory frame.

3.2.5.1   Flip Angle

As a result of the forced precession, the bulk magnetization is tipped away from the z'-axis, creating a measurable transverse component $\vec{M}_{x'y'}$. The flip angle

α is defined as the smaller angle between $\vec{M}$ and the z-axis. Clearly, based on Eq. (3.82), the value of α at the end of an RF pulse is given by

$$\alpha = \int_0^{\tau_p} \omega_1(t)dt = \int_0^{\tau_p} \gamma B_1^e(t)dt \tag{3.86}$$

In the case of a rectangular pulse,

$$\alpha = \omega_1 \tau_p = \gamma B_1 \tau_p \tag{3.87}$$

As a numerical example, let $\tau_p = 0.1$ ms and $B_1 = 0.6$ G. We then have $\alpha = \frac{\pi}{2}$ for protons.

It is obvious from Eqs. (3.86) and (3.87) that the flip angle depends on both the magnitude of the $\vec{B}_1(t)$ field and the duration of exposure. Normally, the pulse width is chosen based on the frequency selectivity desired, and we can adjust the excitation power to vary the flip angle. For example, for a given τ_p, increasing the pulse intensity by a factor of 2 (namely, setting B_1 to $2B_1$), will double the flip angle according to Eq. (3.87). Another important point to note here is that the shape and form of the pulse envelope function are unimportant as long as the area under $B_1^e(t)$ is the same. In other words, for different $B_1^e(t)$, $\vec{M}$ travels in different trajectories during the excitation period but will end up in the same spatial location if the area under $B_1^e(t)$ is the same.

3.2.5.2   Calculation of $\vec{M}$ after an α Pulse

Before we describe how to calculate the effect of an RF pulse through the use of a rotation operator, it is useful to make clear several notations.

(a)   If an RF pulse rotates $\vec{M}$ about the $\vec{B}_1$ field in the rotating frame by an angle α, we commonly call the pulse an α pulse. Clearly, a 90° or $\frac{\pi}{2}$ pulse rotates $\vec{M}$ by 90°; likewise, a 180° or π pulse rotates $\vec{M}$ by 180°. Sometimes, it is necessary to make the axis of rotation explicit. Assume that the $\vec{B}_1$ field in the rotating frame points in a direction specified by (φ, θ), as shown in Fig. 3.9; we call the corresponding $\vec{B}_1$ field an $\alpha_{(\varphi,\theta)}$ pulse. In practice, it is usually assumed that $\theta = 0$ and the pulse is simply written as α_φ. Two popular choices of φ are 0 or 90°, corresponding to a $\alpha_{x'}$ pulse and a $\alpha_{y'}$ pulse, respectively.

(b)   We use $t = 0_-$ and $t = 0_+$ to represent the time instants immediately before and after a pulse, respectively.

(c)   We will use $\longrightarrow$ as a general spin processing operator. For example,

$$M_{x'}(0_-) \xrightarrow{\alpha_{x'}} M_{x'}(0_+) \tag{3.88}$$

means that an $\alpha_{x'}$ pulse transforms $M_{x'}(0_-)$ to $M_{x'}(0_+)$.

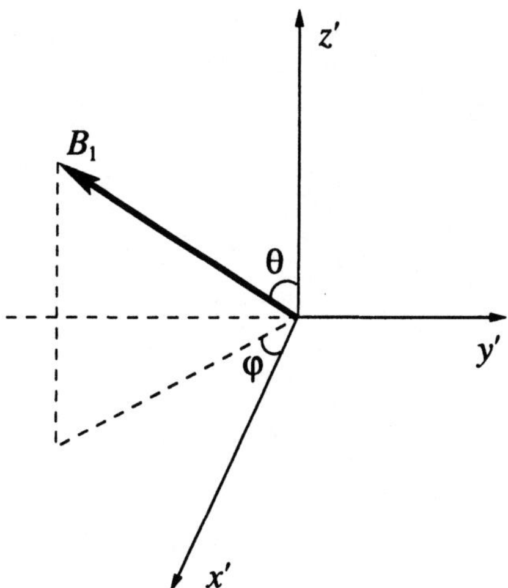

Figure 3.9 A tilted RF field with an initial phase angle φ and a tilt angle θ.

With these clarifications, let us first consider the effect of an $\alpha_{x'}$ pulse. Based on Eq. (3.82), we have

$$\begin{cases} M_{x'}(0_+) = 0 \\ M_{y'}(0_+) = M_z^0 \sin \alpha \\ M_{z'}(0_+) = M_z^0 \cos \alpha \end{cases} \tag{3.89}$$

if the spin system was at thermal equilibrium before the pulse. Under a more general prepulse condition, the postpulse magnetization is given by

$$\begin{cases} M_{x'}(0_+) = M_{x'}(0_-) \\ M_{y'}(0_+) = M_{y'}(0_-) \cos \alpha + M_{z'}(0_-) \sin \alpha \\ M_{z'}(0_+) = -M_{y'}(0_-) \sin \alpha + M_{z'}(0_-) \cos \alpha \end{cases} \tag{3.90}$$

Similarly to Eq. (3.20), we define a rotation operator about the x'-, y'-, and z'-axis, respectively, as

$$\mathbf{R}_{x'}(\alpha) = \begin{bmatrix} 1 & 0 & 0 \\ 0 & \cos \alpha & \sin \alpha \\ 0 & -\sin \alpha & \cos \alpha \end{bmatrix} \tag{3.91}$$

$$\mathbf{R}_{y'}(\alpha) = \begin{bmatrix} \cos \alpha & 0 & -\sin \alpha \\ 0 & 1 & 0 \\ \sin \alpha & 0 & \cos \alpha \end{bmatrix} \tag{3.92}$$

and

$$\mathbf{R}_{z'}(\alpha) = \begin{bmatrix} \cos \alpha & \sin \alpha & 0 \\ -\sin \alpha & \cos \alpha & 0 \\ 0 & 0 & 1 \end{bmatrix} \tag{3.93}$$

As illustrated in Fig. 3.10, $\mathbf{R}_{x'}$, $\mathbf{R}_{y'}$, and $\mathbf{R}_{z'}$ specify a clockwise rotation as observed against the x'-, y'-, and z'-axis, respectively.

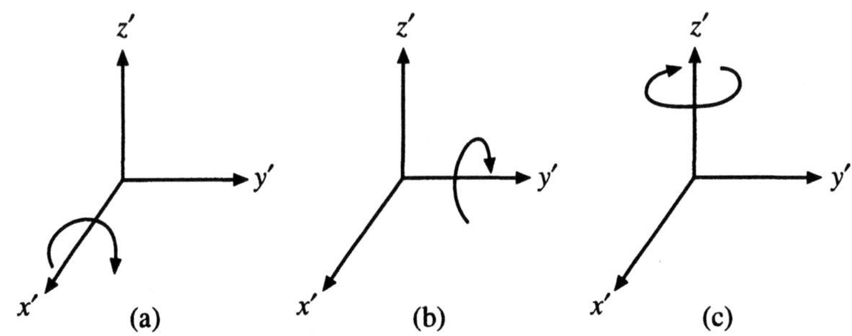

Figure 3.10   Graphical representation of (a) $\mathbf{R}_{x'}$, (b) $\mathbf{R}_{y'}$, and (c) $\mathbf{R}_{z'}$.

With the matrix operators defined in Eqs. (3.91), (3.92), and (3.93), the effect of an α pulse applied along the x'- or y'-axis can be calculated as follows:

$$\vec{M}_{\text{rot}}(0_+) \xrightarrow{\alpha_{x'}} \mathbf{R}_{x'}(\alpha)\vec{M}_{\text{rot}}(0_-) \tag{3.94a}$$

$$\vec{M}_{\text{rot}}(0_+) \xrightarrow{\alpha_{-x'}} \mathbf{R}_{-x'}(\alpha)\vec{M}_{\text{rot}}(0_-) = \mathbf{R}_{x'}(-\alpha)\vec{M}_{\text{rot}}(0_-) \tag{3.94b}$$

$$\vec{M}_{\text{rot}}(0_+) \xrightarrow{\alpha_{y'}} \mathbf{R}_{y'}(\alpha)\vec{M}_{\text{rot}}(0_-) \tag{3.94c}$$

$$\vec{M}_{\text{rot}}(0_+) \xrightarrow{\alpha_{-y'}} \mathbf{R}_{-y'}(\alpha)\vec{M}_{\text{rot}}(0_-) = \mathbf{R}_{y'}(-\alpha)\vec{M}_{\text{rot}}(0_-) \tag{3.94d}$$

where it is understood that $\vec{M}_{\text{rot}} = [M_{x'}, M_{y'}, M_{z'}]^T$.

The effect of an α_φ pulse can be represented by three cascaded spin rotations: $-\varphi_{z'}\alpha_{x'}\varphi_{z'}$. Or in terms of the rotation matrices, we have[7]

$$\vec{M}_{\text{rot}}(0_+) = \mathbf{R}_{z'}(\varphi)\mathbf{R}_{x'}(\alpha)\mathbf{R}_{z'}(-\varphi)\vec{M}_{\text{rot}}(0_-) \tag{3.95}$$

which gives the following postpulse magnetizations:

$$M_{x'}(0_+) = M_{x'}(0_-)(\cos\alpha\sin^2\varphi + \cos^2\varphi) + M_{y'}(0_-)\sin^2\frac{\alpha}{2}\sin 2\varphi$$
$$-M_{z'}(0_-)\sin\alpha\sin\varphi \tag{3.96a}$$

$$M_{y'}(0_+) = M_{x'}(0_-)\sin^2\frac{\alpha}{2}\sin 2\varphi + M_{y'}(0_-)(\cos\alpha\cos^2\varphi + \sin^2\varphi)$$
$$+M_{z'}(0_-)\sin\alpha\cos\varphi \tag{3.96b}$$

$$M_{z'}(0_+) = M_{x'}(0_-)\sin\alpha\sin\varphi - M_{y'}(0_-)\sin\alpha\cos\varphi$$
$$+M_{z'}(0_-)\cos\alpha \tag{3.96c}$$

---

[7]Note that the operator precedence is from right to left.

The effect of an $\alpha_{(\varphi,\theta)}$ pulse can be calculated in an analogous manner. Specifically, it can be shown that

$$\vec{M}_{\mathrm{rot}}(0_+) = \mathbf{R}_{z'}(\varphi)\mathbf{R}_{y'}(\hat{\theta})\mathbf{R}_{x'}(\alpha)\mathbf{R}_{y'}(-\hat{\theta})\mathbf{R}_{z'}(-\varphi)\vec{M}_{\mathrm{rot}}(0_-) \qquad (3.97)$$

where $\hat{\theta} = -\frac{\pi}{2} + \theta$. The resulting magnetization is given by

$$\begin{aligned}
M_{x'}(0_+) = {} & M_{x'}(0_-)[\cos\alpha(\sin^2\varphi + \cos^2\varphi\cos^2\theta) + \cos^2\varphi\sin^2\theta] \\
& + M_{y'}(0_-)[\sin^2\tfrac{\alpha}{2}\sin 2\varphi\sin^2\theta + \sin\alpha\cos\theta] \\
& + M_{z'}(0_-)[\sin^2\tfrac{\alpha}{2}\sin 2\theta\cos\varphi - \sin\alpha\sin\varphi\sin\theta] \qquad (3.98\mathrm{a})
\end{aligned}$$

$$\begin{aligned}
M_{y'}(0_+) = {} & M_{x'}(0_-)[\sin^2\tfrac{\alpha}{2}\sin 2\varphi\sin^2\theta - \sin\alpha\cos\theta] \\
& + M_{y'}(0_-)[\cos\alpha(\cos^2\varphi + \sin^2\varphi\cos^2\theta) + \sin^2\varphi\sin^2\theta] \\
& + M_{z'}(0_-)[\sin^2\tfrac{\alpha}{2}\sin 2\theta\sin\varphi + \sin\alpha\cos\varphi\sin\theta] \qquad (3.98\mathrm{b})
\end{aligned}$$

$$\begin{aligned}
M_{z'}(0_+) = {} & M_{x'}(0_-)[\sin\alpha\sin\varphi\sin\theta + \sin^2\tfrac{\alpha}{2}\cos\varphi\sin 2\theta] \\
& + M_{y'}(0_-)[-\sin\alpha\cos\varphi\sin\theta + \sin^2\tfrac{\alpha}{2}\sin\varphi\sin 2\theta] \\
& + M_{z'}(0_-)[\cos\alpha\sin^2\theta + \cos^2\theta] \qquad (3.98\mathrm{c})
\end{aligned}$$

The postpulse magnetization can also be expressed in the laboratory frame. According to Eq. (3.60), we have

$$\begin{bmatrix} M_x(0_+) \\ M_y(0_+) \\ M_z(0_+) \end{bmatrix} = \begin{bmatrix} \cos\omega_0\tau_p & \sin\omega_0\tau_p & 0 \\ -\sin\omega_0\tau_p & \cos\omega_0\tau_p & 0 \\ 0 & 0 & 1 \end{bmatrix} \begin{bmatrix} M_{x'}(0_+) \\ M_{y'}(0_+) \\ M_{z'}(0_+) \end{bmatrix} \qquad (3.99)$$

by noting that

$$\begin{bmatrix} \cos\omega_0\tau_p & -\sin\omega_0\tau_p & 0 \\ \sin\omega_0\tau_p & \cos\omega_0\tau_p & 0 \\ 0 & 0 & 1 \end{bmatrix}^{-1} = \begin{bmatrix} \cos\omega_0\tau_p & \sin\omega_0\tau_p & 0 \\ -\sin\omega_0\tau_p & \cos\omega_0\tau_p & 0 \\ 0 & 0 & 1 \end{bmatrix} \qquad (3.100)$$

where τ_p is the pulse duration and it is assumed that the rotating reference frame was set in motion immediately before the pulse is applied.

3.2.5.3 Examples

Through the next three examples, we show how to use the formulas in the preceding section for calculating the excitation effects.

■ Example 3.6

Assume that a spin system was at thermal equilibrium when an RF pulse was applied. Calculate the resulting magnetization if the RF pulse is (a) a $90_{x'}$ pulse and (b) a $45_{y'}$ pulse.

The prepulse magnetization value is

$$\begin{bmatrix} M_{x'}(0_-) \\ M_{y'}(0_-) \\ M_{z'}(0_-) \end{bmatrix} = \begin{bmatrix} 0 \\ 0 \\ M_z^0 \end{bmatrix}$$

After a $90_{x'}$ pulse, we have

$$\begin{bmatrix} M_{x'}(0_+) \\ M_{y'}(0_+) \\ M_{z'}(0_+) \end{bmatrix} = \mathbf{R}_{x'}(90^\circ) \begin{bmatrix} M_{x'}(0_-) \\ M_{y'}(0_-) \\ M_{z'}(0_-) \end{bmatrix}$$

$$= \begin{bmatrix} 1 & 0 & 0 \\ 0 & 0 & 1 \\ 0 & -1 & 0 \end{bmatrix} \begin{bmatrix} 0 \\ 0 \\ M_z^0 \end{bmatrix}$$

$$= \begin{bmatrix} 0 \\ M_z^0 \\ 0 \end{bmatrix}$$

Similarly, the magnetization after a $45_{y'}$ pulse is given by

$$\begin{bmatrix} M_{x'}(0_+) \\ M_{y'}(0_+) \\ M_{z'}(0_+) \end{bmatrix} = \mathbf{R}_{y'}(45^\circ) \begin{bmatrix} M_{x'}(0_-) \\ M_{y'}(0_-) \\ M_{z'}(0_-) \end{bmatrix}$$

$$= \begin{bmatrix} \frac{\sqrt{2}}{2} & 0 & -\frac{\sqrt{2}}{2} \\ 0 & 1 & 0 \\ -\frac{\sqrt{2}}{2} & 0 & \frac{\sqrt{2}}{2} \end{bmatrix} \begin{bmatrix} 0 \\ 0 \\ M_z^0 \end{bmatrix}$$

$$= \begin{bmatrix} -\frac{\sqrt{2}}{2} M_z^0 \\ 0 \\ \frac{\sqrt{2}}{2} M_z^0 \end{bmatrix}$$

■ Example 3.7

In this example, we derive the following relationship:

$$M_{x'y'} \xrightarrow{\pi_\varphi} M_{x'y'}^* e^{-i2\varphi} \tag{3.101}$$

which describes the effect of a 180°_φ pulse.

According to Eq. (3.95), we have

$$\mathbf{R}_\varphi(\pi) = \mathbf{R}_{z'}(\varphi)\mathbf{R}_{x'}(\pi)\mathbf{R}_{z'}(-\varphi)$$

For simplicity, consider only the transverse magnetization. Then, we have

$$\mathbf{R}_\varphi(\pi) = \begin{bmatrix} \cos\varphi & \sin\varphi \\ -\sin\varphi & \cos\varphi \end{bmatrix} \begin{bmatrix} 1 & 0 \\ 0 & -1 \end{bmatrix} \begin{bmatrix} \cos\varphi & -\sin\varphi \\ \sin\varphi & \cos\varphi \end{bmatrix}$$

$$= \begin{bmatrix} \cos\varphi & \sin\varphi \\ -\sin\varphi & \cos\varphi \end{bmatrix} \begin{bmatrix} \cos\varphi & -\sin\varphi \\ -\sin\varphi & -\cos\varphi \end{bmatrix}$$

$$= \begin{bmatrix} \cos^2\varphi - \sin^2\varphi & -2\cos\varphi\sin\varphi \\ -2\cos\varphi\sin\varphi & \sin^2\varphi - \cos^2\varphi \end{bmatrix}$$

$$= \begin{bmatrix} \cos 2\varphi & -\sin 2\varphi \\ -\sin 2\varphi & -\cos 2\varphi \end{bmatrix} \tag{3.102}$$

This equation implies that

$$M_{x'}(0_+) = M_{x'}(0_-)\cos 2\varphi - M_{y'}(0_-)\sin 2\varphi$$
$$M_{y'}(0_+) = -M_{x'}(0_-)\sin 2\varphi - M_{y'}(0_-)\cos 2\varphi$$

Therefore,

$$\begin{aligned} M_{x'y'}(0_+) &= M_{x'}(0_+) + iM_{y'}(0_+) \\ &= M_{x'}(0_-)\cos 2\varphi - M_{y'}(0_-)\sin 2\varphi \\ &\quad - iM_{x'}(0_-)\sin 2\varphi - iM_{y'}(0_-)\cos 2\varphi \\ &= [M_{x'}(0_-) - iM_{y'}(0_-)](\cos 2\varphi - i\sin 2\varphi) \\ &= M_{x'y'}^*(0_-)e^{-i2\varphi} \end{aligned} \tag{3.103}$$

which proves Eq. (3.101). Based on the result, it is easy to show

$$M_{x'y'} \xrightarrow{\pi_{x'}} M_{x'y'}^* \tag{3.104a}$$

$$M_{x'y'} \xrightarrow{\pi_{y'}} -M_{x'y'}^* \tag{3.104b}$$

noting that $\varphi = 0$ and $\pi/2$, respectively, for $\pi_{x'}$ and $\pi_{y'}$.

■ Example 3.8

Assume a spin system has two isochromats at thermal equilibrium condition with resonance frequency ω_0 and $\omega_0 + \delta\omega_0$. We calculate the effect of the excitation sequence $90^\circ_{x'} - \tau - 90^\circ_{y'}$ with $\tau = \frac{\pi}{4}\frac{1}{\delta\omega_0}$.

Ignoring any off-resonance effect (to be discussed in Section 3.2.6), we find that the effect of the first $90^\circ_{x'}$ on both isochromats is the same, resulting in

$$\begin{cases} M_{1,x'} = 0 \\ M_{1,y'} = M^0_{1,z} \\ M_{1,z'} = 0 \end{cases} \quad \text{and} \quad \begin{cases} M_{2,x'} = 0 \\ M_{2,y'} = M^0_{2,z} \\ M_{2,z'} = 0 \end{cases}$$

During the time delay, $\vec{M}_1$ stays the same (ignoring any relaxation effects), but $\vec{M}_2$ precesses at an angular frequency of $\delta\omega_0$ in the rotating frame. As a result, $\vec{M}_2$ takes the following value immediately before the second pulse:

$$\begin{cases} M_{2,x'} = \sin(\delta\omega_0\tau)M^0_{2,z} = \sin\frac{\pi}{4}M^0_{2,z} = \frac{\sqrt{2}}{2}M^0_{2,z} \\ M_{2,y'} = \cos(\delta\omega_0\tau)M^0_{2,z} = \cos\frac{\pi}{4}M^0_{2,z} = \frac{\sqrt{2}}{2}M^0_{2,z} \\ M_{2,z'} = 0 \end{cases}$$

The second pulse is applied along the y'-axis and, therefore, has no effect on the first isochromat because it has been lying along the y'-axis since the first pulse. Consequently, the final value for $\vec{M}_1$ after the two pulses is

$$\begin{bmatrix} M_{1,x'}(0_+) \\ M_{1,y'}(0_+) \\ M_{1,z'}(0_+) \end{bmatrix} = \begin{bmatrix} 0 \\ M^0_{1,z} \\ 0 \end{bmatrix}$$

For the second isochromat, the magnetization vector will be flipped 90° around the y'-axis, giving rise to the following postpulse value:

$$\begin{bmatrix} M_{2,x'}(0_+) \\ M_{2,y'}(0_+) \\ M_{2,z'}(0_+) \end{bmatrix} = \begin{bmatrix} \cos 90^\circ & 0 & -\sin 90^\circ \\ 0 & 1 & 0 \\ \sin 90^\circ & 0 & \cos 90^\circ \end{bmatrix} \begin{bmatrix} \frac{\sqrt{2}}{2}M^0_{2,z} \\ \frac{\sqrt{2}}{2}M^0_{2,z} \\ 0 \end{bmatrix}$$

$$= \begin{bmatrix} 0 \\ \frac{\sqrt{2}}{2}M^0_{2,z} \\ \frac{\sqrt{2}}{2}M^0_{2,z} \end{bmatrix}$$

3.2.6 Off-Resonance Excitations

Most excitations are assumed to be on-resonance. However, in practice, if magnetic field inhomogeneities and chemical-shift effects are not negligible, excitations rarely are exactly on-resonance for all the isochromats. When the excitation field is off-resonance for a certain isochromat, the effective magnetic field that the isochromat sees in the rotating frame is

$$
\begin{aligned}
\vec{B}_{\text{eff}} &= \left(B_0 - \frac{\omega_{\text{rf}}}{\gamma} \right) \vec{k}' + B_1^e(t)\vec{i}' \\
&= \frac{\Delta\omega_0}{\gamma}\vec{k}' + B_1^e(t)\vec{i}'
\end{aligned}
\tag{3.105}
$$

where $\Delta\omega_0 = \omega_0 - \omega_{\text{rf}}$ measures the degree of off-resonance.

Equation (3.105) suggests that the effective field has two components: the usual B_1 component pointing along the x'-axis and a residual component $\Delta\omega_0/\gamma$ pointing along the z'-axis, as shown in Fig. 3.11a. Intuitively, based on the above discussion one can predict a precession of $\vec{M}_{\text{rot}}$ about $\vec{B}_{\text{eff}}$. A more rigorous analysis can be obtained by directly solving the following Bloch equation:

$$
\begin{cases}
\dfrac{dM_{x'}}{dt} = \Delta\omega_0 M_{y'} \\[2mm]
\dfrac{dM_{y'}}{dt} = -\Delta\omega_0 M_{x'} + \gamma B_1^e(t) M_{z'} \\[2mm]
\dfrac{dM_{z'}}{dt} = -\gamma B_1^e(t) M_{y'}
\end{cases}
\tag{3.106}
$$

which governs the motion of $\vec{M}$ during the RF pulse. Unfortunately, a closed-form solution to the above equations is not available for an arbitrary envelope function $B_1^e(t)$. To illustrate the difference between on-resonance and off-resonance excitations, we consider a simple case with a rectangular pulse for which $B_1^e(t) = B_1 \Pi(\frac{t-\tau_p/2}{\tau_p})$. For this pulse, a closed-form solution to the Bloch equation indeed exists, which is given by

$$
\begin{cases}
M_{x'}(t) = M_z^0 \sin\theta \cos\theta[1 - \cos(\omega_{\text{eff}}t)] \\[2mm]
M_{y'}(t) = M_z^0 \sin\theta \sin(\omega_{\text{eff}}t) \\[2mm]
M_{z'}(t) = M_z^0[\cos^2\theta + \sin^2\theta \cos(\omega_{\text{eff}}t)]
\end{cases}
\qquad 0 \le t \le \tau_p
\tag{3.107}
$$

where

$$
\omega_{\text{eff}} = \sqrt{\Delta\omega_0^2 + \omega_1^2}
\tag{3.108}
$$

and

$$
\theta = \arctan\left(\frac{\omega_1}{\Delta\omega_0} \right)
\tag{3.109}
$$

The magnetization components along each axis immediately after the pulse are given by

$$\begin{cases} M_{x'}(0_+) = M_{x'}(\tau_p) = M_z^0 \sin\theta\cos\theta(1 - \cos\alpha) \\ M_{y'}(0_+) = M_{y'}(\tau_p) = M_z^0 \sin\theta\sin\alpha \\ M_{z'}(0_+) = M_{z'}(\tau_p) = M_z^0(\cos^2\theta + \sin^2\theta\cos\alpha) \end{cases} \quad (3.110)$$

where $\alpha = \omega_{\text{eff}}\tau_p$ is now the flip angle about the axis of the effective magnetic field.

Note that the transverse magnetization immediately after the pulse is no longer along the y'-axis as in the case of on-resonance excitation but has a phase shift φ_0 from the y'-axis toward the x'-axis, which is given by

$$\tan\varphi_0 = \frac{M_x(0_+)}{M_y(0_+)} = \frac{\sin\theta\cos\theta(1 - \cos\alpha)}{\sin\theta\sin\alpha}$$

$$= \frac{(1 - \cos\alpha)}{\sin\alpha}\frac{\Delta\omega_0}{\omega_{\text{eff}}} = \tan\frac{\alpha}{2}\frac{\Delta\omega_0}{\omega_{\text{eff}}} \quad (3.111)$$

It is evident from Eq. (3.111) that the phase shift φ_0 increases almost linearly with the frequency shift $\Delta\omega_0$. This phase shift can be problematic for some MRI applications. In addition, the magnitude of the transverse magnetization given by

$$M_{x'y'}(0_+) = \sqrt{M_{x'}^2(0_+) + M_{y'}^2(0_+)}$$

$$= M_z^0 \sin\theta\sqrt{\sin^2\alpha + (1 - \cos\alpha)^2\cos^2\theta} \quad (3.112)$$

decreases as the frequency offset increases.

3.2.7 Frequency Selectivity of an RF Pulse

From the discussion in Section 3.2.6, we know that for a spin system with more than one resonance frequency, an RF pulse of the form $B_1 e^{-i\omega_{\text{rf}}t}$ for $0 \le t \le \tau_p$ will excite not only $\vec{M}(\omega_{\text{rf}})$ but other isochromats as well. An important question that one often encounters is: How will a pulse of the general form $B_1^e(t)e^{-i\omega_{\text{rf}}t}$ affect the various isochromats of a spin system? To give an exact answer to this question, we need to resort to the Bloch equation. However, a closed-form solution to the Bloch equation is not available under this general situation. In this section, we describe an approximate approach based on Fourier analysis.

It is well known that Fourier analysis of a time function reveals its spectral content. Specifically, let

$$\{\mathcal{F}B_1^e\}(\omega) = \int_{-\infty}^{\infty} B_1^e(t)e^{i\omega t}dt = \mathcal{F}^{-1}\{B_1^e(t)\} \quad (3.113)$$

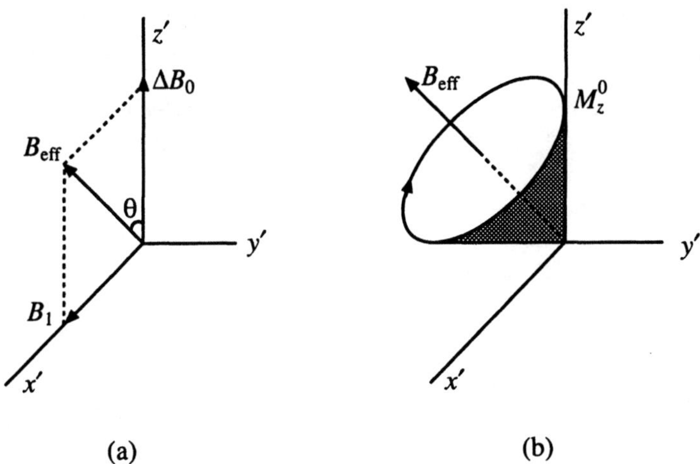

Figure 3.11   Off-resonance excitation: (a) effective field in the rotating frame, and (b) precession of $\vec{M}_{\text{rot}}$ about the effective field.

We have

$$B_1^e(t) = \frac{1}{2\pi} \int_{-\infty}^{\infty} \{\mathcal{F}B_1^e\}(\omega)e^{-i\omega t}d\omega \tag{3.114}$$

and

$$B_1(t) = \frac{1}{2\pi} \int_{-\infty}^{\infty} \{\mathcal{F}B_1^e\}(\omega)e^{-i(\omega+\omega_{rf})t}d\omega \tag{3.115}$$

In signal processing, $\{\mathcal{F}B_1^e\}(\omega)$ is interpreted as the frequency spectrum of the pulse envelope function. It is more insightful here to view it as the amplitude of a clockwise rotating vector specified by $e^{-i(\omega+\omega_{rf})t}$. In other words, Eq. (3.115) decomposes $B_1(t)$ into a continuum of clockwise-rotating microvectors with amplitudes $\{\mathcal{F}B_1^e\}(\omega)d\omega$ in the complex plane. Similarly, we can decompose the bulk magnetization vectors in terms of its isochromats as

$$\vec{M} = \int_{-\infty}^{\infty} \vec{M}(\omega)d\omega \tag{3.116}$$

To establish a link between the isochromats and the micro-B_1 vectors, we further assume that the spin system behaves like a linear system;[8] namely, the excitation effect of $B_1(t)$ is equal to the sum of the excitation effects of individual component $\{\mathcal{F}B_1^e\}(\omega)d\omega e^{-i(\omega+\omega_{rf})t}$. Since $\{\mathcal{F}B_1^e\}(\omega)d\omega e^{-i(\omega+\omega_{rf})t}$ is a fictitious pulse of infinite length but of infinitesimal strength, it will, in steady

---

[8] The *linear system* assumption is not valid for a nuclear spin system *during excitation*. Therefore, the excitation property of an RF pulse derived from Fourier analysis is not accurate.

state, excite only the on-resonance isochromat $\vec{M}(\omega + \omega_{\text{rf}})$ if the relaxation effects can be ignored.[9] Therefore, the frequency excitation property of an RF pulse of the form $B_1^e(t)e^{-i\omega_{\text{rf}}t}$ is fully characterized by $\{\mathcal{F}B_1^e\}(\omega)$ under conditions of Fourier analysis. To be more specific, $\{\mathcal{F}B_1^e\}(\omega)d\omega$ is the excitation field that acts on $\vec{M}(\omega + \omega_{\text{rf}})$. Since $\{\mathcal{F}B_1^e\}(\omega)$ is a complex-valued function, we can rewrite it as $\{\mathcal{F}B_1^e\}(\omega) = |\{\mathcal{F}B_1^e\}(\omega)|e^{i\varphi(\omega)}$. Therefore, the on-resonance magnetic field that each isochromat sees has a phase shift $\varphi(\omega)$ from the x'-axis.[10] As a result, there is a phase dispersal among the isochromats when they flip down to the transverse plane, as expected from the discussion in Section 3.2.6. In addition, the flip angle is different for different isochromats. According to Eq. (3.86), the flip angle for the $\vec{M}(\omega_{\text{rf}})$ isochromat is given by

$$\alpha(0) = \gamma \int_0^{\tau_p} B_1^e(\tau)d\tau \tag{3.117}$$

Based on the linearity assumption, the flip angle for other isochromats is given by

$$\alpha(\omega) = \frac{|\{\mathcal{F}B_1^e\}(\omega)|}{|\{\mathcal{F}B_1^e\}(0)|}\alpha(\omega_{\text{rf}}) \tag{3.118}$$

Knowing $\alpha(\omega)$ and $\varphi(\omega)$, we can calculate the resulting postpulse magnetization for each isochromat according to Eq. (3.96).

As an example, let us examine the excitation property of a rectangular pulse whose envelope function is $B_1^e(t) = B_1\Pi(\frac{t-\tau_p/2}{\tau_p})$. From the results in Example 2.3, we have

$$\{\mathcal{F}B_1^e\}(\omega) = B_1\tau_p\text{sinc}\left(\tfrac{1}{2}\omega\tau_p\right)e^{i\omega\tau_p/2} \tag{3.119}$$

Therefore, the frequency excitation property is characterized by the following equations:

$$\frac{\alpha(\omega)}{\alpha(0)} = \text{sinc}\left(\tfrac{1}{2}\omega\tau_p\right) \tag{3.120a}$$

$$\varphi(\omega) = \tfrac{1}{2}\omega\tau_p \tag{3.120b}$$

Note that we allow flip angle α to take negative values instead of advancing φ by $180°$. Clearly, the two ways are equivalent for describing the spin motion.

Before concluding this section, an observation from Eq. (3.120a) is in order. If we treat the sinc function to be zero beyond the first zero crossing on both

---

[9] This is a valid assumption if the duration of $B_1^e(t)$ is short relative to the spin relaxation times. For those pulses, the Fourier prediction is rather accurate. For longer pulses, the Fourier prediction is less accurate because the relaxation effects cannot be ignored; consequently, the spin system cannot be treated as a linear system due to spin interactions.

[10] Since $\varphi(0) = 0$, $\vec{M}(\omega_{\text{rf}})$ will always flip around the x'-axis.

sides, a rectangular pulse of the above form will excite nuclear spins resonating over a frequency range $|\omega - \omega_{\mathrm{rf}}| < 2\pi/\tau_p$. Therefore, a short rectangular pulse of $\tau_p = 1 \ \mu s$ will excite nuclei resonating over a frequency bandwidth of 10^3 kHz centered around the excitation frequency ω_{rf}. These short rectangular pulses (approximating a δ-function) are called *hard* or *nonselective* pulses, since they are designed to excite "everything" in the spin system. On the other hand, a rectangular RF pulse of $\tau_p = 10$ ms will produce excitation over a narrow frequency bandwidth of 100 Hz. Such long pulses are called *selective* pulses because they selectively excite nuclei resonating in the selected frequency range. In practice, based on the asymptotic property of the Fourier transform, better frequency selectivity can be achieved by utilizing smoother pulses, such as the Gaussian or sinc pulses, rather than the rectangular pulse. For this reason, long selective pulses are often called *soft* pulses. The design of an RF pulse with good frequency selectivity is an important subject of MRI and is still an active area of research. We will return to this topic when we discuss the signal localization in Chapter 5.

3.3   Free Precession and Relaxation

After a magnetized spin system has been perturbed from its thermal equilibrium state by an RF pulse, it will, according to the laws of thermodynamics, return to this state, provided the external force is removed and sufficient time is given. This process is characterized by a precession of $\vec{M}$ about the B_0 field, called *free precession*; a recovery of the longitudinal magnetization M_z, called *longitudinal relaxation*; and the destruction of the transverse magnetization M_{xy}, called *transverse relaxation*. Both relaxation processes are often ascribed to the existence of time-dependent microscopic magnetic fields that surround a nucleus as a result of the random thermal motions present in an object. But the exact mechanisms by which these relaxation events occur for an arbitrary spin system are far too diverse and complex to be properly covered here. The interested reader is referred to the text by Abragam [1]. In this section, we give only a phenomenological description of the relaxation process using the Bloch equation. The effect of spin relaxations on image appearance (contrast) is dependent on the excitation scheme used for data acquisition, an important topic to be discussed in Chapter 7.

Phenomenologically, the transverse and longitudinal relaxations are described by a first-order process. Specifically, in the Larmor-rotating frame, we have

$$\begin{cases} \dfrac{dM_{z'}}{dt} = -\dfrac{M_{z'} - M_z^0}{T_1} \\[2mm] \dfrac{dM_{x'y'}}{dt} = -\dfrac{M_{x'y'}}{T_2} \end{cases} \qquad (3.121)$$

These equations are directly derived from the rotating frame Bloch equation in Eq. (3.75) in which the first term drops out because $\vec{B}_{\mathrm{eff}} = (B_0 - \omega_0/\gamma)\vec{k}' = 0$.

Solving Eq. (3.121), we obtain the following time evolution for the transverse and longitudinal magnetization components:

$$\begin{cases} M_{x'y'}(t) = M_{x'y'}(0_+)e^{-t/T_2} \\ M_{z'}(t) = M_z^0\left(1 - e^{-t/T_1}\right) + M_{z'}(0_+)e^{-t/T_1} \end{cases} \tag{3.122}$$

where $M_{x'y'}(0_+)$ and $M_{z'}(0_+)$ are the magnetizations on the transverse plane and along the z-axis immediately after an RF pulse, and M_z^0 is, as before, the longitudinal magnetization at thermal equilibrium.

An important point about this phenomenological description is that both the decay of the transverse magnetization and the recovery of the longitudinal magnetization after an RF perturbation follow an exponential function. This exponential description, especially for the transverse relaxation, applies only to spin systems with weak spin-spin interactions, as is the case with spins residing in liquid state molecules. For solids and macromolecules, the mechanisms for transverse relaxation are more complicated. For many biological applications of MRI, however, we deal almost exclusively with "slowly" relaxing spins for which the phenomenological description is often appropriate.

Another point worth noting is that T_1 and T_2 are not defined as the times at which longitudinal and transverse relaxations are completed. To see this point more clearly, consider the T_1 and T_2 relaxations after a 90° pulse, which produces $M_{x'y'}(0_+) = M_z^0$ and $M_{z'}(0_+) = 0$. By some simple arithmetic, we can easily verify, based on Eq. (3.122), that

$$\begin{cases} M_{z'}(T_1) \approx 63\% M_z^0 \\ M_{x'y'}(T_2) \approx 37\% M_{x'y'}(0_+) \end{cases} \tag{3.123}$$

Therefore, $M_{z'}$ will regain 63% of its thermal equilibrium value after a time interval T_1, but $M_{x'y'}$ will lose 63% of its initial value after a time interval T_2, as illustrated in Fig. 3.12. The values of T_1 and T_2 depend on the tissue composition, structure, and surroundings. For a given spin system, T_1 is always longer than T_2. As an example, T_1 is about 300 to 2000 ms, and T_2 is about 30 to 150 ms in biological tissues.

The combined effect of free precession and relaxation can be seen by putting the magnetization vector back to the laboratory frame. Specifically, applying the transformation rule in Eq. (3.64) to Eq. (3.122), we obtain

$$M_{xy}(t) = M_{xy}(0_+)e^{-t/T_2}e^{-i\omega_0 t} \tag{3.124a}$$

$$M_z(t) = M_z^0\left(1 - e^{-t/T_1}\right) + M_z(0_+)e^{-t/T_1} \tag{3.124b}$$

where

$$M_{xy}(0_+) = M_{x'y'}(0_+)e^{-i\omega_0 \tau_p} \tag{3.125}$$

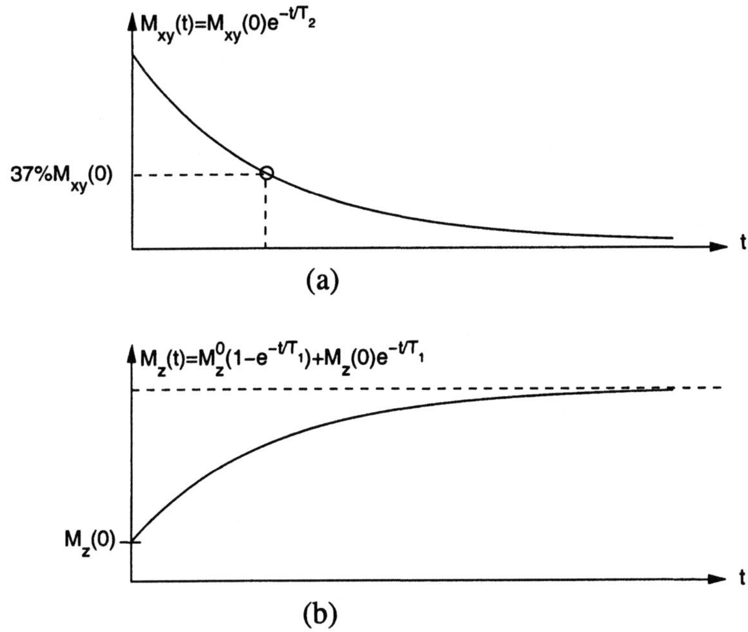

Figure 3.12 Relaxation curves.

is the "initial" transverse magnetization observed in the laboratory frame by the signal detection system. The time delay term is included because we reset the time to zero at the end of the pulse ($t = \tau_p$) to describe the relaxation effects.

Equation (3.124) gives an "exact" phenomenological description of how transverse and longitudinal magnetization evolves after an RF pulse as time progresses. Specifically, it is clear from Eq. (3.124a) that in the laboratory frame the evolution of the transverse magnetization is characterized by an exponential decay e^{-t/T_2} and a precession about the B_0 field $e^{-i\omega_0 t}$. The length of the free precession period is dependent on the T_2 value. For biological tissues, T_2 is on the order of tens of milliseconds, which enables detection of MR signals during this period. It is also worth noting that while $\vec{M}$ spirals back to the z-axis, its magnitude is not preserved because of the relaxation processes, as illustrated in Fig. 3.13. This behavior is different from that of $\vec{M}$ during the excitation period, when $\vec{M}$ spirals down from the z-axis with a fixed magnitude.[11]

---

[11]Relaxation is normally ignored during the excitation period for most RF pulses.

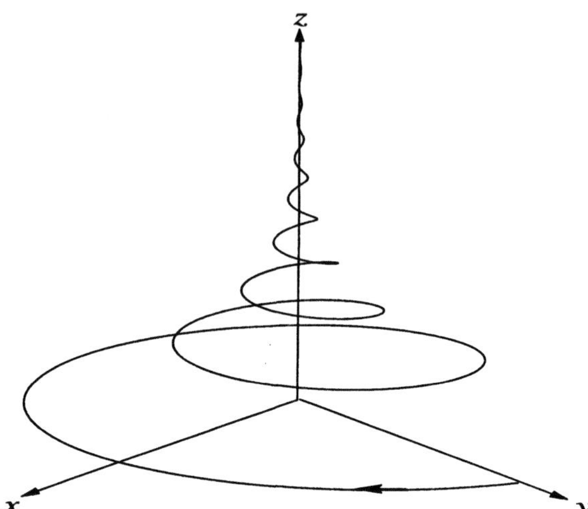

Figure 3.13 The trajectory of the tip of $\vec{M}$ during the relaxation period as observed in the laboratory frame.

3.4 Signal Detection

We know from the foregoing discussion that by placing an object in an external magnetic field $\vec{B}_0$ and stimulating it with another alternating or oscillating magnetic field $\vec{B}_1(t)$, we can induce a macroscopic magnetism in the form of a rotating magnetization in the object. This is the so-called NMR phenomenon. The next question is how to detect this magnetism, or more specifically, how to convert this rotating magnetization to electrical signals. We address this question in this section. We begin with a brief review of the basic physical principles of signal detection and then describe the concept of signal demodulation and quadrature detection. Emphasis is placed on deriving mathematical expressions of the activated signal in terms of various variables characterizing the spin system and the excitation conditions.

3.4.1 Basic Detection Principles

MR signal detection is based on the well-known Faraday law of electromagnetic induction and the principle of reciprocity. The Faraday law of induction states that time-varying magnetic flux through a conducting loop (a receiver coil) will induce in the coil an electromagnetic force (or voltage) that is equal to the rate at which the magnetic flux through the coil is changing. There are many daily-life examples of this law in action. That the power generators convert mechanical rotation of a permanent magnet into household electricity is one such example.

In MRI, the bulk magnetization is precessing at a radio frequency and any conducting loop resonating at the frequency can be used as a receiver coil. In fact, in many circumstances, the same RF coil used for excitation is also used for detection. The detection sensitivity of a receiver coil is determined through the principle of reciprocity [13]. Specifically, assume that $\vec{B}_r(r)$ is the laboratory frame magnetic field at location r produced by a hypothetical unit direct current flowing in the coil. Then, the magnetic flux through the coil by $\vec{M}(r,t)$ is given by

$$\Phi(t) = \int_{\text{object}} \vec{B}_r(r) \cdot \vec{M}(r,t)dr \qquad (3.126)$$

Then, according to the Faraday law of induction, the voltage $V(t)$ induced in the coil is

$$V(t) = -\frac{\partial \Phi(t)}{\partial t} = -\frac{\partial}{\partial t}\int_{\text{object}} \vec{B}_r(r) \cdot \vec{M}(r,t)dr \qquad (3.127)$$

The voltage $V(t)$ induced in the receiver coil is often regarded as the raw NMR signal. Therefore, Eq. (3.127) is the most basic formula of MR signal detection, which embodies the Faraday law of induction and the principle of reciprocity. From this formula we can quantitatively determine how various factors in an NMR experiment affect the received MR signal. In the ensuing section, we use this formula to derive some commonly used signal expressions.

3.4.2   Signal Expressions

The term *signal* can mean various things in MRI. It refers sometimes to the transverse magnetization, sometimes to the induced voltage signal, and sometimes to the induced voltage after some processing. This section shows what form the signal takes at different stages of the signal detection module.

Let us begin by rewriting Eq. (3.127) in scalar form as

$$V(t) = -\frac{\partial}{\partial t}\int_{\text{object}} [B_{r,x}(r)M_x(r,t) + B_{r,y}(r)M_y(r,t)$$
$$+ B_{r,z}(r)M_z(r,t)]dr \qquad (3.128)$$

where the following vector decomposition is assumed:

$$\vec{B}_r = B_{r,x}\vec{i} + B_{r,y}\vec{j} + B_{r,z}\vec{k} \qquad (3.129)$$

Since $M_z(r,t)$ is a slowly varying function compared to the free precession of the M_x and M_y components, the last term in Eq. (3.128) can be ignored, yielding

$$V(t) = -\int_{\text{object}} \left[B_{r,x}(r)\frac{\partial M_x(r,t)}{\partial t} + B_{r,y}(r)\frac{\partial M_y(r,t)}{\partial t} \right] dr \qquad (3.130)$$

Equation (3.130) indicates that the induced voltage is a function of only M_x and M_y. This is why it is normally known that MR signals are dependent on the transverse magnetization.

To develop this expression further, we rewrite $B_{r,x}$ and $B_{r,y}$ as

$$\begin{cases} B_{r,x} = |B_{r,xy}(r)| \cos \phi_r(r) \\ B_{r,y} = |B_{r,xy}(r)| \sin \phi_r(r) \end{cases} \tag{3.131}$$

where $\phi_r(r)$ is the reception phase angle. If the reception field at location r points along the x-axis, then $\phi_r(r) = 0$. On the other hand, if the field points along the y-axis, $\phi_r(r) = \pi/2$. For other cases, $\phi_r(r)$ takes a value between 0 and 2π.

To evaluate the time derivative of M_x and M_y as required by Eq. (3.130), we invoke the free precession equation, Eq. (3.124), from which we can obtain

$$M_x(r,t) = |M_{xy}(r,0)| e^{-t/T_2(r)} \cos[-\omega(r)t + \phi_e(r)] \tag{3.132a}$$

$$M_y(r,t) = |M_{xy}(r,0)| e^{-t/T_2(r)} \sin[-\omega(r)t + \phi_e(r)] \tag{3.132b}$$

where $\phi_e(r)$ is the initial phase shift introduced by RF excitation. Similarly to $\phi_r(r)$, $\phi_e(r)$ takes a value between 0 and 2π depending on the direction of $\vec{M}_{xy}(r,0)$. Specifically, $\phi_e(r) = 0$ if $\vec{M}_{xy}(r,0)$ lies along the x-axis, or $\phi_e(r) = \pi/2$ if $\vec{M}_{xy}(r,0)$ lies along the y-axis.

From Eq. (3.132), one immediately obtains

$$\begin{aligned} \frac{\partial M_x(r,t)}{\partial t} = {}& \omega(r)|M_{xy}(r,0)| e^{-t/T_2(r)} \sin[-\omega(r)t + \phi_e(r)] \\ & - \frac{1}{T_2(r)} |M_{xy}(r,0)| e^{-t/T_2(r)} \cos[-\omega(r)t + \phi_e(r)] \end{aligned} \tag{3.133a}$$

$$\begin{aligned} \frac{\partial M_y(r,t)}{\partial t} = {}& -\omega(r)|M_{xy}(r,0)| e^{-t/T_2(r)} \cos[-\omega(r)t + \phi_e(r)] \\ & - \frac{1}{T_2(r)} |M_{xy}(r,0)| e^{-t/T_2(r)} \sin[-\omega(r)t + \phi_e(r)] \end{aligned} \tag{3.133b}$$

For most applications, free precession is at a much faster rate than relaxation, namely,

$$\omega(r) \gg 1/T_2(r) \tag{3.134}$$

Hence, the second terms in the equations above can be ignored, yielding

$$\frac{\partial M_x(r,t)}{\partial t} = \omega(r)|M_{xy}(r,0)| e^{-t/T_2(r)} \sin[-\omega(r)t + \phi_e(r)] \tag{3.135a}$$

$$\frac{\partial M_y(r,t)}{\partial t} = -\omega(r)|M_{xy}(r,0)| e^{-t/T_2(r)} \cos[-\omega(r)t + \phi_e(r)] \tag{3.135b}$$

Substituting Eqs. (3.131) and (3.135) into Eq. (3.130) with some simplifications, we obtain

$$V(t) = -\int_{\text{object}} \omega(\boldsymbol{r})|B_{r,xy}(\boldsymbol{r})||M_{xy}(\boldsymbol{r},0)|e^{-t/T_2(\boldsymbol{r})}$$

$$\sin[-\omega(\boldsymbol{r})t + \phi_e(\boldsymbol{r}) - \phi_r(\boldsymbol{r})]d\boldsymbol{r} \tag{3.136}$$

or

$$V(t) = \int_{\text{object}} \omega(\boldsymbol{r})|B_{r,xy}(\boldsymbol{r})||M_{xy}(\boldsymbol{r},0)|e^{-t/T_2(\boldsymbol{r})}$$

$$\cos\left[-\omega(\boldsymbol{r})t + \phi_e(\boldsymbol{r}) - \phi_r(\boldsymbol{r}) + \frac{\pi}{2}\right]d\boldsymbol{r} \tag{3.137}$$

Equation (3.136) or (3.137) is a basic signal expression that explicitly shows the dependence of a detected voltage signal on the laboratory frame transverse magnetization $M_{xy}(\boldsymbol{r},0)$, the free precession frequency $\omega(\boldsymbol{r})$, and the detection sensitivity of the receiver coil $B_{r,xy}(\boldsymbol{r})$.

The voltage signal $V(t)$ is a high-frequency signal because the transverse magnetization vector precesses at the Larmor frequency, as observed at the laboratory frame. This can pose unnecessary problems for electronic circuitries in later processing stages. In practice, $V(t)$ is moved to a low-frequency band using what is known as the *phase-sensitive detection* (PSD) method, or *signal demodulation* method. Signal demodulation consists of multiplying $V(t)$ by a reference sinusoidal signal and then low-pass-filtering it to remove the high-frequency component. Referring to Fig. 3.14a and assuming that the reference signal is $2\cos\omega_0 t$, we have

$$2V(t)\cos\omega_0 t = 2\int_{\text{object}} \omega(\boldsymbol{r})|B_{r,xy}(\boldsymbol{r})||M_{xy}(\boldsymbol{r},0)|e^{-t/T_2(\boldsymbol{r})}$$

$$\cos\left[-\omega(\boldsymbol{r})t + \phi_e(\boldsymbol{r}) - \phi_r(\boldsymbol{r}) + \frac{\pi}{2}\right]\cos\omega_0 t\, d\boldsymbol{r}$$

$$= \int_{\text{object}} \omega(\boldsymbol{r})|B_{r,xy}(\boldsymbol{r})||M_{xy}(\boldsymbol{r},0)|e^{-t/T_2(\boldsymbol{r})}$$

$$\cos\left[-\omega(\boldsymbol{r})t - \omega_0 t + \phi_e(\boldsymbol{r}) - \phi_r(\boldsymbol{r}) + \frac{\pi}{2}\right]d\boldsymbol{r}$$

$$+ \int_{\text{object}} \omega(\boldsymbol{r})|B_{r,xy}(\boldsymbol{r})||M_{xy}(\boldsymbol{r},0)|e^{-t/T_2(\boldsymbol{r})}$$

$$\cos\left[-\omega(\boldsymbol{r})t + \omega_0 t + \phi_e(\boldsymbol{r}) - \phi_r(\boldsymbol{r}) + \frac{\pi}{2}\right]d\boldsymbol{r} \tag{3.138}$$

Removing the first component by low-pass filtering will result in a low-frequency signal, which is the output of the PSD system. Denoting this signal

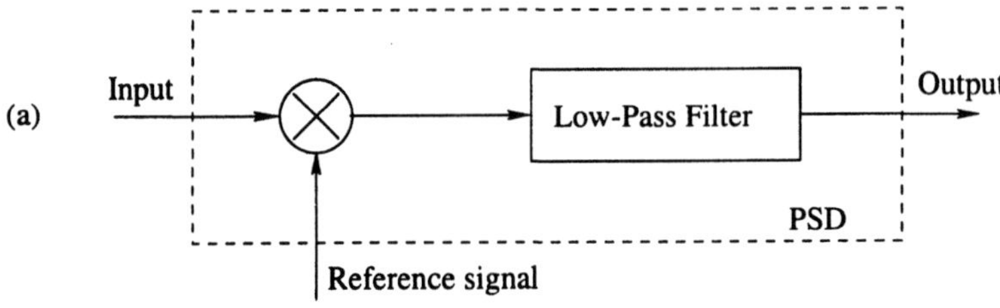

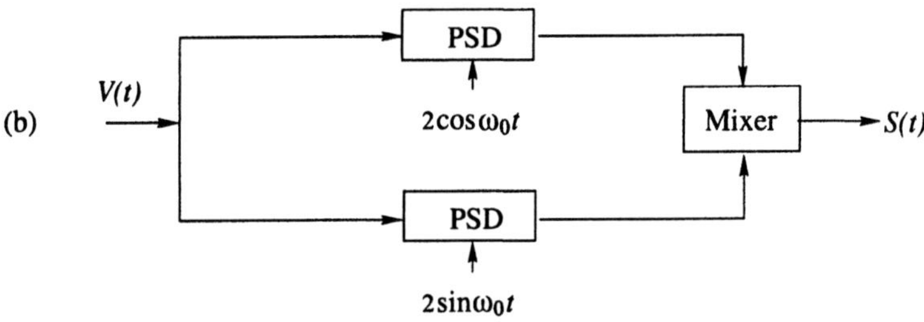

Figure 3.14 Phase-sensitive detection.

as $V_{\text{psd}}(t)$, we have

$$V_{\text{psd}}(t) = \int_{\text{object}} \omega(\boldsymbol{r})|B_{r,xy}(\boldsymbol{r})||M_{xy}(\boldsymbol{r},0)|c^{-t/T_2(\boldsymbol{r})}$$

$$\cos\left[-\omega(\boldsymbol{r})t + \omega_0 t + \phi_e(\boldsymbol{r}) - \phi_r(\boldsymbol{r}) + \frac{\pi}{2}\right] d\boldsymbol{r} \qquad (3.139)$$

It is often convenient to express $\omega(\boldsymbol{r})$ as

$$\omega(\boldsymbol{r}) = \omega_0 + \Delta\omega(\boldsymbol{r}) \qquad (3.140)$$

where $\Delta\omega(\boldsymbol{r})$ is the spatially dependent resonance frequency in the rotating frame. Then, we have

$$V_{\text{psd}}(t) = \int_{\text{object}} [\omega_0 + \Delta\omega(\boldsymbol{r})]|B_{r,xy}(\boldsymbol{r})||M_{xy}(\boldsymbol{r},0)|e^{-t/T_2(\boldsymbol{r})}$$

$$\cos\left[-\Delta\omega(\boldsymbol{r})t + \phi_e(\boldsymbol{r}) - \phi_r(\boldsymbol{r}) + \frac{\pi}{2}\right] d\boldsymbol{r} \qquad (3.141)$$

In practice, $\Delta\omega(\boldsymbol{r}) \ll \omega_0$, and Eq. (3.141) can be further simplified to

$$V_{\text{psd}}(t) = \omega_0 \int_{\text{object}} |B_{r,xy}(\boldsymbol{r})||M_{xy}(\boldsymbol{r},0)|e^{-t/T_2(\boldsymbol{r})}$$

$$\cos\left[-\Delta\omega(\boldsymbol{r})t + \phi_e(\boldsymbol{r}) - \phi_r(\boldsymbol{r}) + \frac{\pi}{2}\right] d\boldsymbol{r} \qquad (3.142)$$

which is a general expression for signals from a single PSD. Since $\Delta\omega(r)$ is the precession frequency in the rotating frame, $V_{\text{psd}}(t)$ is often regarded as the signal detected in the rotating frame. A notable drawback of this detection scheme is that we cannot determine from the signal whether the isochromat is precessing clockwise ($\Delta\omega > 0$) or counterclockwise ($\Delta\omega < 0$). To overcome this problem, a second PSD system is used with reference signal $2\sin\omega_0 t$, which has a 90° phase shift relative to the first. It is easy to show that the output from this detection system is

$$V_{\text{psd}}(t) = \omega_0 \int_{\text{object}} |B_{r,xy}(r)||M_{xy}(r,0)|e^{-t/T_2(r)}$$

$$\sin\left[-\Delta\omega(r)t + \phi_e(r) - \phi_r(r) + \frac{\pi}{2}\right] dr \qquad (3.143)$$

In this way, we are detecting the rotating magnetization with two "detectors," which are orthogonal to each other. This detection scheme, known as *quadrature detection*, is commonly used in modern MRI systems. The two outputs from such a system are often put in a complex form, as shown in Fig. 3.14b, with one output being treated as the real part and the other as the imaginary part.

Specifically, let

$$S(t) = S_R(t) + iS_I(t) \qquad (3.144)$$

with $S_R(t)$ being the output from the first PSD given in Eq. (3.142) and $S_I(t)$ being the output from the second PSD given in Eq. (3.143). Then,

$$S(t) = \omega_0 \int_{\text{object}} |B_{r,xy}(r)||M_{xy}(r,0)|e^{-i[\Delta\omega(r)t - \phi_e(r) + \phi_r(r) - \pi/2]}dr$$

$$(3.145)$$

Invoking the earlier-established complex notation that

$$\begin{cases} B_{r,xy} = B_{r,x} + iB_{r,y} \\ M_{xy} = M_x + iM_y \end{cases} \qquad (3.146)$$

we have

$$|B_{r,xy}(r)|e^{-i\phi_r(r)} = B_{r,xy}^*(r) \qquad (3.147a)$$

$$|M_{xy}(r,0)|e^{i\phi_e(r)} = M_{xy}(r,0) \qquad (3.147b)$$

where $B_{r,xy}^*$ is the complex conjugate of $B_{r,xy}$. With Eq. (3.147), Eq. (3.145) can be written as

$$S(t) = \omega_0 e^{i\pi/2} \int_{\text{object}} B_{r,xy}^*(r)M_{xy}(r,0)e^{-i\Delta\omega(r)t}dr \qquad (3.148)$$

The scaling constant $\omega_0 e^{i\pi/2}$ in Eq. (3.148) is often omitted, resulting in the following popular signal expression:

$$S(t) = \int_{\text{object}} B_{r,xy}^*(r)M_{xy}(r,0)e^{-i\Delta\omega(r)t}dr \qquad (3.149)$$

Furthermore, if the receiver coil has a homogeneous reception field over the region of interest, as is often assumed, the signal expression in Eq. (3.149) can be further simplified to

$$S(t) = \int_{\text{object}} M_{xy}(\boldsymbol{r}, 0)e^{-i\Delta\omega(\boldsymbol{r})t}d\boldsymbol{r} \qquad (3.150)$$

Note that in the preceding derivation, it is implicitly assumed that the object sees a static inhomogeneous magnetic field during the free precession period. Expressing the field distribution as

$$B(\boldsymbol{r}) = B_0 + \Delta B(\boldsymbol{r}) \qquad (3.151)$$

we have

$$\Delta\omega(\boldsymbol{r}) = \gamma\Delta B(\boldsymbol{r}) \qquad (3.152)$$

and Eq. (3.150) becomes

$$S(t) = \int_{\text{object}} M_{xy}(\boldsymbol{r}, 0)e^{-i\gamma\Delta B(\boldsymbol{r})t}d\boldsymbol{r} \qquad (3.153)$$

If the inhomogeneous field is time-varying, that is, ΔB is a function of both space and time, then all the foregoing signal expressions need to be modified accordingly. Specifically, denoting the inhomogeneous field component as $\Delta B(\boldsymbol{r}, t)$, $\Delta\omega(\boldsymbol{r})t$ should be replaced by $\gamma \int_0^t \Delta B(\boldsymbol{r}, \tau)d\tau$. For example, Eq. (3.148) should be rewritten as

$$S(t) = \omega_0 e^{i\pi/2} \int_{\text{object}} B_{r,xy}^*(\boldsymbol{r}) M_{xy}(\boldsymbol{r}, 0)e^{-i\gamma \int_0^t \Delta B(\boldsymbol{r}, \tau)d\tau}d\boldsymbol{r} \qquad (3.154)$$

■ **Example 3.9**

We calculate the signal generated by an α pulse in this example.

Assume that the object has a thermal equilibrium magnetization $M_z^0(\boldsymbol{r})$. The transverse magnetization generated by the pulse is

$$M_{xy}(\boldsymbol{r}, t = 0_+) = M_z^0(\boldsymbol{r})\sin\alpha e^{i\phi_e(\boldsymbol{r})}$$

Substituting the result into Eq. (3.153) yields

$$S(t) = \sin\alpha \int_{\text{object}} M_z^0(\boldsymbol{r})e^{i\phi_e(\boldsymbol{r})}e^{-i\gamma\Delta B(\boldsymbol{r})t}d\boldsymbol{r}$$

which is the desired expression for the signal generated by an arbitrary α pulse in the presence of an inhomogeneous static field.

Exercises

3.1   For the following nuclei, does their spin quantum number take an integral, half-integral, or zero value? For each case, discuss whether the nucleus is NMR-active.

    (a) ^{1}H, ^{2}H

    (b) ^{16}O, ^{17}O

    (c) ^{12}C, ^{13}C

    (d) ^{31}P, ^{23}Na

3.2   In the absence of an external magnetic field, a bulk object exhibits no net nuclear magnetism because:

    (a)   Nuclear magnetic moments for all nuclei are zero.

    (b)   Nuclear magnetic moments cancel out each other.

    (c)   The bulk magnetization vector is too small to be detected.

    (d)   All of the above.

3.3   What are the primary functions of the static magnetic field $\vec{B}_0$ in MR imaging?

3.4   What is the Zeeman splitting phenomenon?

3.5   Why is MRI known as a low-sensitivity imaging technique?

3.6   What is the primary function of the oscillating $\vec{B}_1(t)$ field?

3.7   What is the resonance condition?

3.8   Why does a spin system often have more than one resonance frequency? If you place a cup of water in a perfectly homogeneous magnetic field, do you expect to detect more than one resonance frequency from the protons? Why?

3.9   What is an isochromat?

3.10   Justify the last two equations in Eq. (3.57).

3.11   Given a fixed flip angle, the larger the $\vec{M}$ the stronger the $\vec{B}_1$ needed because a stronger force is required to flip a larger $\vec{M}$. True or false?

3.12　Briefly discuss how one can selectively elicit the NMR phenomenon from one spin system of a biological sample (such as protons) without affecting the others (such as ^{31}P)?

3.13　Justify that the two representations of nuclear precession in Eq. (3.25) and Eq. (3.16) are equivalent.

3.14　Prove the following relationships for the rotation matrices $\mathbf{R}_{x'}(\alpha)$, $\mathbf{R}_{y'}(\alpha)$, and $\mathbf{R}_{z'}(\alpha)$:

(a)　$\mathbf{R}_{x'}^{-1}(\alpha) = \mathbf{R}_{x'}(-\alpha) = \mathbf{R}_{-x'}(\alpha)$

(b)　$\mathbf{R}_{y'}^{-1}(\alpha) = \mathbf{R}_{y'}(-\alpha) = \mathbf{R}_{-y'}(\alpha)$

(c)　$\mathbf{R}_{z'}^{-1}(\alpha) = \mathbf{R}_{z'}(-\alpha) = \mathbf{R}_{-z'}(\alpha)$

3.15　In which plane does the receiver coil pick up the activated MR signal? Is the received signal dependent on the time evolution of the longitudinal component after an RF pulse? Why?

3.16　Calculate and sketch $\vec{B}_{1,\mathrm{rot}}(t)$ assuming that

$$\vec{B}_1(t) = B_1 \cos(\omega_{\mathrm{rf}}t + \pi/4)\vec{i} - B_1 \sin(\omega_{\mathrm{rf}}t + \pi/4)\vec{j}$$

3.17　The bulk magnetization of a proton spin system is flipped 90° by a rectangular RF pulse of width 1.0 ms.

(a)　What is the magnitude of the B_1 field required?

(b)　How many precession cycles take place in the laboratory frame during the pulse, assuming $B_0 = 0.5$, 1.0, and 1.5 T, respectively.

3.18　Assume that $\vec{B}_1(t) = B_1 \cos \omega_{\mathrm{rf}}t\,\vec{i} - B_1 \sin \omega_{\mathrm{rf}}t\,\vec{j}$ is a stationary vector in the ω_{rf}-rotating frame, namely, $\vec{B}_{1,\mathrm{rot}}(t) = B_1\vec{i}'$. Derive an expression for $\vec{B}_1(t)$ such that

(a)　$\vec{B}_{1,\mathrm{rot}}(t) = B_1\vec{j}'$

(b)　$\vec{B}_{1,\mathrm{rot}}(t) = B_1\vec{i}' + B_1\vec{j}'$

3.19　Derive the closed-form solution given in Eq. (3.82) for the Bloch equation for on-resonance excitation with an arbitrary pulse.

3.20　Calculate and depict the bulk magnetization vector of a spin system relative to the prepulse reference frame after a $90°_{x'}$ pulse. Assume that the

Larmor frequency of the spin system is 10 MHz, the pulse lasts 1.0 ms, and the prepulse condition is $M_{x'}(0_-) = M_{y'}(0_-) = 0$ and $M_{z'}(0_-) = M_z^0$.

3.21   Calculate the resulting magnetization in the laboratory frame immediately after a $90^\circ_{x'}$ pulse with duration of τ and 2τ, respectively.

3.22   Assume that a spin system with a single resonance component was at thermal equilibrium. Calculate the transverse magnetization resulting from the following excitation sequences:

(a) $90^\circ_{x'}, 90^\circ_{y'}$

(b) $90^\circ_{x'}, -\tau - 90^\circ_{y'}$

(c) $45^\circ_{x'}, 90^\circ_{y'}$

(d) $30^\circ_{x'}, (-15^\circ_{z'}) 80^\circ_{x'}, 15^\circ_{z'}$

3.23   Calculate the effects of the following excitation sequences on a spin system with two isochromats at resonance frequencies ω_0 and $\omega_0 - \delta\omega_0$. It is assumed that the spin system is at thermal equilibrium and $\tau = \frac{\pi}{3}$.

(a) $90^\circ_{x'}, -\tau - 180^\circ_{y'}$

(b) $45^\circ_{x'}, -\tau/2 - 90^\circ_{y'}$

3.24   Derive the closed-form solution given in Eq. (3.107) for the Bloch equation for off-resonance excitation with a rectangular pulse.

3.25   Prove the relationships given in Eq. (3.57).

3.26   Prove the result in Eq. (3.60).

3.27   Assume that a known RF pulse $\vec{B}_1(t) = B_1 \cos(\omega_0 t)\vec{i} - B_1 \sin(\omega_0 t)\vec{j}$ flips the bulk magnetization vector onto the y'-axis (of the rotating frame) immediately after the pulse. Modify this $\vec{B}_1$ field such that the bulk magnetization vector ends up in the following positions immediately after the pulse:

(a)   Lying along the $-y'$-axis

(b)   Lying along the x'-axis

(c)   Lying along the $-x'$-axis

(d)   Lying along a vector 45° away from the y'-axis toward the x' in the transverse plane

3.28　Specify two pulses that will convert $M_{x'y'}$ to $M_{x'y'}^*$ and $-M_{x'y'}^*$, respectively.

3.29　Use a vector model to schematically show the effects of a $90^\circ_{x'}$, $90^\circ_{-x'}$, $90^\circ_{y'}$, $90^\circ_{-y'}$, $180^\circ_{x'}$, $180^\circ_{y'}$ pulse on the bulk magnetization vector originally pointing along the z'-axis.

3.30　The excitation property of an RF pulse is derived from the *inverse* Fourier transform of its envelope function. How is it related to the *forward* transform?

3.31　An RF pulse applied along the x'-axis for 100 μs flips an "on-resonance" magnetization by 90° onto the y'-axis. How much magnetization is tipped onto the (x', y')-plane if the excitation is "off-resonance" by 10 kHz?

3.32　Describe what is meant by "hard" and "soft" pulses.

3.33　The frequency distribution of an RF pulse can presumably be calculated from its Fourier transform. Compare the situation pertaining to Problem 3.31 with the result you expect from the Fourier transform.

3.34　A spin system has three isochromats with resonance frequencies at ω_0, $\omega_0 + \Delta$, and $\omega_0 - \Delta$, where $\omega_0 = 42$ MHz and $\Delta = 0.25$ kHz. We next assume that an RF pulse defined by $B_1(t) = B_1^e(t)e^{-i\omega_0 t}$, where the Fourier transform of $B_1^e(t)$ is given in the following figure, will flip the isochromats by 90°, 67.5°, and 67.5°, respectively. Calculate the flip angles of all the isochromats for the following pulses based on the Fourier theory.

(a)　$B_1^e(2t)e^{-i\omega_0 t}$

(b)　$2B_1^e(2t)e^{-i\omega_0 t}$

(c)　$B_1^e(t/2)e^{-i\omega_o t}$

(d)　$\frac{1}{2}B_1^e(t/2)e^{-i\omega_0 t}$

(e)　$2B_1^e(2t)e^{-i(\omega_0+\Delta)t}$

(f)　$2B_1^e(2t)e^{-i(\omega_0-\Delta)t}$

(g)　$\frac{1}{2}B_1^e(t/2)e^{-i(\omega_0+\Delta)t}$

(h)　$\frac{1}{2}B_1^e(t/2)e^{-i(\omega_0-\Delta)t}$

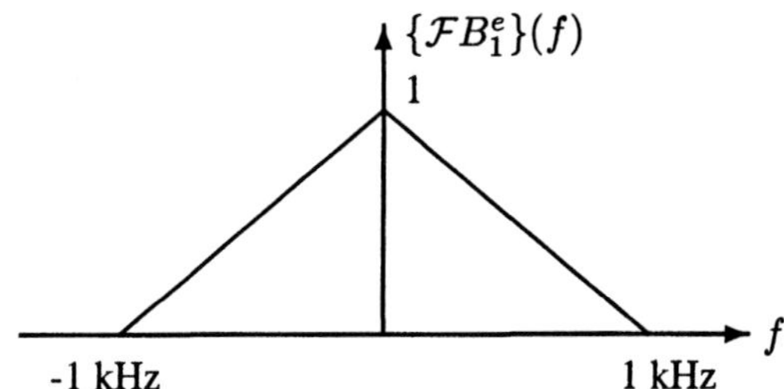

3.35   Design an RF pulse that will selectively excite a 10 kHz wide frequency band centered at 42 MHz with 45° flip angle for a spin system of protons.

3.36   After an RF pulse, M_{xy} decays to zero and M_z returns to M_z^0. During this relaxation process, the amount of M_{xy} lost is equal to the amount of M_z that is gained. True or false?

3.37   During the *excitation* period, the magnitude of $\vec{M}(t)$ stays constant while $\vec{M}(t)$ spirals down. Give an example to demonstrate that this statement is not true during the *relaxation* period when $\vec{M}(t)$ spirals up.

3.38   How long does it take for the longitudinal magnetization M_z of a spin system with longitudinal relaxation time constant T_1 to recover 63% of its thermal equilibrium value after (a) a 90° pulse and (b) a 75° pulse?

3.39   A spin system is excited by a $180°_{x'} - \tau - 90°_{x'}$ sequence with $\tau \sim 2T_1$.

  (a)   Plot the time evolution of the $M_{z'}$ component in the τ time interval.

  (b)   Calculate the magnitude of $M_{x'y'}$ immediately after the $90°_{x'}$ pulse and plot its time evolution after this pulse.

3.40   An imaging sequence often involves a series of excitation pulses to generate signals to cover k-space. Since a 90° pulse completely rotates any available M_z component onto the transverse plane, magnetization along the z-axis is always zero immediately after a 90° pulse in any imaging sequence with 90° excitation pulses. True or false?

3.41   Why is forced precession much slower than free precession?

Chapter 4

Signal Characteristics

The great mystery of the spin echo was what made the spins get back in phase again? Was echo a challenge to the basic concepts of irreversibility? Was there a Maxwell demon at work producing the refocusing?

Charles P. Slichter

In this chapter, we examine in detail time signals observed from a nuclear spin system after pulse excitations. We classify these signals into three major categories: free induction decays (FID), RF echoes, and gradient echoes. For each type of signal, we describe its excitation requirements, general characteristics, and mathematical expression.

4.1 Basic Assumptions

Let us state some general assumptions underlying the discussion throughout this chapter.

First, we assume that an RF pulse is applied instantaneously so that the pulse interval is treated as zero. If precise timing of the occurrence of a signal is desired, finite pulse intervals need to be properly accounted for, but this is rarely the case in practice.

Second, we ignore any imperfections in excitation and reception so that any phase shift due to off-resonance effects and nonuniform B_r weighting on the received signal are omitted. Under this assumption, we can use the simplified signal expression in Eq. (3.150). Furthermore, for notational convenience, we will replace $\Delta\omega$ by ω so that ω now represents the precessional frequency in the rotating frame. Consequently, Eq. (3.150) can be written as

$$S(t) = \int_{\text{object}} M_{xy}(\boldsymbol{r}, 0_+) e^{-t/T_2(\boldsymbol{r})} e^{-i\omega(\boldsymbol{r})t} d\boldsymbol{r} \qquad (4.1)$$

Third, for a heterogeneous spin system, we introduce a spin spectral density function $\rho(\omega)$ to characterize its frequency distribution. Specifically, let $dM(\omega)$ be the isochromatic bulk magnetization.[1] Then,

$$dM(\omega) = \rho(\omega) d\omega \qquad (4.2)$$

and

$$M = \int_{-\infty}^{\infty} \rho(\omega) d\omega \qquad (4.3)$$

Having $\rho(\omega)$, Eq. (4.1) can be rewritten as

$$S(t) = \int_{-\infty}^{\infty} \rho(\omega) e^{-t/T_2(\omega)} e^{-i\omega t} d\omega \qquad (4.4)$$

Note that $\rho(\omega)$ is not identical to the frequency spectrum of $S(t)$. For distinction, we use $\hat{\rho}(\omega)$ to represent the frequency spectrum of a time signal. By definition,

$$S(t) = \frac{1}{2\pi} \int_{-\infty}^{\infty} \hat{\rho}(\omega) e^{-i\omega t} d\omega \qquad (4.5)$$

Therefore, $\rho(\omega) = 2\pi \hat{\rho}(\omega)$ only when T_2 relaxation is omitted.

In practice, $\rho(\omega)$ can take various forms, depending on $M_z(\boldsymbol{r})$ and $B(\boldsymbol{r})$. We describe two of them for later use. First, for a spin system with N isochromats at frequency ω_n, the spectral density function consists of N delta functions located at ω_n. More specifically,

$$\rho(\omega) = \sum_{n=1}^{N} M_{z,n}^0 \delta(\omega - \omega_n) \qquad (4.6)$$

where $M_{z,n}^0$ is the thermal equilibrium value for the bulk magnetization of resonance frequency ω_n. Second, when a sample is placed in a special inhomogeneous magnetic field with a Lorentzian distribution, the resulting spectral density function takes the following form:

$$\rho(\omega) = M_z^0 \frac{(\gamma \Delta B_0)^2}{(\gamma \Delta B_0)^2 + (\omega - \omega_0)^2} \qquad (4.7)$$

---

[1] For notational convenience, we simply use $M_x(\omega)$, $M_y(\omega)$, and $M_z(\omega)$ to denote isochromatic magnetization components.

■ **Example 4.1**

Determine $\rho(\omega)$ for a simple case, in which a sample with spin concentration $c(x) = \rho_0 \Pi(x)$ is placed in an inhomogeneous field $B(x) = B_0 + x^2$.

We first calculate the time signal after a 90° pulse. Pick an isochromat at an arbitrary location x. Its resonance frequency is

$$\omega(x) = \gamma(B_0 + x^2)$$

and its magnetization is

$$M_z^0 = c(x)dx$$

The infinitesimal signal generated by this isochromat after a 90° pulse is

$$dS(t) = c(x)dx\,e^{-t/T_2}e^{-i\omega t} = c(x)e^{-t/T_2}e^{-i\gamma(B_0+x^2)t}dx \qquad (4.8)$$

The full-fledged time signal from the entire sample is

$$S(t) = \int_{-\infty}^{\infty} dS(t) = \int_{-1/2}^{1/2} \rho_0 e^{-t/T_2}e^{-i\gamma(B_0+x^2)t}dx \qquad (4.9)$$

By variable substitution, Eq. (4.9) can be rewritten as

$$S(t) = \int_{\omega_0-\gamma/4}^{\omega_0+\gamma/4} \frac{\rho_0}{2\sqrt{|\omega - \omega_0|/\gamma}}e^{-t/T_2}e^{-i\omega t}d\omega \qquad (4.10)$$

Therefore, the spin spectral density function is

$$\rho(\omega) = \begin{cases} \dfrac{\rho_0}{2\sqrt{|\omega-\omega_0|/\gamma}} & |\omega - \omega_0| < \gamma/4 \\ 0 & \text{otherwise} \end{cases} \qquad (4.11)$$

4.2   Free Induction Decays

Free induction decays (FID) arise from the action of a single pulse on a nuclear spin system. "Free" refers to the fact that the signal is generated by the free precession of the bulk magnetization vector about the $\vec{B}_0$ field; "induction" indicates that the signal was produced based on Faraday's law of electromagnetic induction; and "decay" reflects the characteristic decrease with time of the signal amplitude.

FID signals are the most basic form of transient signals from a spin system after a pulse excitation. They are also the mother signal for other forms of MR signals described later in this chapter. Mathematically, an FID signal resulting from an α pulse takes the following form:

$$S(t) = \sin \alpha \int_{-\infty}^{\infty} \rho(\omega) e^{-t/T_2(\omega)} e^{-i\omega t} d\omega \qquad t \geq 0 \qquad (4.12)$$

Clearly, the spectral density function $\rho(\omega)$ determines the characteristics of an FID signal. For example, the FID signal of a spin system with a single spectral component resonating at frequency ω_0 can be expressed as

$$S(t) = M_z^0 \sin \alpha e^{-t/T_2} e^{-i\omega_0 t} \qquad t \geq 0 \qquad (4.13)$$

Two basic parameters of an FID signal are its amplitude and decay rate. Regardless of the spectral distribution of a spin system, the FID signal reaches its maximum amplitude at $t = 0$, whose value is given by

$$A_f = \sin \alpha \int_{-\infty}^{\infty} \rho(\omega) d\omega = M_z^0 \sin \alpha \qquad (4.14)$$

Hence, the maximum amplitude of an FID signal depends on both the flip angle and the thermal equilibrium value of the bulk magnetization.

The decay rate of an FID signal is strongly tied to the underlying spectral distribution. In the case of a single spectral component, the FID signal bears a characteristic T_2 decay, as indicated in Eq. (4.13). This situation occurs when both the sample and the magnetic field to which the sample is exposed are perfectly homogeneous. When the magnetic field is inhomogeneous, the FID signal decays at a much faster rate. To illustrate this point, consider two proton isochromats, one at 1 T and the other at 1.01 T. Their precessional frequencies will be 42 and 42.42 MHz, respectively. Then, in 1 μs, isochromat 1 will have made 42 turns while isochromat 2 will have made 42.42 turns. In this short time span, the first isochromat will be almost a half (0.42) turn behind the second, or nearly 180° out of phase. If we look at a large number of isochromats, a random phase relationship will be established in this process. As a consequence, their magnetic moments will cancel each other, leading to a loss of the bulk magnetization or a decay in the detected signal.

To characterize the signal decay in the presence of field inhomogeneity, a new time constant T_2^* is frequently used. More specifically, if the field inhomogeneity lends itself to a Lorentzian distribution, as described by Eq. (4.7), the FID signal becomes

$$S(t) = \sin \alpha \int_{-\infty}^{\infty} M_z^0 \frac{(\gamma \Delta B_0)^2}{(\gamma \Delta B_0)^2 + (\omega - \omega_0)^2} e^{-t/T_2} e^{-i\omega t} d\omega$$

$$= \sin \alpha \int_{-\infty}^{\infty} \left[M_z^0 \frac{(\gamma \Delta B_0)^2}{(\gamma \Delta B_0)^2 + \omega^2} e^{-i\omega t} d\omega \right] e^{-t/T_2} e^{-i\omega_0 t}$$

$$= \pi M_z^0 \gamma \Delta B_0 \sin \alpha e^{-\gamma \Delta B_0 t} e^{-t/T_2} e^{-i\omega_0 t}$$

$$= \pi M_z^0 \gamma \Delta B_0 \sin \alpha e^{-t/T_2^*} e^{-i\omega_0 t} \qquad t \geq 0 \qquad (4.15)$$

where

$$\frac{1}{T_2^*} = \frac{1}{T_2} + \gamma \Delta B_0 \tag{4.16}$$

Although Eq. (4.16) is widely used in the MR literature, it is valid only restrictively for Lorentzian spectral density functions. For other types of spectral density function, the envelope function of an FID signal will not be an exponential function, and T_2^* should be interpreted as the effective time constant of an approximating exponential. To illustrate the effect of different spectral distributions on the characteristics of an FID signal, some examples are shown in Fig. 4.1.

To summarize, an FID signal is the transient response of a spin system after a pulse excitation. The magnitude of the signal is dependent on a number of parameters, in particular, the flip angle, the total number of spins in the sample, and the magnetic field strength. How long an FID signal persists in practice depends mainly on the degree of field inhomogeneity, which is characterized by the T_2^* decay.

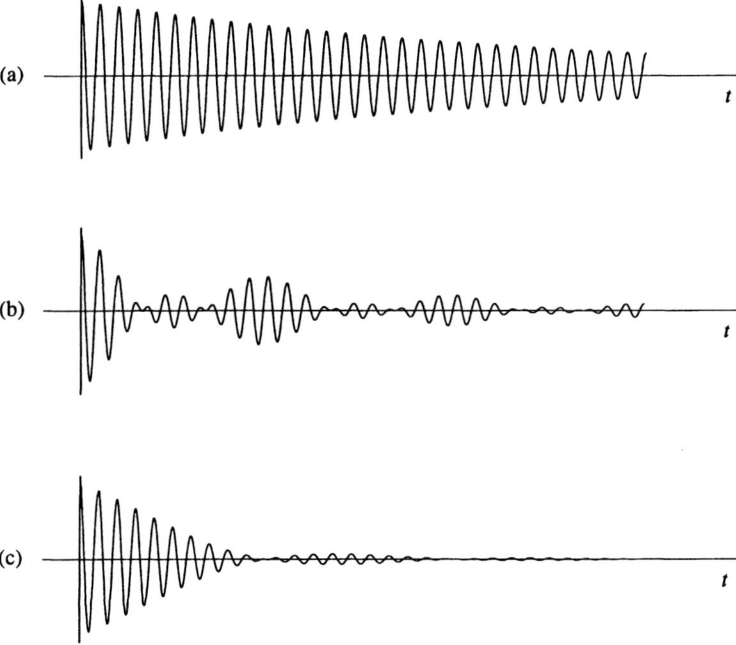

Figure 4.1   Simulated FID signals from a spin system with (a) one isochromat, (b) three isochromats, and (c) a continuum of isochromats. Note that the decaying pattern of the signals changes for different spectral distributions.

■ **Example 4.2**

In this example, we take a close look at the frequency spectrum of an FID signal. First, consider the case of a single spectral component. According to Eq. (4.13), the FID signal can be written as

$$S(t) = Ae^{-t/T_2}e^{-i\omega_0 t} \qquad t \geq 0$$

where A is a scaling constant. Its frequency spectrum is given by

$$\hat{\rho}(\omega) = \mathcal{F}\{S(t)\} = \int_0^\infty Ae^{-t/T_2}e^{-i\omega_0 t}e^{-i\omega t}\,dt$$

$$= \frac{AT_2}{1 + T_2^2(\omega + \omega_0)^2} - i\frac{AT_2^2(\omega + \omega_0)}{1 + T_2^2(\omega + \omega_0)^2}$$

The real and imaginary parts of $\hat{\rho}(\omega)$ are called absorption-mode and dispersion-mode components, respectively. Several notable features of $\hat{\rho}(\omega)$ are summarized as follows:

(a) The absorption-mode spectrum given by

$$\Re\{\hat{\rho}(\omega)\} = \frac{AT_2}{1 + T_2^2(\omega + \omega_0)^2} \tag{4.17}$$

has a Lorentzian line shape, as shown in Fig. 4.2.

(b) The full width at half-maximum (FWHM), also called the line width, of the absorption-mode spectrum is $1/(\pi T_2)$.

(c) The magnitude spectrum given by

$$|\hat{\rho}(\omega)| = \frac{AT_2}{\sqrt{1 + T_2^2(\omega + \omega_0)^2}} \tag{4.18}$$

has a non-Lorentzian line shape.

(d) The line width of the magnitude spectrum is $\sqrt{3}/(\pi T_2)$. In other words, the magnitude spectrum is a factor of $\sqrt{3}$ broader than the absorption-mode counterpart.

For FID signals with more than one spectral component, the absorption-mode spectrum is a summation of Lorentzian lines whose locations and line widths are directly related to the isochromat resonance frequencies and relaxation times, respectively. An example of such a spectrum is shown in Fig. 4.3.

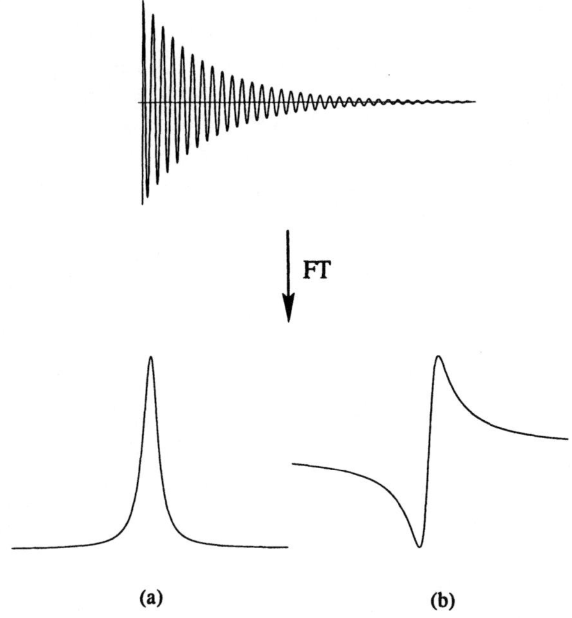

Figure 4.2   (a) FID signal of a single spectral component, (b) absorption-mode spectrum, and (c) dispersion-mode spectrum .

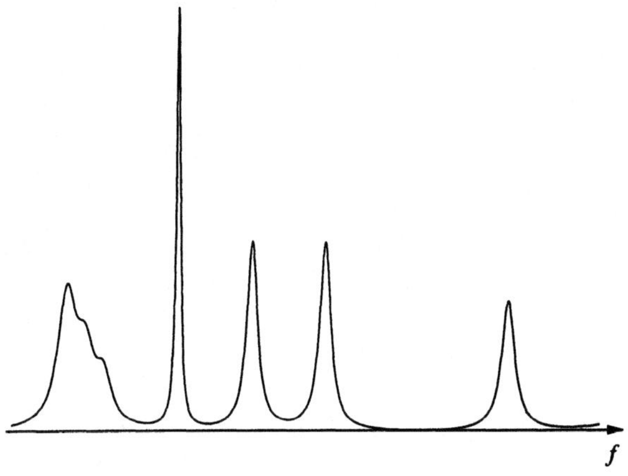

Figure 4.3   Simulated ^{31}P absorption-mode spectrum.

4.3   RF Echoes

In this section, we discuss another form of MR signal, known as *echo*. A feature distinguishing an echo signal from an FID signal is the "two-sidedness" of an echo signal, one side of which is from the refocusing phase of a transverse magnetization and the other side from the dephasing period. Such a two-sided signal is essential for symmetric coverage of k-space, as will become evident in Chapter 5.

An echo signal can be generated either by multiple RF pulses or by magnetic field gradient reversal. Signals of the former type are called *RF echoes* and the latter *gradient echoes*. RF echoes were discovered by Erwin L. Hahn in 1950. Since then, the concept of realigning incoherent magnetization vectors by refocusing RF pulses has been widely used in various types of NMR experiments. This section is devoted to a description of RF echoes. However, echo phenomena in multiple pulse excitations are extremely rich—as a popular saying goes, it is easier to generate an echo than to ignore it in multiple-pulse MR experiments. The ensuing discussion focuses on echoes from multiple RF pulses. Gradient echoes are discussed in Section 4.4.

4.3.1   Two-Pulse Echo

To generate an RF echo, at least two pulses are necessary. We begin with a simple two-pulse excitation scheme consisting of a 90° pulse followed by a time delay τ and then a 180° pulse. This excitation scheme is denoted as

$$90° - \tau - 180° \tag{4.19}$$

The echo signal thus generated is called a *spin echo* (SE).

To see intuitively how a spin echo is formed, we follow the action of the applied pulses and the evolution of the transverse magnetization. For simplicity, we assume that the 90° pulse is applied along the x'-axis and the 180° is applied along the y'-axis, and further that the sample has two isochromats with precessional frequencies ω_s (slow) and ω_f (fast) in the rotating frame. Under the condition of negligible off-resonance effects, the $90°_{x'}$ pulse rotates both magnetization vectors onto the y'-axis, as shown in Fig. 4.4a. After the pulse, these vectors precess about the z-axis. Since one is precessing relatively faster than the other, they progressively lose phase coherence as the free precession continues. After a time interval τ, the two vectors fan out in the transverse plane by a phase angle $(\omega_f - \omega_s)\tau$, as shown in Fig. 4.4b. At this point, the $180°_{y'}$ pulse flips the two vectors over to the other side of the transverse plane, as shown in Fig. 4.4c. As a consequence, the faster vector is now lagging behind the slower by the same phase angle with which it was leading prior to the $180°_{y'}$ pulse. Since both vectors will continue to precess clockwise at angular frequencies ω_f and ω_s (assuming that the magnetic field inhomogeneity is time-invariant), the faster isochromat

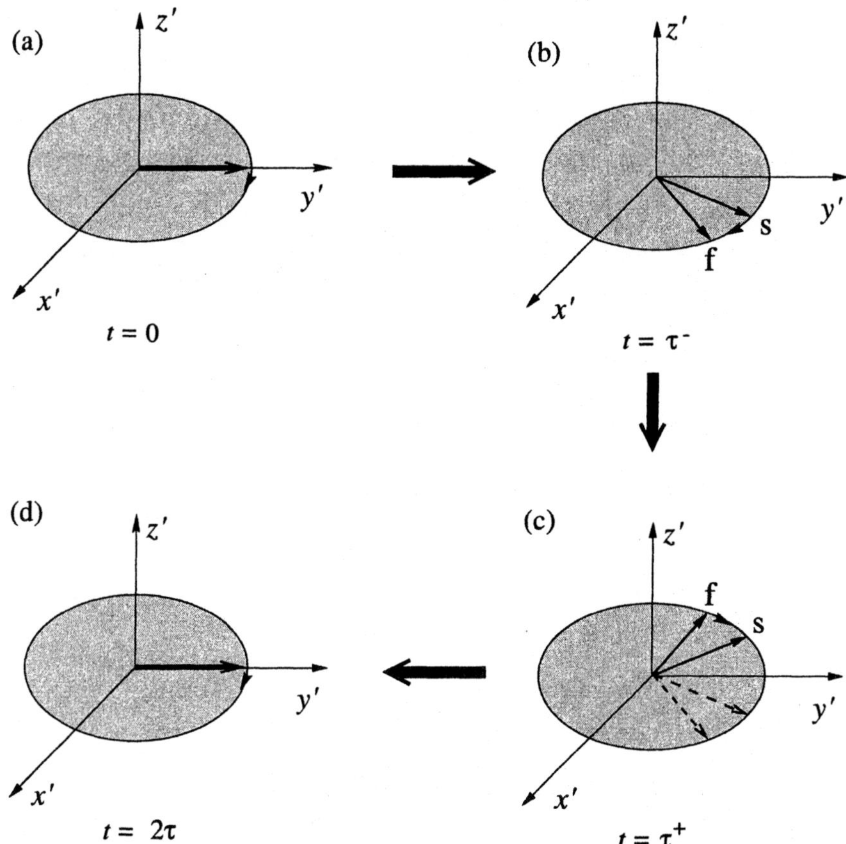

Figure 4.4   Vector diagram illustrating the refocusing of isochromats in a spin-echo experiment.

will "catch" the slower after a time interval τ, thus recreating a phase coherence between the two vectors at time $t = 2\tau$, as shown in Fig. 4.4d.

Although Fig. 4.4 shows the rephasing process of only two isochromats, the analysis can be extended to an arbitrary number of them. In fact, because of the existence of a large number of isochromats in a real sample, a total dephasing normally occurs by the time the $180^\circ_{y'}$ pulse is applied. This means that the transverse magnetization $M_{x'y'}$ completely vanishes and the FID signal disappears at $t = \tau$. After the $180^\circ_{y'}$ pulse, $M_{x'y'}$ grows gradually and reaches the maximum value at $t = 2\tau$, as shown in Fig. 4.5. If we ignore the T_2 relaxation, the mechanism responsible for the loss of the phase coherence among the isochromats during the free precession period before the $180^\circ_{y'}$ is the same as that responsible for the recovery of the phase coherence after the pulse. Therefore, $M_{x'y'}$ as a function of time possesses the following property:

$$|M_{x'y'}(\tau - t)| = |M_{x'y'}(\tau + t)| \qquad 0 \leq t \leq \tau \qquad (4.20)$$

which implies that $|M_{x'y'}(t)|$ has a mirror symmetry about the time point $t = \tau$. With the transverse magnetization $M_{x'y'}$ being completely destroyed by dephasing at $t = \tau$, the rebirth of $M_{x'y'}(t)$ for $t > \tau$ is a consequence of the refocusing power of the 180°. For this reason, $M_{x'y'}(t)$ for $t > \tau$ is frequently referred to as the recalled (rephased) transverse magnetization, of which the rephasing part ($\tau < t < 2\tau$) is responsible for one side of the echo signal and the subsequent dephasing part ($t > 2\tau$) is responsible for the other side.

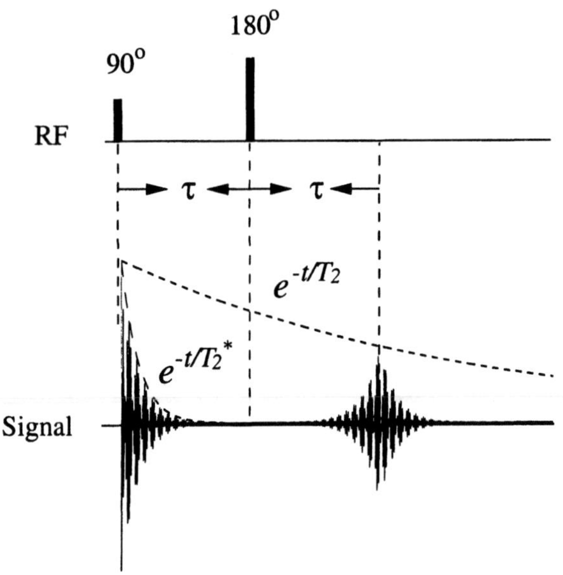

Figure 4.5 Formation of a spin echo signal by a $90° - \tau - 180°$ pulse sequence. The application of a 90° pulse produces the FID, which quickly disappears as the spins dephase. The application of a 180° pulse at a time τ after the 90° pulse produces an echo at a time 2τ after the 90° pulse.

We next derive the echo signal in a more rigorous fashion. For generality, we consider the following two-pulse sequence:

$$\alpha_1 - \tau - \alpha_2 \qquad (4.21)$$

To simplify the discussion, we assume that both pulses are applied along the y'-axis. For pulses applied in different directions, the derivation needs to be modified accordingly. This is left for the reader. Two transforms are used in the following analysis. First, the effect of an $\alpha_{y'}$-pulse is calculated using the following transform:

$$\begin{bmatrix} M_{x'} \\ M_{y'} \\ M_{z'} \end{bmatrix} \xrightarrow{\alpha_{y'}} \begin{bmatrix} M_{x'}\cos\alpha - M_{z'}\sin\alpha \\ M_{y'} \\ M_{x'}\sin\alpha + M_{z'}\cos\alpha \end{bmatrix} \tag{4.22}$$

Second, the effect of a τ delay is described by

$$\begin{bmatrix} M_{x'} \\ M_{y'} \\ M_{z'} \end{bmatrix} \xrightarrow{\tau} \begin{bmatrix} (M_{x'}\cos\omega\tau + M_{y'}\sin\omega\tau)e^{-\tau/T_2} \\ (-M_{x'}\sin\omega\tau + M_{y'}\cos\omega\tau)e^{-\tau/T_2} \\ M_z^0(1 - e^{-\tau/T_1}) + M_{z'}e^{-\tau/T_1} \end{bmatrix} \tag{4.23}$$

where ω is the precessional frequency in the rotating frame.

Consider an arbitrary isochromat of frequency ω initially at the thermal equilibrium state. We have after the α_1 pulse

$$M_{x'}(\omega, 0_+) = -M_z^0(\omega)\sin\alpha_1$$
$$M_{y'}(\omega, 0_+) = 0$$
$$M_{z'}(\omega, 0_+) = M_z^0(\omega)\cos\alpha_1$$

After the τ delay, the magnetization components take the following set of values:

$$M_{x'}(\omega, \tau) = -M_z^0(\omega)\sin\alpha_1\cos\omega\tau e^{-\tau/T_2} \tag{4.24a}$$

$$M_{y'}(\omega, \tau) = M_z^0(\omega)\sin\alpha_1\sin\omega\tau e^{-\tau/T_2} \tag{4.24b}$$

$$\begin{aligned} M_{z'}(\omega, \tau) &= M_z^0(\omega)(1 - e^{-\tau/T_1}) + M_z^0(\omega)\cos\alpha_1 e^{-\tau/T_1} \\ &= M_z^0(\omega)[1 - (1 - \cos\alpha_1)e^{-\tau/T_1}] \end{aligned} \tag{4.24c}$$

The α_2 has no effect on the y'-component but transforms the x'- and z'-components to the following set of values:

$$\begin{aligned} M_{x'}(\omega, \tau_+) = &-M_z^0(\omega)\sin\alpha_1\cos\alpha_2\cos\omega\tau e^{-\tau/T_2} \\ &-M_z^0(\omega)[1 - (1 - \cos\alpha_1)e^{-\tau/T_1}]\sin\alpha_2 \end{aligned} \tag{4.25a}$$

$$\begin{aligned} M_{z'}(\omega, \tau_+) = &\ M_z^0(\omega)[1 - (1 - \cos\alpha_1)e^{-\tau/T_1}]\cos\alpha_2 \\ &-M_z^0(\omega)\sin\alpha_1\sin\alpha_2\cos\omega\tau e^{-\tau/T_2} \end{aligned} \tag{4.25b}$$

The x'-component in Eq. (4.25a) can be rewritten as

$$\begin{aligned} M_{x'}(\omega, \tau_+) = &- M_z^0(\omega)\sin\alpha_1\cos^2\frac{\alpha_2}{2}\cos\omega\tau e^{-\tau/T_2} \\ &+ M_z^0(\omega)\sin\alpha_1\sin^2\frac{\alpha_2}{2}\cos\omega\tau e^{-\tau/T_2} \\ &- M_z^0(\omega)[1 - (1 - \cos\alpha_1)e^{-\tau/T_1}]\sin\alpha_2 \end{aligned} \tag{4.26}$$

Similarly, the y'-component in Eq. (4.24b) can be rewritten as

$$M_{y'}(\omega, \tau_+) = M_z^0(\omega) \sin \alpha_1 \cos^2 \frac{\alpha_2}{2} \sin \omega \tau e^{-\tau/T_2}$$

$$+ M_z^0(\omega) \sin \alpha_1 \sin^2 \frac{\alpha_2}{2} \sin \omega \tau e^{-\tau/T_2} \tag{4.27}$$

Consequently, the transverse magnetization immediately after the second pulse can be written as

$$M_{x'y'}(\omega, \tau_+) = M_z^0(\omega) \sin \alpha_1 \left(\sin^2 \frac{\alpha_2}{2} e^{-i\omega\tau} - \cos^2 \frac{\alpha_2}{2} e^{i\omega\tau} \right) e^{-\tau/T_2}$$

$$- M_z^0(\omega)[1 - (1 - \cos \alpha_1)e^{-\tau/T_1}] \sin \alpha_2 \tag{4.28}$$

Free precession of this vector about the z'-axis after the pulse is described by

$$M_{x'y'}(\omega, t) = M_{x'y'}(\omega, \tau_+) e^{-(t-\tau)/T_2} e^{-i\omega(t-\tau)}$$

$$= M_z^0(\omega) \sin \alpha_1 \left(-\cos^2 \frac{\alpha_2}{2} e^{-i\omega\tau} + \sin^2 \frac{\alpha_2}{2} e^{i\omega\tau} \right) e^{-t/T_2} e^{-i\omega(t-\tau)}$$

$$- M_z^0(\omega)[1 - (1 - \cos \alpha_1)e^{-\tau/T_1}] \sin \alpha_2 e^{-(t-\tau)/T_2} e^{-i\omega(t-\tau)}$$

$$= M_z^0(\omega) \sin \alpha_1 \sin^2 \frac{\alpha_2}{2} e^{-t/T_2} e^{-i\omega(t-2\tau)}$$

$$- M_z^0(\omega) \sin \alpha_1 \cos^2 \frac{\alpha_2}{2} e^{-t/T_2} e^{-i\omega t}$$

$$- M_z^0(\omega)[1 - (1 - \cos \alpha_1)e^{-\tau/T_1}] \sin \alpha_2 e^{-(t-\tau)/T_2} e^{-i\omega(t-\tau)} \tag{4.29}$$

for $t > \tau$. For an ensemble of a large number of isochromats, the second and third terms in Eq. (4.29) represent a purely dephasing component because the phase angle among the isochromats becomes larger as time progresses. These two components contribute to the FID signal formed from the second pulse. On the contrary, spins in the first term are rephasing gradually and achieve complete phase coherence at $t = 2\tau$. Therefore, this component will produce an echo signal, which can be expressed as

$$S(t) = \sin \alpha_1 \sin^2 \frac{\alpha_2}{2} \int_{-\infty}^{\infty} \rho(\omega) e^{-t/T_2(\omega)} e^{-i\omega(t-T_E)} d\omega \tag{4.30}$$

for $|t - T_E| \leq T_{acq}/2$, where

$$\begin{aligned} T_E = 2\tau : \quad & \text{echo time} \\ T_{acq} : \quad & \text{data acquisition interval} \end{aligned}$$

It is clear from Eq. (4.30) that the echo peaks at $t = T_E$, and its value is given by

$$A_E = \sin \alpha_1 \sin^2 \frac{\alpha_2}{2} \int_{-\infty}^{\infty} \rho(\omega) e^{-T_E/T_2(\omega)} d\omega \tag{4.31}$$

Ignoring the frequency dependence of T_2, we get

$$A_{\mathrm{E}} = M_z^0 \sin \alpha_1 \sin^2 \frac{\alpha_2}{2} e^{-T_{\mathrm{E}}/T_2} \qquad (4.32)$$

which explicitly shows the T_2-weighting on the echo amplitude. Clearly, A_{E} reaches its maximum value $M_z^0 e^{-T_{\mathrm{E}}/T_2}$ when $\alpha_1 = 90°$ and $\alpha_2 = 180°$. This value is still a factor of e^{-T_{E}/T_2} smaller than the maximum value of the initial FID. This signal loss occurs because the loss of phase coherence in the magnetic moments resulting from random field fluctuations cannot be recovered by a refocusing RF pulse.

In summary, an echo signal is formed as a result of the refocusing of a large number of dephased isochromats; it peaks when the isochromats reach a new phase coherence. Typically, an echo signal is a two-sided signal consisting of two "mirrored" FIDs. Although each side of an echo carries a T_2^*-decay, the amplitude of a spin echo is T_2-weighted. This feature is useful for generating a T_2-weighted image contrast, as discussed in Chapter 7.

■ **Example 4.3**

We calculate the echo signal from the following sequences:

    (a) $90°_{y'} - \tau - 90°_{y'}$

    (b) $90°_{y'} - \tau - 180°_{y'}$

    (c) $90°_{x'} - \tau - 180°_{y'}$

For the first and second sequences, we can obtain the echo signal expression from Eq. (4.30) by simply setting α_1 and α_2 to the given values. Specifically, in the first case, $\alpha_1 = \alpha_2 = 90°$, and therefore

$$S_1(t) = \frac{1}{2} \int_{-\infty}^{\infty} \rho(\omega) e^{-t/T_2(\omega)} e^{-i\omega(t-T_{\mathrm{E}})} d\omega \qquad (4.33)$$

In the second case, setting $\alpha_1 = 90°$ and $\alpha_2 = 180°$ gives

$$S_2(t) = \int_{-\infty}^{\infty} \rho(\omega) e^{-t/T_2(\omega)} e^{-i\omega(t-T_{\mathrm{E}})} d\omega \qquad (4.34)$$

Equations (4.33) and (4.34) indicate that the echo signals generated by sequences (a) and (b) are identical apart from the scaling constant. The amplitude of $S_1(t)$ is reduced by half compared to $S_2(t)$ because the refocusing $90°$ pulse only partially rephased the spins.

The echo signal generated by the third sequence is different from $S_2(t)$ because the magnetization is refocused along the positive direction of the y'-axis, as shown in Fig. 4.4. Noting that $S_2(t)$ represents an echo signal formed along the positive direction of the x'-direction, we can obtain the echo expression of the third sequence by phase-shifting $S_2(t)$ by $\frac{\pi}{2}$. That is,

$$S_3(t) = i \int_{-\infty}^{\infty} \rho(\omega) e^{-t/T_2(\omega)} e^{-i\omega(t-T_{\rm E})} d\omega \qquad (4.35)$$

4.3.2   Three-Pulse Echoes

In this section we analyze echoes from a three-pulse sequence denoted as

$$\alpha_1 - \tau_1 - \alpha_2 - \tau_2 - \alpha_3 \qquad (4.36)$$

In general, up to five echoes can be generated by a three-pulse sequence: three conventional spin echoes (SE), one secondary spin echo, and one stimulated echo (STE), as shown in Fig. 4.6.

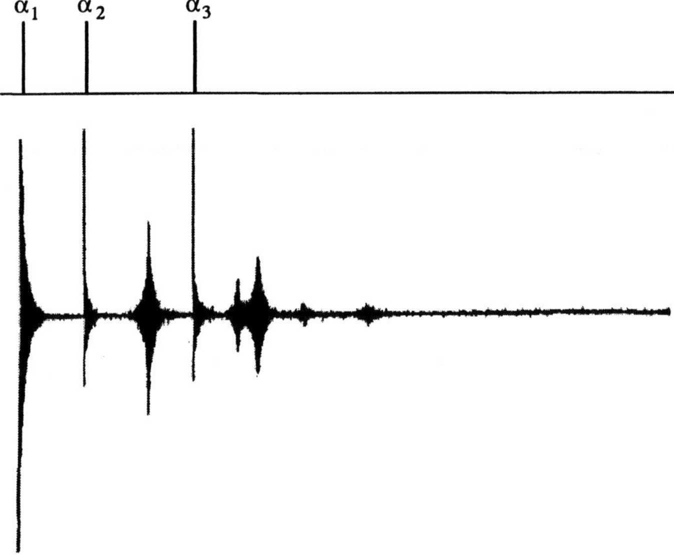

Figure 4.6   A train of three RF pulses generates three primary spin echoes, one secondary spin echo, and one stimulated echo.

The three conventional SEs are produced by each possible pair of RF pulses. Specifically, the FID generated by the first pulse is refocused by the second pulse to produce the first SE at $t = 2\tau_1$ and by the third pulse to produce the third SE at $t = 2(\tau_1 + \tau_2)$, while the FID generated by the second pulse is refocused by the third pulse to produce the second SE at $t = \tau_1 + 2\tau_2$. Simply put, SE_1 results from the action of pulses α_1 and α_2, SE_2 from the action of pulses α_2 and α_3, and SE_3 from the action of pulses α_1 and α_3. Under the assumption that $\tau_2 > 2\tau_1$, SE_1 takes place between the second and the third pulses, and it is "mirrored" by the third pulse to yield a secondary echo signal at $t = 2\tau_2$ (or $\tau_2 - \tau_1$ after the third pulse). The echo that arises from the combined effect of all three pulses is called a *stimulated echo*.

To clearly understand the occurrence of the stimulated echo, let us temporarily set $\alpha_1 = \alpha_2 = \alpha_3 = 90°$. After the first pulse, the equilibrium magnetization M_z^0 is flipped entirely onto the transverse plane. If τ_1 is on the order of T_2 or less, we will have appreciable transverse magnetization at the time τ_1. Consequently, the second $90°$ pulse, in addition to inducing the first SE, will produce a longitudinal magnetization. For the duration of τ_2 after the second pulse, this magnetization is "stored" along the z'-axis while it is going through the longitudinal relaxation process. The third $90°$ pulse, which comes at the end of the τ_2 interval, simply rotates this stored longitudinal magnetization back to the transverse plane. Since the intrinsic properties of the isochromats have not been altered by the magnetization gymnastics, they will precess at the same speed and direction following the third pulse as they did prior to the second pulse. In addition, this magnetization was influenced by the inhomogeneous field only during the τ_1 interval. Therefore, the constructive interference among these isochromat vectors will reach the maximum at $t = \tau_1$ after the third pulse, and thus the stimulated echo is formed.

Next, we analytically derive the five echoes from the generic three-pulse sequence in Eq. (4.36). For simplicity, we again assume that all the pulses are applied along the y'-axis. Making use of the results of a two-pulse sequence obtained in Section 4.3.1, particularly in Eqs. (4.29) and (4.25a), we have after the α_2-pulse

$$M_{x'y'}(\omega, t) = M_{x'y'}(\omega, \tau_{1+})e^{-i\omega(t-\tau_1)}$$

$$= M_z^0(\omega)\sin\alpha_1\left(-\cos^2\frac{\alpha_2}{2}e^{-i\omega\tau_1} + \sin^2\frac{\alpha_2}{2}e^{i\omega\tau_1}\right)e^{-t/T_2}e^{-i\omega(t-\tau_1)}$$

$$-M_z^0(\omega)[1 - (1-\cos\alpha_1)e^{-\tau_1/T_1}]\sin\alpha_2 e^{-(t-\tau_1)/T_2}e^{-i\omega(t-\tau_1)}$$

$$= M_z^0(\omega)\sin\alpha_1\sin^2\frac{\alpha_2}{2}e^{-t/T_2}e^{-i\omega(t-2\tau_1)}$$

$$-M_z^0(\omega)\sin\alpha_1\cos^2\frac{\alpha_2}{2}e^{-t/T_2}e^{-i\omega t}$$

$$-M_z^0(\omega)[1 - (1-\cos\alpha_1)e^{-\tau_1/T_1}]\sin\alpha_2 e^{-(t-\tau_1)/T_2}e^{-i\omega(t-\tau_1)} \quad (4.37a)$$

$$M_{z'}(\omega, t)$$

$$= M_z^0(\omega)[1 - (1-\cos\alpha_2)e^{-(t-\tau_1)/T_1} - (1-\cos\alpha_1)\cos\alpha_2 e^{-t/T_1}]$$

$$-M_z^0(\omega)\sin\alpha_1\sin\alpha_2\cos\omega\tau_1 e^{-\tau_1/T_2}e^{-(t-\tau_1)/T_1} \quad (4.37b)$$

for $t > \tau_1$. As discussed in Section 4.3.1, the first term in Eq. (4.37a) produces the first echo of the sequence. Based on Eq. (4.37), we have at the end of the τ_2 delay

$$
\begin{aligned}
M_{x'}&(\omega, \tau_1 + \tau_2) \\
&= -M_z^0(\omega)\sin\alpha_1\cos^2\frac{\alpha_2}{2}\cos\omega\tau_1\cos\omega\tau_2 e^{-(\tau_1+\tau_2)/T_2} \\
&\quad + M_z^0(\omega)\sin\alpha_1\sin^2\frac{\alpha_2}{2}\cos\omega\tau_1\cos\omega\tau_2 e^{-(\tau_1+\tau_2)/T_2} \\
&\quad - M_z^0(\omega)[1-(1-\cos\alpha_1)e^{-\tau_1/T_1}]\sin\alpha_2\cos\omega\tau_2 e^{-\tau_2/T_2} \\
&\quad + M_z^0(\omega)\sin\alpha_1\cos^2\frac{\alpha_2}{2}\sin\omega\tau_1\sin\omega\tau_2 e^{-(\tau_1+\tau_2)/T_2} \\
&\quad + M_z^0(\omega)\sin\alpha_1\sin^2\frac{\alpha_2}{2}\sin\omega\tau_1\sin\omega\tau_2 e^{-(\tau_1+\tau_2)/T_2} \\
&= -M_z^0(\omega)\sin\alpha_1\cos^2\frac{\alpha_2}{2}\cos\omega(\tau_1+\tau_2)e^{-(\tau_1+\tau_2)/T_2} \\
&\quad + M_z^0(\omega)\sin\alpha_1\sin^2\frac{\alpha_2}{2}\cos\omega(\tau_2-\tau_1)e^{-(\tau_1+\tau_2)/T_2} \\
&\quad - M_z^0(\omega)[1-(1-\cos\alpha_1)e^{-\tau_1/T_1}]\sin\alpha_2\cos\omega\tau_2 e^{-\tau_2/T_2} \quad (4.38)
\end{aligned}
$$

$$
\begin{aligned}
M_{y'}&(\omega, \tau_1 + \tau_2) \\
&= M_z^0(\omega)\sin\alpha_1\cos^2\frac{\alpha_2}{2}\cos\omega\tau_1\sin\omega\tau_2 e^{-(\tau_1+\tau_2)/T_2} \\
&\quad - M_z^0(\omega)\sin\alpha_1\sin^2\frac{\alpha_2}{2}\cos\omega\tau_1\sin\omega\tau_2 e^{-(\tau_1+\tau_2)/T_2} \\
&\quad + M_z^0(\omega)[1-(1-\cos\alpha_1)e^{-\tau_1/T_1}]\sin\alpha_2\sin\omega\tau_2 e^{-\tau_2/T_2} \\
&\quad + M_z^0(\omega)\sin\alpha_1\cos^2\frac{\alpha_2}{2}\sin\omega\tau_1\cos\omega\tau_2 e^{-(\tau_1+\tau_2)/T_2} \\
&\quad + M_z^0(\omega)\sin\alpha_1\sin^2\frac{\alpha_2}{2}\sin\omega\tau_1\cos\omega\tau_2 e^{-(\tau_1+\tau_2)/T_2} \\
&= M_z^0(\omega)\sin\alpha_1\cos^2\frac{\alpha_2}{2}\sin\omega(\tau_1+\tau_2)e^{-(\tau_1+\tau_2)/T_2} \\
&\quad - M_z^0(\omega)\sin\alpha_1\sin^2\frac{\alpha_2}{2}\sin\omega(\tau_2-\tau_1)e^{-(\tau_1+\tau_2)/T_2} \\
&\quad + M_z^0(\omega)[1-(1-\cos\alpha_1)e^{-\tau_1/T_1}]\sin\alpha_2\sin\omega\tau_2 e^{-\tau_2/T_2} \quad (4.39)
\end{aligned}
$$

and

$$
\begin{aligned}
M_{z'}&(\omega, \tau_1 + \tau_2) \\
&= M_z^0(\omega)[1-(1-\cos\alpha_2)e^{-\tau_2/T_1}-(1-\cos\alpha_1)\cos\alpha_2 e^{-(\tau_1+\tau_2)/T_1}] \\
&\quad - M_z^0(\omega)\sin\alpha_1\sin\alpha_2\cos\omega\tau_1 e^{-\tau_1/T_2}e^{-\tau_2/T_1} \quad (4.40)
\end{aligned}
$$

The α_3 pulse has no effect on the y'-component, and the resulting x'- and z'-components are as follows:

$$M_{x'}[\omega, (\tau_1 + \tau_2)_+]$$

$$
\begin{aligned}
= &-M_z^0(\omega)\sin\alpha_1\cos^2\frac{\alpha_2}{2}\cos\alpha_3\cos\omega(\tau_1+\tau_2)e^{-(\tau_1+\tau_2)/T_2} \\
&+M_z^0(\omega)\sin\alpha_1\sin^2\frac{\alpha_2}{2}\cos\alpha_3\cos\omega(\tau_2-\tau_1)e^{-(\tau_1+\tau_2)/T_2} \\
&-M_z^0(\omega)[1-(1-\cos\alpha_1)e^{-\tau_1/T_1}]\sin\alpha_2\cos\alpha_3\cos\omega\tau_2 e^{-\tau_2/T_2} \\
&-M_z^0(\omega)[1-(1-\cos\alpha_2)e^{-\tau_2/T_1} \\
&\qquad -(1-\cos\alpha_1)\cos\alpha_2 e^{-(\tau_1+\tau_2)/T_1}]\sin\alpha_3 \\
&+M_z^0(\omega)\sin\alpha_1\sin\alpha_2\sin\alpha_3\cos\omega\tau_1 e^{-\tau_1/T_2}e^{-\tau_2/T_1}
\end{aligned}
\tag{4.41}
$$

and

$$M_{z'}[\omega, (\tau_1 + \tau_2)_+]$$

$$
\begin{aligned}
= &\,M_z^0(\omega)[1-(1-\cos\alpha_2)e^{-\tau_2/T_1} \\
&\qquad -(1-\cos\alpha_1)\cos\alpha_2 e^{-(\tau_1+\tau_2)/T_1}]\cos\alpha_3 \\
&-M_z^0(\omega)\sin\alpha_1\sin\alpha_2\sin\alpha_3\cos\omega\tau_1 e^{-\tau_1/T_2}e^{-\tau_2/T_1} \\
&+M_z^0(\omega)\sin\alpha_1\cos^2\frac{\alpha_2}{2}\sin\alpha_3\cos\omega(\tau_1+\tau_2)e^{-(\tau_1+\tau_2)/T_2} \\
&-M_z^0(\omega)\sin\alpha_1\sin^2\frac{\alpha_2}{2}\sin\alpha_3\cos\omega(\tau_2-\tau_1)e^{-(\tau_1+\tau_2)/T_2} \\
&+M_z^0(\omega)[1-(1-\cos\alpha_1)e^{-\tau_1/T_1}]\sin\alpha_2\sin\alpha_3\cos\omega\tau_2 e^{-\tau_2/T_2}
\end{aligned}
$$

$$\tag{4.42}$$

Combining the x'- and y'-components in complex form yields

$$M_{xy}[\omega, (\tau_1 + \tau_2)_+]$$

$$
\begin{aligned}
= &\,M_x(\omega,(\tau_1+\tau_2)_+) + iM_y(\omega,(\tau_1+\tau_2)_+) \\
&-M_z^0(\omega)\sin\alpha_1\cos^2\frac{\alpha_2}{2}\cos^2\frac{\alpha_3}{2}e^{-i\omega(\tau_1+\tau_2)}e^{-(\tau_1+\tau_2)/T_2} \\
&+M_z^0(\omega)\sin\alpha_1\cos^2\frac{\alpha_2}{2}\sin^2\frac{\alpha_3}{2}e^{i\omega(\tau_1+\tau_2)}e^{-(\tau_1+\tau_2)/T_2} \\
&+M_z^0(\omega)\sin\alpha_1\sin^2\frac{\alpha_2}{2}\cos^2\frac{\alpha_3}{2}e^{-i\omega(\tau_2-\tau_1)}e^{-(\tau_1+\tau_2)/T_2} \\
&-M_z^0(\omega)\sin\alpha_1\sin^2\frac{\alpha_2}{2}\sin^2\frac{\alpha_3}{2}e^{i\omega(\tau_2-\tau_1)}e^{-(\tau_1+\tau_2)/T_2} \\
&+\tfrac{1}{2}M_z^0(\omega)\sin\alpha_1\sin\alpha_2\sin\alpha_3 e^{-i\omega\tau_1}e^{-\tau_1/T_2}e^{-\tau_2/T_1} \\
&+\tfrac{1}{2}M_z^0(\omega)\sin\alpha_1\sin\alpha_2\sin\alpha_3 e^{i\omega\tau_1}e^{-\tau_1/T_2}e^{-\tau_2/T_1} \\
&-M_z^0(\omega)[1-(1-\cos\alpha_1)e^{-\tau_1/T_1}]\sin\alpha_2\cos^2\frac{\alpha_3}{2}e^{-i\omega\tau_2}e^{-\tau_2/T_2} \\
&+M_z^0(\omega)[1-(1-\cos\alpha_1)e^{-\tau_1/T_1}]\sin\alpha_2\sin^2\frac{\alpha_3}{2}e^{i\omega\tau_2}e^{-\tau_2/T_2} \\
&-M_z^0(\omega)[1-(1-\cos\alpha_2)e^{-\tau_2/T_1} - \\
&\qquad (1-\cos\alpha_1)\cos\alpha_2 e^{-(\tau_1+\tau_2)/T_1}]\sin\alpha_3
\end{aligned}
\tag{4.43}
$$

During the free precession period after the third pulse, the transverse magnetization is

$$M_{x'y'}(\omega, t) = M_{x'y'}[\omega, (\tau_1 + \tau_2)_+]e^{-(t-\tau_1-\tau_2)/T_2}e^{-i\omega(t-\tau_1-\tau_2)} \qquad (4.44)$$

for $t \geq \tau_1 + \tau_2$. Substituting Eq. (4.43) into Eq. (4.44), we can see that the second, fourth, sixth, and eighth components in Eq. (4.43) will each produce an echo signal, while the remaining five components form an FID signal. The echo formed between the second and third pulses and the four echoes formed after the third pulses are as follows:

$$S_1(t) = A_1 \int_{-\infty}^{\infty} \rho(\omega)e^{-t/T_2(\omega)}e^{-i\omega(t-2\tau_1)}d\omega \qquad (4.45a)$$

$$S_2(t) = A_2 \int_{-\infty}^{\infty} \rho(\omega)e^{-t/T_2(\omega)}e^{-i\omega(t-2\tau_1)}d\omega \qquad (4.45b)$$

$$S_3(t) = A_3 \int_{-\infty}^{\infty} \rho(\omega)e^{-t/T_2(\omega)}e^{-i\omega(t-2\tau_2)}d\omega \qquad (4.45c)$$

$$S_4(t) = A_4 \int_{-\infty}^{\infty} \rho(\omega)e^{-t/T_2(\omega)}e^{-i\omega[t-(\tau_1+2\tau_2)]}d\omega \qquad (4.45d)$$

$$S_5(t) = A_5 \int_{-\infty}^{\infty} \rho(\omega)e^{-t/T_2(\omega)}e^{-i\omega[t-2(\tau_1+\tau_2)]}d\omega \qquad (4.45e)$$

where

$$A_1 = \sin\alpha_1 \sin^2\frac{\alpha_2}{2} \qquad (4.46a)$$

$$A_2 = \frac{1}{2}\sin\alpha_1 \sin\alpha_2 \sin\alpha_3 e^{-\tau_2/T_1} \qquad (4.46b)$$

$$A_3 = -\sin\alpha_1 \sin^2\frac{\alpha_2}{2}\sin^2\frac{\alpha_3}{2} \qquad (4.46c)$$

$$A_4 = [1 - (1 - \cos\alpha_1)e^{-\tau_1/T_1}]\sin\alpha_2 \sin^2\frac{\alpha_3}{2} \qquad (4.46d)$$

$$A_5 = \sin\alpha_1 \cos^2\frac{\alpha_2}{2}\sin^2\frac{\alpha_3}{2} \qquad (4.46e)$$

The preceding signal expressions indicate that all the echoes are formed along the x'-axis except for echo 3, which is formed along the $-x'$-axis. By tracing back the pathway for the formation of each echo, it is easy to see that echo 1 is a spin echo formed as a result of the action of pulses 1 and 2; echo 2 is a stimulated echo formed from the combined effect of all three pulses; echo 3 is a secondary echo formed as a result of the action of pulse 3 on the first echo; and echoes 4 and 5 are also spin echoes formed as a result of the action of pulse 3 on the FID signals from pulses 2 and 1, respectively.

It is often convenient to write an echo signal in the following general form:

$$S(t) = A_E \int_{-\infty}^{\infty} \rho(\omega)e^{-t/T_2(\omega)}e^{-i\omega(t-T_E)}d\omega \qquad (4.47)$$

The amplitude and echo time of the five echoes generated by the three-pulse sequence are summarized in Table 4.1.

Table 4.1   Echoes from a Three-Pulse Sequence

Echo Type	Echo Time	Echo Amplitude[a]
Primary	$2\tau_1$	$\sin\alpha_1 \sin^2\frac{\alpha_2}{2} e^{-2\tau_1/T_2}$
Stimulated	$2\tau_1 + \tau_2$	$\frac{1}{2}\sin\alpha_1 \sin\alpha_2 \sin\alpha_3 e^{-\tau_2/T_1} e^{-2\tau_1/T_2}$
Secondary	$2\tau_2$	$-\sin\alpha_1 \sin^2\frac{\alpha_2}{2} \sin^2\frac{\alpha_3}{2} e^{-2\tau_2/T_2}$
SE	$\tau_1 + 2\tau_2$	$[1 - (1 - \cos\alpha_1)e^{-\tau_1/T_1}]\sin\alpha_2 \sin^2\frac{\alpha_3}{2} e^{-(\tau_1+2\tau_2)/T_2}$
SE	$2(\tau_1 + \tau_2)$	$\sin\alpha_1 \cos^2\frac{\alpha_2}{2} \sin^2\frac{\alpha_3}{2} e^{-2(\tau_1+\tau_2)/T_2}$

[a] M_z^0 is normalized to 1.

■ Example 4.4

Stimulated echoes find many useful applications in imaging and localized spectroscopy. This example takes a closer look at the stimulated echo of the three-pulse sequence in Fig. 4.6.

Following the echo pathway, one can see that the stimulated echo comes from the z-component, $-M_z^0 \sin\alpha_1 \sin\alpha_2 \cos\omega\tau_1 e^{-\tau_1/T_2}$, in Eq. (4.27). This magnetization was previously in the transverse plane and then stored as a longitudinal magnetization by the α_2 pulse. During the subsequent τ_2 delay, the magnetization retains its earlier phase evolution history accumulated while it was in the transverse plane. This phenomenon is called *phase memory*. When this magnetization is converted back to a transverse magnetization by the α_3 pulse, this phase memory will be rewound, which leads to the formation of the stimulated echo.

As shown in Table 4.1, a stimulated echo bears both T_1 and T_2 weightings. To generate a maximum stimulated echo signal, one should set $\alpha_1 = \alpha_2 = \alpha_3 = 90°$. In this case, $A_{\text{ste}} = \frac{1}{2}M_z^0$.

4.3.3 Extended Phase Graphs

Although the Bloch equation is a useful tool for analyzing echoes from multiple excitation pulses, it is rather tedious and not very intuitive. In this section, we describe another formalism called *extended phase graphs*.

Consider an α pulse applied along the y'-axis. The magnetizations $M_{x'}^{+}$, $M_{y'}^{+}$, and $M_{z'}^{+}$ immediately after the pulse are given by

$$\begin{cases} M_{x'}^{+} = M_{x'} \cos\alpha - M_{z'} \sin\alpha \\ M_{y'}^{+} = M_{y'} \\ M_{z'}^{+} = M_{x'} \sin\alpha + M_{z'} \cos\alpha \end{cases} \tag{4.48}$$

Using the complex notation $M_{x'y'} = M_{x'} + iM_{y'}$ and $M_{x'y'}^{*} = M_{x'} - iM_{y'}$, we get

$$M_{x'y'}^{+} = M_{x'y'} \cos^2\frac{\alpha}{2} - M_{x'y'}^{*} \sin^2\frac{\alpha}{2} - M_{z'} \sin\alpha \tag{4.49a}$$

$$M_{z'}^{+} = M_{z'} \cos\alpha + \frac{1}{2}(M_{x'y'} + M_{x'y'}^{*}) \sin\alpha \tag{4.49b}$$

The decomposition above, originally due to Woessner [268], offers an interesting interpretation of the effect of a pulse with an arbitrary flip angle. This interpretation provides an intuitive insight into how an echo signal is formed. Specifically, with this decomposition, a pulse separates the rotating (transverse) magnetization into two parts. One part is proportional to the prepulse value ($M_{x'y'}$), and the other part is proportional to its complex conjugate ($M_{x'y'}^{*}$). Noting that

$$M_{x'y'} \xrightarrow{\ 0°\ } M_{x'y'} \tag{4.50a}$$

$$M_{x'y'} \xrightarrow{\ 180°_{y'}\ } -M_{x'y'}^{*} \tag{4.50b}$$

the decomposition in Eq. (4.49a) can be interpreted as saying that the fraction of the prepulse magnetization that experiences a 180°-like pulse is $\sin^2\frac{\alpha}{2}$, and the fraction remaining unchanged is $\cos^2\frac{\alpha}{2}$. The phase reversal introduced by the 180°-like pulse allows that portion of the spins to regain phase coherence and form a spin echo. Another echo formation mechanism occurs through the action of the pulse on $M_{z'}$. According to Eq. (4.49b), the $M_{z'}$ after a pulse also includes a term proportional to $M_{x'y'}$ and a term proportional to $M_{x'y'}^{*}$. When these terms are flipped back onto the transverse plane, the $M_{x'y'}^{*}$ term will rephase and form what is known as the stimulated echo.

An extended phase graph, in essence, is a graphical representation of both the Woessner decomposition and the subsequent phase evolution of the magnetization components, so that each echo formation mechanism can be revealed pictorially. To see how to construct such a phase graph, first recall that the free precession of a transverse magnetization is described by $e^{-i(\phi_0 + \omega t)}$; thus, its phase evolution can be represented by a tilted line corresponding to $\phi = \phi_0 + \omega t$, as shown in Fig 4.7a. On the other hand, a longitudinal component is stationary during the free precession period (ignoring T_1 relaxation) and its phase evolution is a horizontal line ($\phi = \phi_0$), as shown in Fig. 4.7b, where ϕ_0 is the prepulse phase.

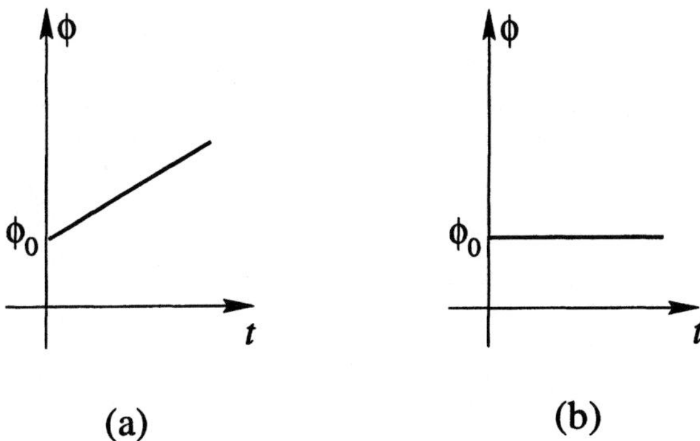

Figure 4.7 Phase plots during a free precession period for (a) a transverse magnetization, and (b) a longitudinal magnetization.

Second, to incorporate the Woessner decomposition into the phase graph, we represent an RF pulse simply by a vertical line at which point of time a magnetization is split into several magnetization components. Specifically, according to Eq. (4.49), a transverse magnetization is split into four branches as described by

$$
M_{x'y'} \xrightarrow{\alpha}
\begin{cases}
M^+_{x'y'} = M_{x'y'} \cos^2 \frac{\alpha}{2} \\[4pt]
M^+_{x'y'} = -M^*_{x'y'} \sin^2 \frac{\alpha}{2} \\[4pt]
M^+_{z'} = \frac{1}{2} M_{x'y'} \sin \alpha \\[4pt]
M^+_{z'} = \frac{1}{2} M^*_{x'y'} \sin \alpha
\end{cases}
\tag{4.51}
$$

and a longitudinal component is split into two branches corresponding to

$$
M_{z'} \xrightarrow{\alpha}
\begin{cases}
M^+_{x'y'} = -M_{z'} \sin \alpha \\[4pt]
M^+_{z'} = M_{z'} \cos \alpha
\end{cases}
\tag{4.52}
$$

Equations (4.51) and (4.52), called the *branching rules* of an extended phase graph, are shown pictorially in Fig. 4.8.

To construct an extended phase graph, we also need to know where to start. Let us assume that a spin system is at the thermal equilibrium state initially, when a pulse sequence is applied. Then, an extended phase graph will start with a point in the origin and generate various branches and subbranches, according to the above branching rule. However, one can generate an extended phase graph from any set of initial conditions for $M_{x'y'}$ and $M_{z'}$ using the same principle if the values of $M_{x'y'}$ and $M_{z'}$ are known. In practice, the former case is usually assumed; therefore, an extended phase graph is a tree rooted at the origin with a number of tilted and horizontal branches.

In an extended phase graph, all the connecting branches from the root to an end point form a path of phase evolution. An echo is said to occur whenever a

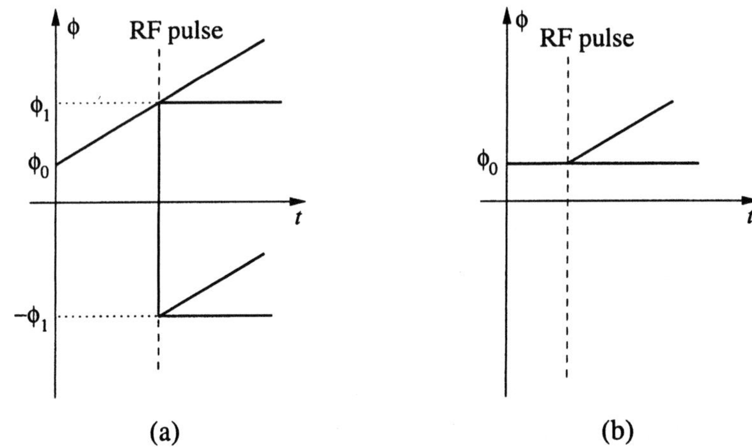

Figure 4.8 Branching rule of an extended phase graph. (a) A transverse magnetization is split into four branches, and (b) a longitudinal magnetization is split into two branches.

phase path crosses the zero line (horizontal axis) during a free precession period. To see this more clearly, we construct an extended phase graph for a three-pulse sequence discussed earlier in Section 4.3.2. The result is shown in Fig. 4.9, where to differentiate rotating (transverse) components from static (longitudinal) components, tilted branches are drawn in solid lines and horizontal branches in dashed lines. Note also that the relaxation effects as well as the weighting coefficients for the different branches resulting from the Woessner decomposition in Eq. (4.49) are not included in an extended phase graph. If the amplitude of an echo signal is desired, it is necessary to introduce those weighting factors into the phase path, which is left as an exercise for the reader.

Based on the extended phase graph, one can easily calculate the maximum number of echo signals that can be generated by a number of pulses. Let T_n be the total number of tilted branches and H_n be the total number of horizontal branches after the nth pulse. According to the branching rule described earlier, one can derive that

$$\begin{cases} T_n = 2T_{n-1} + H_{n-1} \\ H_n = 2T_{n-1} + H_{n-1} \end{cases} \quad n > 1 \qquad (4.53)$$

with initial conditions $T_1 = 1$ and $H_1 = 1$. These recursions can be simplified to

$$T_n = 3T_{n-1} \qquad (4.54)$$

whose solution is

$$T_n = 3^{n-1} \qquad (4.55)$$

Based on the tree structure of an extended phase graph, one can see that the total number of echoes generated by T_n is

$$N_E(n) = \frac{T_n - 1}{2} = \frac{3^{n-1} - 1}{2} \tag{4.56}$$

Note that N_E given in Eq. (4.56) represents the maximum number of echo signals that can be created after the nth pulse, and it is useful for predicting how many signals can be detected at the end of the sequence. But it is not the total number of echoes generated by the sequence. For example, for $n = 3$, $N_E = 4$, which is the number of echoes that emerge after the third pulse; the total number of echoes generated by the entire sequence is actually 5, as discussed in Section 4.3.2. If it is necessary to calculate the maximum total number of echoes that can be generated by a sequence of N pulses, we simply sum up all $N_E(n)$ for

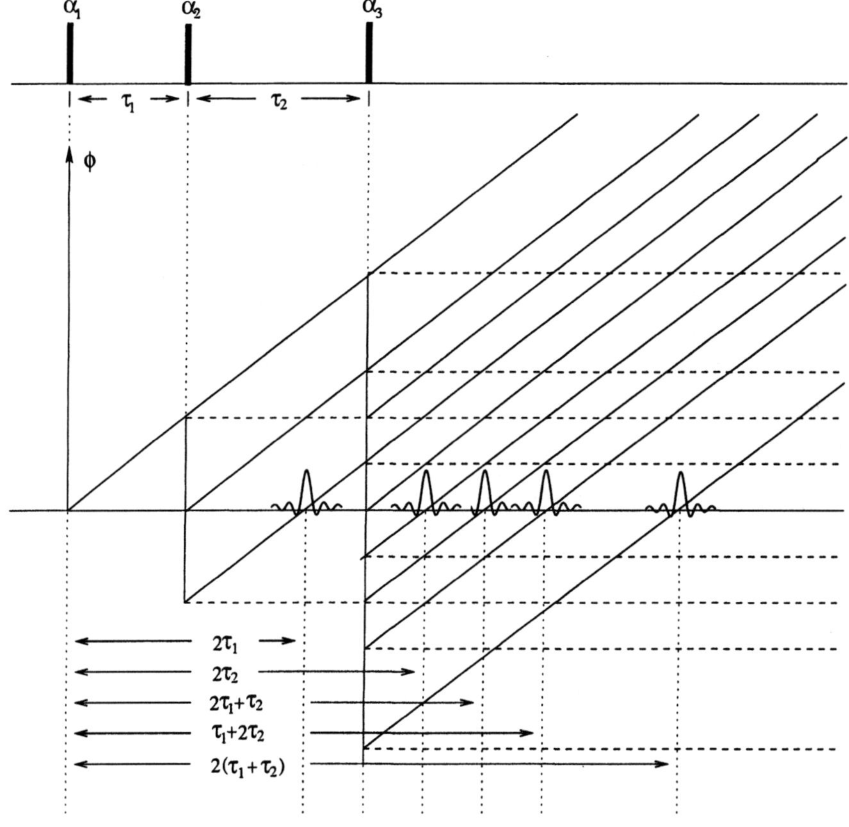

Figure 4.9 Extended phase graph for a three-pulse sequence.

$n = 1, 2, \ldots, N$. Namely,

$$\sum_{n=1}^{N} N_E(n) = \frac{1}{2} \left(\frac{3^N - 1}{2} - N \right) \tag{4.57}$$

4.3.4 The CPMG Echo Train

When a spin system is excited by a 90° pulse followed by a sequence of 180° pulses, a train of spin echoes will be generated. Suppose that the 90° pulse is applied at $t = 0$ and the 180° pulses at $(2n - 1)\tau$ for $n = 1, 2, \ldots, N$. A train of N echoes will be formed at $t = 2n\tau$, and the echo amplitudes are weighted by

$$E_n = e^{-2n\tau/T_2} \tag{4.58}$$

Formation of these echoes can be predicted easily using the extended phase graph as shown in Fig. 4.10. One can easily see from the phase graph that all the later echoes formed at $t = 2n\tau$ for $n > 1$ are secondary echoes of the primary echo at $t = 2\tau$. In other words, any echo except for the first in the echo train is an echo of the preceding echo. Because of the simple relationship for the echo amplitudes in Eq. (4.58), this multiple-echo sequence is an efficient way to measure T_2 values.

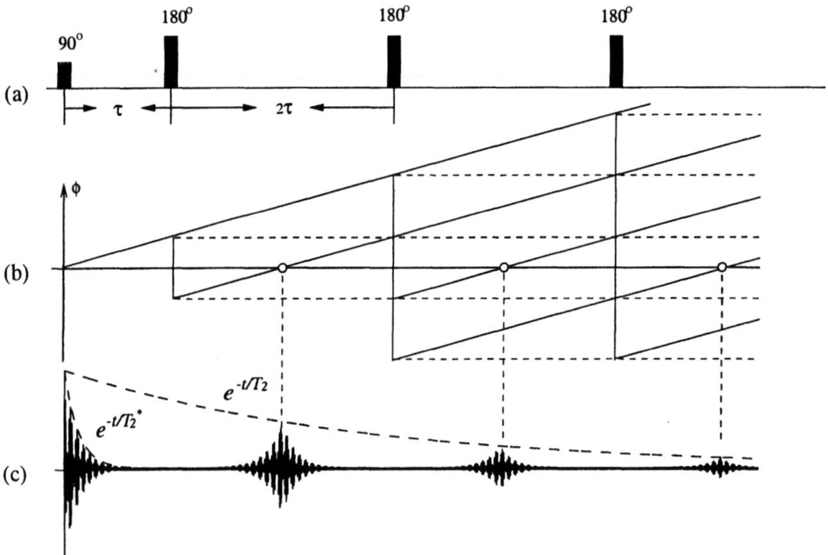

Figure 4.10 Formation of a train of spin echoes by multiple 180° pulses: (a) pulse sequence, (b) extended phase graph, and (c) resulting echo signals.

In the original excitation sequence proposed by Carr and Purcell in 1954, all the RF pulses were applied along the same axis. To reduce cumulative phase errors from any imperfection in the repetitive 180° pulses, Meiboom and Gill proposed a modification in 1958 that applied the refocusing pulses in a direction orthogonal to that of the excitation pulse. For example, if the 90° pulse is applied along the x'-axis, the 180° would be applied along the $\pm y'$-axis. This sequence, subsequently known as the CPMG (Carr–Purcell–Meiboom–Gill) sequence, is widely used in practice. One of its applications in fast imaging is discussed in Chapter 9.

4.4 Gradient Echoes

Another form of echo signal frequently used in MRI is generated using time-varying gradient magnetic fields. Such an echo is referred to as a *gradient echo* to distinguish it from a spin echo or a stimulated echo. The key concept underlying gradient-echo formation is that a gradient field can dephase and rephase a signal in a controlled fashion so that one or multiple echo signals can be created. To grasp this mechanism, let us first formally define a gradient field.

4.4.1 Gradient Fields

A gradient field $\vec{B}_G$ in the context of MRI is a special kind of inhomogeneous field whose z-component varies linearly along a specific direction called the *gradient direction*. Specifically, $\vec{B}_G$ is called an x-gradient field if

$$B_{G,z} = G_x x \tag{4.59}$$

and G_x is called the x-gradient. Similarly, $\vec{B}_G$ is called a y-gradient field if

$$B_{G,z} = G_y y \tag{4.60}$$

or a z-gradient field if

$$B_{G,z} = G_z z \tag{4.61}$$

As discussed in Section 1.2.2, the gradient system consists of three gradient coils referred to as the x-gradient, y-gradient, and z-gradient coils, respectively, which in the ideal case produce an x-gradient field, a y-gradient field, and a z-gradient field. It is important to note that for each case, the magnetic field produced by a gradient coil also has components in the x-direction ($B_{G,x}$) and y-direction ($B_{G,y}$). However, these components are often ignored because the B_0 field is so strong in the z-direction. For this reason, $B_{G,z}$ itself is often loosely referred to as the gradient field,[2] and $B_{G,z}$ and B_G are used interchangeably when there is no confusion.

---

[2] Such a gradient field does not exist according to the Maxwell equations.

With this understanding, the overall magnetic field in the presence of a gradient field in the region of interest can be expressed as

$$\vec{B} = (B_0 + B_{G,z})\vec{k} \tag{4.62}$$

where $B_{G,z}$ is as defined in Eq. (4.59), Eq. (4.60), or Eq. (4.61) when one gradient coil is turned on. When all three gradient coils are turned on simultaneously,

$$B_{G,z} = G_x x + G_y y + G_z z \tag{4.63}$$

and consequently

$$\vec{B} = (B_0 + G_x x + G_y y + G_z z)\vec{k} \tag{4.64}$$

The three gradients are often grouped into a gradient vector $\vec{G}$ such that

$$\vec{G} = (G_x, G_y, G_z) = G_x\vec{i} + G_y\vec{j} + G_z\vec{k} \tag{4.65}$$

and the direction of $\vec{G}$ is called the *gradient direction* of $\vec{B}_G$ or $\vec{B}$. In this vector notation, Eq. (4.63) can be rewritten as

$$B_{G,z} = \vec{G} \cdot r \tag{4.66}$$

It is important to note here the difference between the gradient direction of $B_{G,z}$ and the direction of the gradient field itself. Although $\vec{G}$ can be made to point along the x-, y-, z-, or an arbitrary direction by turning on G_x, G_y, and G_z individually or simultaneously, the direction of B_G is usually unknown and irrelevant. To illustrate this point, let us consider an inhomogeneous field defined by

$$\vec{B}_G(x, y, z) = (-3x + y + 2z)\vec{i} + (x - 2y - 3z)\vec{j} + (2x - 3y + 5z)\vec{k}$$

Clearly, as a vector quantity, B_G points in different directions at different spatial locations. The z-component of MRI importance is

$$B_{G,z} = 2x - 3y + 5z$$

and its gradients along the three Cartesian directions are given by

$$G_x = \frac{\partial B_{G,z}}{\partial x} = 2$$

$$G_y = \frac{\partial B_{G,z}}{\partial y} = -3$$

$$G_z = \frac{\partial B_{G,z}}{\partial z} = 5$$

The overall gradient of the "field" variation is

$$\vec{G} = \nabla B_{G,z} = G_x\vec{i} + G_y\vec{j} + G_z\vec{k} = 2\vec{i} - 3\vec{j} + 5\vec{k}$$

which points in the direction of a vector defined by $v = (2, -3, 5)$, as shown in Fig. 4.11. That is to say, $B_{G,z}(x, y, z)$ varies linearly along the direction of v.

Note also that $\vec{G}$ is, in general, a function of time. If $\vec{G}$ is a constant in the time interval of interest, we call the gradient field a static field. Otherwise, we have a time-varying gradient field. Both types of gradient field are widely used in various MRI applications.

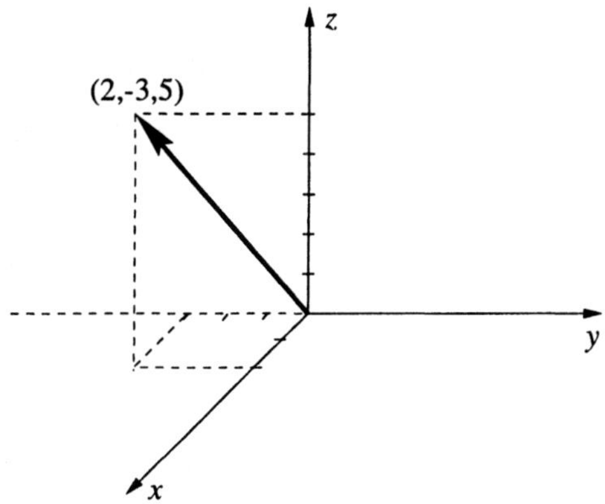

Figure 4.11   Direction of $\vec{G} = 2\vec{i} - 3\vec{j} + 5\vec{k}$.

4.4.2   Formation of Gradient Echoes

For simplicity, we consider the pulse sequence in Fig. 4.12. After the application of an α-degree RF pulse (a gradient echo is often used in combination with small flip angle excitation for fast imaging), a negative x-gradient is turned on. As a result, spins in different x-positions will acquire different phases, which can be expressed in the rotating frame as

$$\phi(x, t) = \gamma \int_0^t -G_x x d\hat{t} = -\gamma G_x x t \qquad 0 \leq t \leq \tau \qquad (4.67)$$

Equation (4.67) indicates that the loss of spin phase coherence becomes progressively worse as time elapses after the excitation pulse. The resulting signal decay is sometimes characterized by another time constant T_2^{**}. After a time $\tau > 3T_2^{**}$, the signal decays to zero. At this point in time, however, if a positive gradient of the same strength is applied, the transverse magnetization components will gradually rephase, resulting in a regrowth of the signal. Specifically, the spin

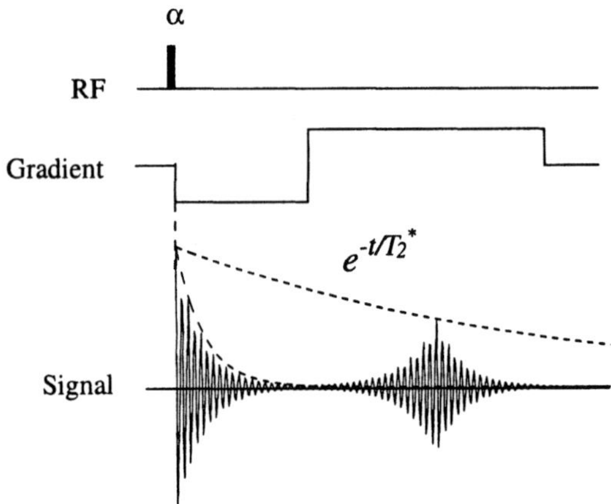

Figure 4.12 Gradient-echo pulse sequence. After the application of a small-flip-angle pulse, a negative x-gradient is turned on to dephase the spins, which are then rephased by a subsequent positive x-gradient.

phase angle in the rotating frame is now given by

$$\phi(x,t) = -\gamma G_x x \tau + \gamma \int_\tau^t G_x x \, d\hat{t}$$

$$= -\gamma G_x x \tau + \gamma G_x x (t - \tau) \qquad \tau \le t \le 2\tau \qquad (4.68)$$

As shown in the phase plot in Fig. 4.13, the phase dispersal introduced by the negative gradient is gradually reduced over time after the positive gradient is turned on at $t = \tau$. After a time τ, the spin phase ϕ is zero for any x value, which means that all the spins have rephased, and therefore an echo signal is formed. This analysis can be extended to the case of unequal dephase and rephase gradients. The echo time in the case may not be equal to 2τ.

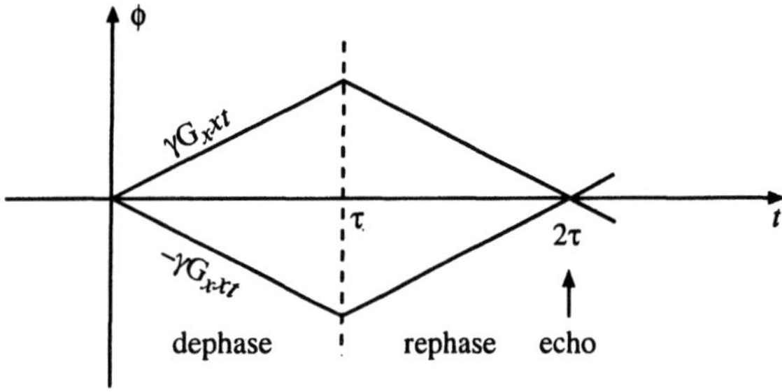

Figure 4.13 Phase progression of spins at $x = -x_1, 0$, and x_1.

In the preceding discussion, we have assumed that the $\vec{B}_0$ field is perfectly homogeneous. In the presence of $\vec{B}_0$ inhomogeneities, the spins will not be completely rephased by the gradient reversal. Consequently, the amplitude of a gradient echo carries a T_2^*-weighting (instead of a T_2-weighting). This is one of the key differences between a gradient echo and an RF echo.

As the CPMG echo train, a gradient-echo train can also be created from one FID signal by repetitive gradient switching as shown in Fig. 4.14. The number of echoes that can be created is limited by T_2^* and by the speed of gradient switching. Modern MR scanners permit up to 64 such echoes to be obtained, which enables the formation of a two-dimensional image with single excitation.

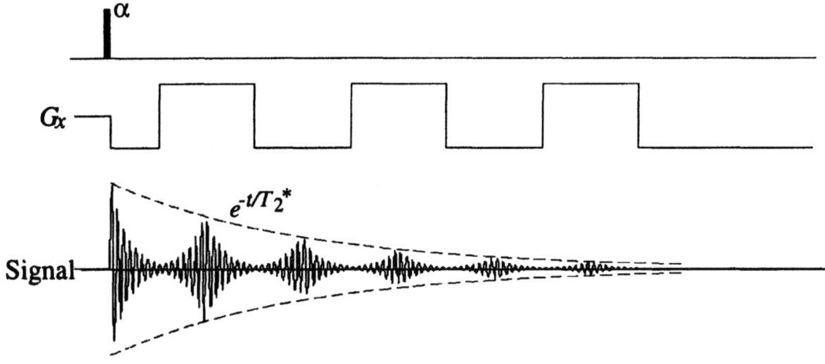

Figure 4.14 Echo train formed using switching gradients.

Exercises

4.1 An FID signal lasts as long as the transverse magnetization. True or false?

4.2 Find a mathematical expression for an FID signal with N spectral components.

4.3 An FID signal of a single spectral component can be expressed as

$$S(t) = Ae^{-t/T_2}e^{-i\omega_0 t} \qquad t \geq 0$$

(a) Show that the line width of the absorption-mode spectrum and the magnitude-mode spectrum is $1/(\pi T_2)$ and $\sqrt{3}/(\pi T_2)$, respectively.

(b) Evaluate the area under the absorption-mode spectrum. That is,

$$\int_{-\infty}^{\infty} \frac{AT_2}{1 + T_2^2(\omega + \omega_0)^2} d\omega$$

4.4 A hypothetical two-sided FID signal of a single spectral component can be expressed as

$$S(t) = Ae^{-|t|/T_2}e^{-i\omega_0 t}$$

(a) Find the absorption-mode, dispersion-mode, and magnitude-mode spectra of this signal.

(b) Compare the line width of the absorption-mode and magnitude-mode spectra.

(c) Compare the line width and area of the absorption-mode spectrum to those of a one-sided FID signal defined in Problem 4.3.

4.5 Calculate the effective FID signal from a sample with a constant spin density function under the following condition:

(a) The magnetic field inhomogeneity has a Gaussian distribution. For example, the histogram of the field distribution can be expressed as

$$e^{-\frac{(B-B_0)^2}{2B_0^2}}$$

(b) The magnetic field is described by $B(x) = B_0 x \Pi(x)$.

4.6 Use a vector diagram to show how a spin echo is formed by a $90^{\circ}_{x'} - \tau - 90^{\circ}_{x'}$ sequence.

4.7 What is the echo time for the gradient echo pulse sequence in Fig. 4.12 if the amplitudes of the negative and positive gradients are G_x and $G_x/3$, respectively?

4.8 NMR signals from a macroscopic sample decay faster in an inhomogeneous magnetic field than in a homogeneous field because of

(a) Phase incoherence of the microscopic signals from different locations.

(b) Frequency differences of the microscopic signals from different locations.

(c) Both of the above.

Select your answer and discuss why it is applicable.

4.9 Assume that an $\alpha_{x'}$ pulse generates an FID signal described by $S(t)$. What are the resulting signals if the same pulse is applied along the $-x'$-, y'-, and $-y'$-axes, respectively?

4.10 A sample with a spin concentration function $c(x)$ is placed in an inhomogeneous field $B(x)$. Calculate the spectral density function $\rho(\omega)$ for the following cases:

(a) $c(x) = \rho_0 \Pi(x)$ and $B(x) = B_0 + x$

(b) $c(x) = \rho_0 \Lambda(x)$ and $B(x) = B_0 + x$

(c) $c(x) = \rho_0 \Lambda(x)$ and $B(x) = B_0 + x^2$

4.11 A spin system with a single isochromat at thermal equilibrium is excited by a $90^\circ_{x'}$- and a $90^\circ_{y'}$- pulse, respectively.

(a) Calculate and sketch the bulk magnetization immediately after the pulse for each case in terms of the thermal equilibrium value.

(b) Let $S_1(t)$ and $S_2(t)$ denote the FID signals generated by the two pulses. How is $S_1(t)$ related to $S_2(t)$?

4.12 Derive and compare the echo signals for each pair of excitation sequences:

(a) $90^\circ_{x'} - \tau - 180^\circ_{y'}$ and $90^\circ_{x'} - \tau - 180^\circ_{x'}$

(b) $90^\circ_{x'} - \tau - 90^\circ_{y'}$ and $90^\circ_{x'} - \tau - 90^\circ_{x'}$

4.13 Find the mathematical expressions for the three FID signals generated by the following sequence:

$$\alpha_1 - \tau_1 - \alpha_2 - \tau_2 - \tau_2 - \alpha_3$$

4.14 Show that the effect of an $\alpha_{x'}$ pulse can be expressed as

$$M^+_{x'y'} = M_{x'y'} \cos^2 \frac{\alpha}{2} + M^*_{x'y'} \sin^2 \frac{\alpha}{2} + iM_{z'} \sin \alpha$$

$$M^+_{z'} = M_{z'} \cos^2 \frac{\alpha}{2} - M_{z'} \sin^2 \frac{\alpha}{2} - M_{y'} \sin \alpha$$

4.15 Calculate the locations and amplitudes of all the echoes generated by the following sequence:

$$90^\circ_{y'} - \tau - 180^\circ_{y'} - 2\tau - 180^\circ_{y'} - 3\tau - 180^\circ_{y'}$$

4.16 Draw an extended phase graph for the following excitation sequences, and for each case discuss how many echoes are generated.

(a) $90^\circ - \tau - 90^\circ - 2\tau - 90^\circ$

(b) $90^\circ - \tau - 90^\circ - 1.5\tau - 90^\circ$

(c) $90^\circ - \tau - 90^\circ - 0.5\tau - 90^\circ$

(d) $45^\circ - \tau - 90^\circ - 2\tau - 90^\circ$

(e) $45^\circ - \tau - 180^\circ - 2\tau - 180^\circ$

4.17 Consider a four-pulse sequence $\alpha_1 - \tau_1 - \alpha_2 - \tau_2 - \alpha_3 - \tau_3 - \alpha_4$.

(a)   What is the maximum number of echo signals that can be generated?

(b)   What is the minimum number of echo signals that can be generated?

(c)   Derive the condition for (a) and (b) to occur.

4.18 Let $B_0(x, y, z) = (20 - 2x + 3y + z)$.

(a)   Sketch the iso-field surface corresponding to $B_0 = 10$.

(b)   Calculate the field strength and field gradients along the x-, y-, and z-directions at point $(5, 0, 10)$.

4.19 For the $B_z(x, y, z)$ given below, calculate ∇B_z and discuss which of them are linear gradient field.

(a) $B_z(x, y, z) = 3 - 2x$

(b) $B_z(x, y, z) = 3 - 2x + x^2$

(c) $B_z(x, y, z) = 5 - x - y - z$

4.20   Assume that the gradients of $B_{G,z}$ along the three axes are: $G_x = 1$, $G_y = -3$, and $G_z = 2$. What is the overall $\vec{B}_{G,z}$? What is the value of $\vec{B}_{G,z}$ at spatial location $(3, 1, 0)$?

4.21   Use a vector diagram to illustrate the refocusing of isochromats in a gradient-echo experiment and compare the result to Fig. 4.4.

4.22   Briefly (in one or two sentences) explain why a spin echo is T_2-weighted but a gradient echo is T_2^* weighted.

Chapter 5

Signal Localization

Zeugmatography

P. C. Lauterbur

Based on the discussion in Chapters 3 and 4, we now know how to activate an MR signal from an object. In fact, the experimental protocol is rather simple: we place the object in a main, uniform magnetic field and then excite it with another oscillating magnetic field at the resonance frequency. The signal thus generated, however, is a sum of "local" signals from all parts of the object. For a spatially homogeneous object, this signal is all that we need, since the local signals are the same regardless of their spatial origins. In practice, the objects we deal with are heterogeneous, and it becomes necessary to differentiate local signals from different parts of a given object. This chapter is concerned with spatial localization of these signals.

There are basically two types of spatial localization method: *selective excitation* (or *reception*[1]) and *spatial encoding*. Central to localization methods of both types is the use of a gradient field. Modern MRI systems provide three orthogonal gradients whose shapes and forms can be adjusted independently. To facilitate the understanding of the role of RF pulses and gradient fields in a general imaging scheme, this chapter first describes the basic concepts of slice-selective excitation and spatial information encoding, and then goes on to discuss multidimensional imaging using a popular mathematical formalism known as k-space. Starting in this chapter and continuing in the rest of the book, we will make use of a graphic tool called *pulse sequence* diagram, which details the timing of RF pulses and gradient waveforms in an imaging scheme.

---

[1] Signal localization using surface coils is not covered in this chapter.

5.1   Slice Selection

Slice selection is perhaps the simplest but also the most popular form of selective excitation used in MRI. To selectively excite spins in a slice, two things are essential: a gradient field and a shaped RF pulse. We discuss both of them in this section. Before we do that, let us first describe the parameters used to characterize an arbitrary slice in a three-dimensional object.

5.1.1   Slice Equation

Mathematically, a slice in a three-dimensional object is defined by the following inequality:

$$|\boldsymbol{\mu}_s \cdot \boldsymbol{r} - s_0| < \Delta s/2 \tag{5.1}$$

where $\boldsymbol{\mu}_s$ specifies the slice (or slice-selection) orientation, Δs is the slice thickness as measured in the direction of $\boldsymbol{\mu}_s$, and s_0 is the distance of the slice from the origin, as shown in Fig. 5.1. Bear in mind that the slice direction is defined here as the orthogonal direction of the slice. Sometimes, when it is not necessary to specify the thickness explicitly, one can express the slice equation simply as

$$\boldsymbol{\mu}_s \cdot \boldsymbol{r} = s_0 \tag{5.2}$$

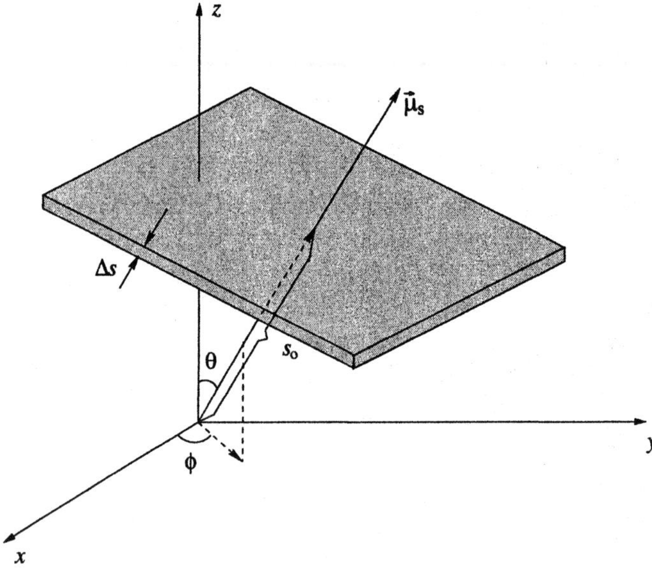

Figure 5.1 Parameters characterizing a slice of arbitrary orientation.

Three special cases of slice selection excite slices along the x-, y-, and z-directions, which are illustrated in Fig. 5.2. The corresponding slice equations are given, respectively, by

$$|x - x_0| < \Delta x/2 \qquad \text{or} \qquad x = x_0 \qquad (5.3a)$$
$$|y - y_0| < \Delta y/2 \qquad \text{or} \qquad y = y_0 \qquad (5.3b)$$
$$|z - z_0| < \Delta z/2 \qquad \text{or} \qquad z = z_0 \qquad (5.3c)$$

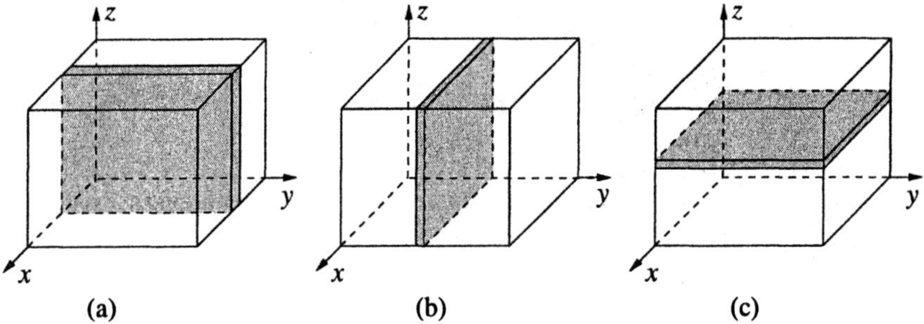

Figure 5.2 Slices selected along the (a) x-direction, (b) y-direction, and (c) z-direction, which are called sagittal, coronal, and transverse slices, respectively.

5.1.2   Slice-Selective Gradients

The need to turn on a gradient field during the excitation period for slice selection is obvious because an RF pulse can only be frequency-selective, and spins at different spatial locations will be excited in the same way if they resonate at the same frequency. Therefore, to make an RF pulse spatially selective, it is necessary to make the spin resonance frequency position-dependent, or most desirably, to vary linearly along the slice-select direction (μ_s). A simple yet effective way to accomplish this is to augment the homogeneous B_0 field with a linear gradient field *during the excitation period*. Such a gradient field is called a *slice-selection* gradient in order to distinguish it from a phase-encoding gradient or frequency-encoding gradient to be introduced later in this chapter.

We next discuss how to design a slice-selection gradient so as to select a slice as shown in Fig. 5.1. Recall from Section 4.4 that a linear gradient field is by definition a magnetic field that points along the z-direction but has an amplitude varying linearly along a particular gradient direction μ_G. Denote the desired slice-selection gradient as

$$G_{ss} = (G_x, G_y, G_z) = G_{ss}\mu_G \qquad (5.4)$$

where $G_{\mathrm{ss}} = \sqrt{G_x^2 + G_y^2 + G_z^2}$ is the overall gradient strength. To render the spin resonance frequency to linearly vary along $\boldsymbol{\mu}_{\mathrm{s}}$, we need to match $\boldsymbol{\mu}_G$ to $\boldsymbol{\mu}_{\mathrm{s}}$. That is,

$$\boldsymbol{\mu}_G = \boldsymbol{\mu}_{\mathrm{s}} \tag{5.5}$$

Expressing $\boldsymbol{\mu}_{\mathrm{s}}$ in terms of the slice orientation angles (ϕ, θ) as

$$\boldsymbol{\mu}_{\mathrm{s}} = (\sin\theta\cos\phi, \sin\theta\sin\phi, \cos\theta) \tag{5.6}$$

we immediately have

$$\begin{cases} G_x = G_{\mathrm{ss}}\sin\theta\cos\phi \\ G_y = G_{\mathrm{ss}}\sin\theta\sin\phi \\ G_z = G_{\mathrm{ss}}\cos\theta \end{cases} \tag{5.7}$$

Equation (5.7) specifies the necessary gradient vector for selecting a slice in an arbitrary direction. Note that the gradient magnitude G_{ss} is not defined in this equation. In principle, any nonzero value for G_{ss} is adequate for discriminating spins along the gradient direction. In practice, however, G_{ss} has to be sufficiently large to select a thin slice. We discuss this topic later in this section in the context of RF pulse truncation.

■ Example 5.1

In this example, we determine an appropriate gradient field for slice selection along the x-, y-, and z-directions.

Consider first the selection of a slice along the x-axis. In this case, $\boldsymbol{\mu}_{\mathrm{s}} = \vec{i}$, and consequently, $\theta = 90°$ and $\phi = 0°$. According to Eq. (5.7), the desired gradient function is

$$G_{\mathrm{ss}} = (G_x, 0, 0)$$

In other words, a nonzero gradient field along the x-direction will enable the selection of a slice orthogonal to the x-axis. Following the same analysis, one can conclude that the desired gradient functions for slice selection along the y- and z-directions are, respectively,

$$G_{\mathrm{ss}} = (0, G_y, 0)$$

and

$$G_{\mathrm{ss}} = (0, 0, G_z)$$

5.1.3 Slice-Selective RF Pulses

After the slice-selection gradient has been chosen, the next step is to translate the desired frequency selectivity established by the slice-selection gradient to the temporal waveform of an RF pulse. Recall from Chapter 3 that an amplitude-modulated RF pulse is characterized by an excitation frequency ω_{rf} and an envelope function $B_1^e(t)$ as[2]

$$B_1(t) = B_1^e(t)e^{-i\omega_{rf}t} \tag{5.8}$$

So, the question now is how to select $B_1^e(t)$ and ω_{rf}. This is the topic of this section.

5.1.3.1 The Fourier Transform Approach

The Fourier transform is the simplest approach for selective pulse design. To illustrate the idea, consider the case shown in Fig. 5.2c. Based on the slice equation given in Eq. (5.3c), it is convenient to define a spatial selection function as

$$p_s(z) = \begin{cases} 1 & |z - z_0| < \Delta z/2 \\ 0 & \text{otherwise} \end{cases} \tag{5.9}$$

which is a "boxcar" function of width Δz centered at $z = z_0$. Using the notation introduced in Chapter 2, we can rewrite $p_s(z)$ as

$$p_s(z) = \Pi\left(\frac{z - z_0}{\Delta z}\right) \tag{5.10}$$

According to the result in Example 5.1, the necessary slice-selection gradient is

$$G_{ss} = (0, 0, G_z) \tag{5.11}$$

In the presence of this gradient, the Larmor frequency at position z is given by

$$\omega(z) = \omega_0 + \gamma G_z z \tag{5.12}$$

or

$$f(z) = f_0 + \gamma G_z z \tag{5.13}$$

Correspondingly, the desired frequency selection function is

$$p(f) = p_s\left(\frac{2\pi f}{\gamma G_z}\right) = \Pi\left(\frac{f - f_c}{\Delta f}\right) \tag{5.14}$$

where

$$f_c = f_0 + \gamma G_z z_0 \tag{5.15}$$

---

[2]The initial phase angle of an RF pulse will not affect its frequency selectivity if it is a constant.

and

$$\Delta f = \gamma G_z \Delta z \tag{5.16}$$

With $p(f)$, one can determine the necessary excitation function $B_1(t)$. The key assumption of the Fourier approach is that $B_1(t)$ is related to $p(f)$ by the Fourier transform. More specifically,

$$B_1(t) \propto \int_{-\infty}^{\infty} p(f)e^{-i2\pi ft} df \tag{5.17}$$

Inserting Eq. (5.14) into Eq. (5.17) and making use of the well-known Fourier transform relationship

$$\text{sinc}(\pi at) \longleftrightarrow \frac{1}{a}\Pi\left(\frac{f}{a}\right) \tag{5.18}$$

we immediately get

$$B_1(t) \propto \Delta f \,\text{sinc}(\pi \Delta ft)e^{-i2\pi f_c t} \tag{5.19}$$

Comparing Eq. (5.19) to Eq. (5.8), we find that the necessary excitation frequency is

$$\omega_{\text{rf}} = 2\pi f_c = \omega_0 + \gamma G_z z_0 \tag{5.20}$$

and the pulse envelope function is

$$B_1^e(t) = A\,\text{sinc}(\pi \Delta ft) \tag{5.21}$$

where A is a constant to be determined by the desired flip angle. Note that the sinc pulse above is not physically realizable because a practical pulse will necessarily start at (or after) $t = 0$ and last only for a finite period of time, say, τ_p. Assume that the pulse is symmetric about the time point $t = \tau_p/2$. The pulse envelope function given in Eq. (5.21) should be modified accordingly to give

$$B_1^e(t) = A\,\text{sinc}\left[\pi \Delta f\left(t - \frac{\tau_p}{2}\right)\right], \qquad 0 \le t \le \tau_p \tag{5.22}$$

The resulting slice-selection profile of the above shifted and truncated pulse (temporarily ignoring the pulse truncation effect) is

$$p(f) = \Pi\left(\frac{f - f_c}{\Delta f}\right)e^{i2\pi(f - f_c)\tau_p/2} \tag{5.23}$$

or

$$p_s(z) = \Pi\left(\frac{z - z_0}{\Delta z}\right)e^{i\gamma G_z(z - z_0)\tau_p/2} \tag{5.24}$$

5.1.3.2 The Bloch Equation Approach

The Fourier method is very simple to use for designing selective pulses, but the resulting envelope function is not accurate because spin systems behave nonlinearly during excitation. To produce more accurate RF pulses, one has to resort to the Bloch equation. Omitting the spin relaxation effects during the excitation period, we can write the Bloch equation in the RF-rotating frame as

$$\frac{\partial \vec{M}_{\text{rot}}(z,t)}{\partial t} = \gamma \vec{M}_{\text{rot}}(z,t) \times \vec{B}_{\text{eff}}(z,t) \tag{5.25}$$

where

$$\vec{B}_{\text{eff}}(t) = B_1^e(t)\vec{i'} + \left(B_0 + G_z z - \frac{\omega_{\text{rf}}}{\gamma} \right)\vec{k'} \tag{5.26}$$

Setting the excitation frequency ω_{rf} to the Larmor frequency of the central slice as described by Eq. (5.20), we have

$$\vec{B}_{\text{eff}}(t) = B_1^e(t)\vec{i'} + G_z(z - z_0)\vec{k'} \tag{5.27}$$

Rewriting Eq. (5.25) in scalar form, we have

$$\begin{cases} \dfrac{dM_{x'}(z,t)}{dt} = \gamma G_z(z - z_0)M_{y'}(z,t) \\[2mm] \dfrac{dM_{y'}(z,t)}{dt} = -\gamma G_z(z - z_0)M_{x'}(z,t) + \gamma B_1^e(t)M_{z'}(z,t) \\[2mm] \dfrac{dM_{z'}(z,t)}{dt} = -\gamma B_1^e(t)M_{y'}(z,t) \end{cases} \tag{5.28}$$

Equation (5.28) are the governing equations for designing amplitude-modulated, slice-selective RF pulses. In general, these equations need to be solved numerically, and a number of numerical algorithms have been proposed for this task. Here, we consider a special case in which a closed-form solution for $B_1^e(t)$ is available. The result will also provide some theoretical justification for the Fourier approach described in the preceding section.

Assume that $M_z(z,t) = M_z^0(z)$ during the excitation, which is true when the tip angle is small. Then, Eq. (5.28) becomes

$$\begin{cases} \dfrac{dM_{x'}(z,t)}{dt} = \gamma G_z(z - z_0)M_{y'}(z,t) \\[2mm] \dfrac{dM_{y'}(z,t)}{dt} = -\gamma G_z(z - z_0)M_{x'}(z,t) + \gamma B_1(t)M_{z'}^0(z) \\[2mm] \dfrac{dM_{z'}(z,t)}{dt} = 0 \end{cases} \tag{5.29}$$

Combining the first two equations in complex form yields

$$\frac{dM_{x'y'}(z,t)}{dt} = \frac{dM_{x'}(z,t)}{dt} + i\frac{dM_{y'}(z,t)}{dt}$$
$$= -i\gamma G_z(z - z_0)M_{x'y'}(z,t) + i\gamma B_1(t)M_z^0(z) \tag{5.30}$$

The solution to Eq. (5.30) under the initial condition $M_{x'y'}(z, 0) = 0$ is[3]

$$M_{x'y'}(z,t) = i\gamma M_z^0(z)e^{-i\gamma G_z(z-z_0)t} \int_0^t B_1(\tau)e^{i\gamma G_z(z-z_0)\tau}d\tau \qquad (5.31)$$

Invoking the earlier assumption that $B_1^e(t)$ is symmetric about $t = \tau_p/2$, we find that the transverse magnetization immediately after the pulse is

$$M_{x'y'}(z,\tau_p) = i\gamma M_z^0(z)e^{-i\gamma G_z(z-z_0)\tau_p/2} \int_{-\tau_p/2}^{\tau_p/2} B_1^e\left(t + \frac{\tau_p}{2}\right) e^{i\gamma G_z(z-z_0)t}dt$$
$$(5.32)$$

Noting that

$$\int_{-\tau_p/2}^{\tau_p/2} B_1^e\left(t + \frac{\tau_p}{2}\right) e^{i\gamma G_z(z-z_0)t}dt = \mathcal{F}^{-1}\left\{B_1^e\left(t + \frac{\tau_p}{2}\right)\right\}\Big|_{f=\frac{\gamma}{2\pi}G_z(z-z_0)}$$
$$(5.33)$$

we can rewrite Eq. (5.32) as

$$\frac{-iM_{x'y'}(z,\tau_p)}{\gamma M_z^0(z)}e^{i\gamma G_z(z-z_0)\tau_p/2} = \mathcal{F}^{-1}\left\{B_1^e\left(t + \frac{\tau_p}{2}\right)\right\}\Big|_{f=\frac{\gamma}{2\pi}G_z(z-z_0)} \qquad (5.34)$$

The left-hand-side term of Eq. (5.34) corresponds to a phase-shifted slice-selection profile. Hence, Eq. (5.34) can be interpreted as saying that the pulse envelope function $B_1^e(t)$ can be determined from the Fourier transform of the desired slice-selection profile. To see this point more clearly, consider exciting a slice defined by $|z - z_0| < \Delta z/2$. The postpulse transverse magnetization can be expressed as

$$M_{x'y'}(z,\tau_p) \propto M_z^0(z)\Pi\left(\frac{z - z_0}{\Delta z}\right) \qquad (5.35)$$

Substituting this result into Eq. (5.34) yields

$$\mathcal{F}^{-1}\left\{B_1^e\left(t + \frac{\tau_p}{2}\right)\right\}\Big|_{f=\frac{\gamma}{2\pi}G_z(z-z_0)} \propto \Pi\left(\frac{z - z_0}{\Delta z}\right) e^{i\gamma G_z(z-z_0)\tau_p/2} \qquad (5.36)$$

Since Eq. (5.36) is derived under the small-tip-angle assumption, we expect the Fourier transform relationship to break down for large-tip-angle excitations. In this regime, direct solution of the Bloch equation may be in order. Nonetheless, experimental results indicate that in many applications the accuracy of the Fourier analysis method remains acceptable for flip angles up to $90°$.

---

[3]Applying the Laplace transform to both sides of Eq. (5.30) gives

$$sM_{x'y'}(z,s) = -i\gamma G_z(z - z_0)M_{x'y'}(z,s) + i\gamma B_1(s)M_z^0(z)$$

Rearrangement yields

$$M_{x'y'}(z,s) = \frac{i\gamma B_1(s)M_z^0(z)}{s + i\gamma G_z(z - z_0)}$$

whose inverse Laplace transform gives the time-domain solution in Eq. (5.31).

5.1.4   Some Practical Considerations

5.1.4.1   Post-Excitation Rephasing

According to both Eq. (5.24) and Eq. (5.34), a linear phase shift $e^{i\gamma G_z(z-z_0)\tau_p/2}$ is introduced across the slice thickness by the slice-selective gradient. If not corrected, this phase shift can lead to an undesirable signal loss. Since the phase shift is a linear function of z, it can be removed by applying a refocusing z-gradient. This procedure is called *post-excitation rephasing*.

Let the rephasing gradient be $G_{r,z}$. The phase angle during the rephasing period is

$$\phi(z,t) = \gamma G_z(z - z_0)\frac{\tau_p}{2} + \gamma G_{r,z}(z - z_0)(t - \tau_p) \qquad t \geq \tau_p \qquad (5.37)$$

Let τ_r be the length of the rephasing period. Then

$$\phi(z, t = \tau_p + \tau_r) = \gamma G_z(z - z_0)\frac{\tau_p}{2} + \gamma G_{r,z}(z - z_0)\tau_r \qquad (5.38)$$

Setting $\phi(z, t = \tau_p + \tau_r) = 0$ yields

$$G_{r,z}\tau_r = -\frac{1}{2}G_z\tau_p \qquad (5.39)$$

Therefore, fixing τ_r, one can determine $G_{r,z}$ or vice versa. For instance, if we want the rephasing period to be half the length of the excitation pulse, namely,

$$\tau_r = t - \tau_p = \frac{\tau_p}{2} \qquad (5.40)$$

then, we have

$$G_{r,z} = -G_z \qquad (5.41)$$

As shown in Fig. 5.3, the rephasing gradient pulse has the opposite polarity of the slice-selection gradient and lasts only half as long for this example.

In general, if $G_{ss} = (G_x, G_y, G_z)$ is used for slice selection, the refocusing gradient $G_r = (G_{r,x}, G_{r,y}, G_{r,z})$ satisfies the following equation:

$$\begin{cases} G_{r,x}\tau_r = -\frac{1}{2}G_x\tau_p \\ G_{r,y}\tau_r = -\frac{1}{2}G_y\tau_p \\ G_{r,z}\tau_r = -\frac{1}{2}G_z\tau_p \end{cases} \qquad (5.42)$$

The relations in Eq. (5.42) are graphically shown in Fig. 5.4.

Note that the rephasing conditions stated in Eqs. (5.39) and (5.42) are not exact, since the amount of spin dephasing during the excitation period was calculated using the Fourier method. In general, the amount of spin dephasing during the excitation period is dependent on the details of the RF pulse and should be calculated from the Bloch equation in order to be precise. Then, the amount of rephasing necessary can be calculated using the same principle discussed above.

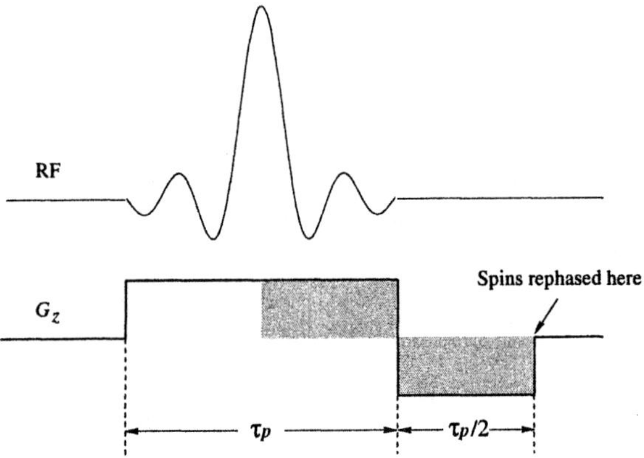

Figure 5.3 Shaped slice-selective RF pulse and the associated gradient waveform for slice selection and refocusing.

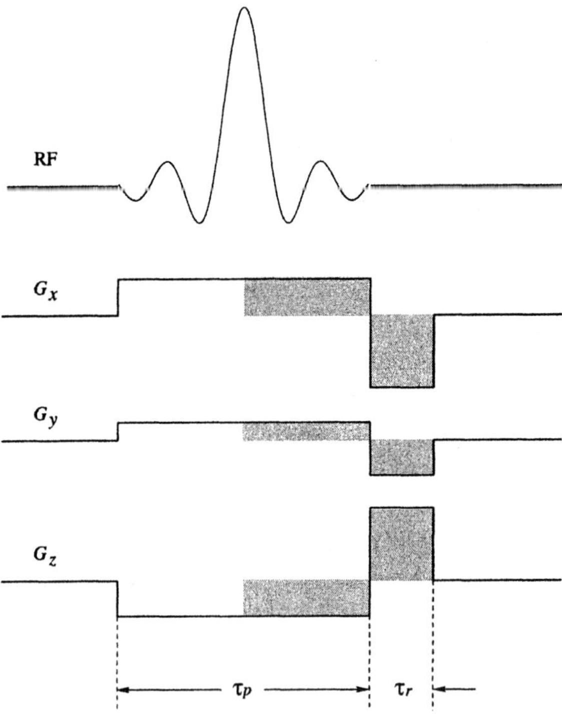

Figure 5.4 Gradient waveforms for slice selection and spin rephasing in general.

5.1.4.2   Pulse Truncation Effects

Equation (5.21) implies that to have a perfect rectangular excitation profile, we need a pulse of infinite length. In practice, the pulse has to be truncated to a finite duration to be useful. As a result, the actual slice profile will deviate from the desired one. Pulse truncation can be characterized mathematically by the multiplication of an infinite pulse with a rectangular window function. For example, corresponding to Eq. (5.22), the truncated sinc pulse can be expressed as

$$\hat{B}_1^e(t) = A\,\text{sinc}\left[\pi\Delta f\left(t - \frac{\tau_p}{2}\right)\right]\Pi\left(\frac{t - \tau_p/2}{\tau_p}\right) \tag{5.43}$$

Omitting the previously discussed phase-shift term, we have the frequency selection profile of the truncated sinc pulse:

$$\hat{p}(f) = \Pi\left(\frac{f - f_c}{\Delta f}\right) * \text{sinc}[\pi(f - f_c)\tau_p] \tag{5.44}$$

Therefore, to a reasonable approximation, the pulse truncation effect is described by the convolution of the ideal selection profile with a sinc function. From the example shown in Fig. 5.5, one can see that pulse truncation results not only in a nonuniform excitation profile across the slice thickness but also in excitation of spins in the neighboring slices to a varying degree. The latter effect is known as the *cross-talk* artifact.

To minimize the pulse truncation effects, it is necessary to pack as many sidelobes into the pulse as possible. If one assumes that n sidelobes on each side

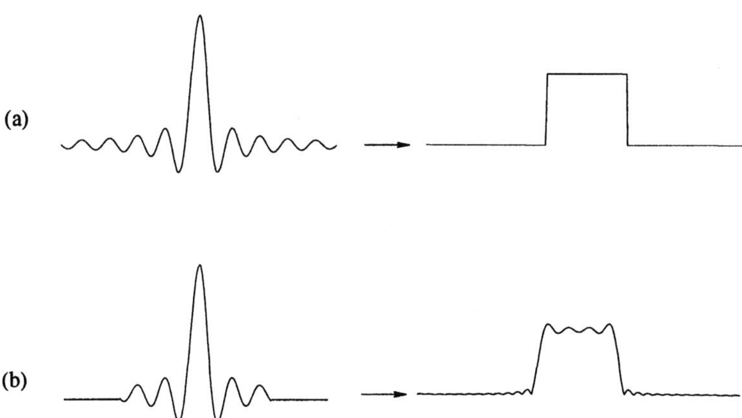

Figure 5.5   Pulse truncation effects: (a) a sinc pulse and the corresponding frequency selection profile, and (b) a truncated sinc pulse and the resulting frequency selection profile.

of the sinc function are kept, it is easy to show that the effective pulse length τ_p is related to the slice-selection gradient G_z and slice thickness Δz by

$$\tau_p = \frac{4n\pi}{\gamma G_z \Delta z} \tag{5.45}$$

Equation (5.45) shows that for a given pulse length τ_p, if the number of sidelobes in the pulse is increased to reduce the cross-talk artifact, G_z must be increased accordingly so as to maintain the same slice thickness Δz. For a given pulse, the effect of different gradient strengths is shown graphically in Fig. 5.6. It is evident from Eq. (5.45) that the thinnest slice that can be selected is limited by the available gradient strength and the allowable pulse length.

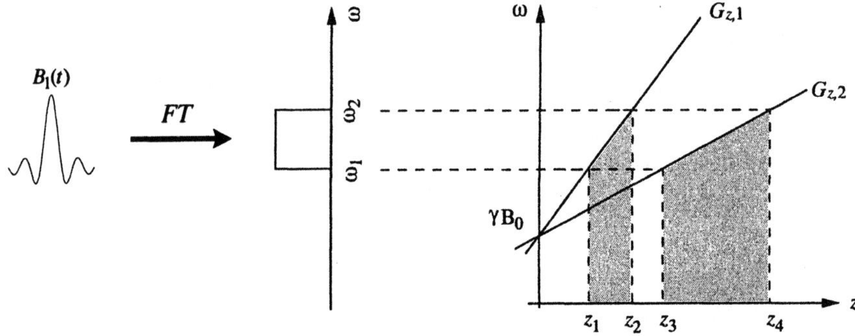

Figure 5.6 Illustration of different gradient strengths mapping the same pulse to slices of different thicknesses. Note that $B_1(t)$ selectively excites spins in $z_1 < z < z_2$ in the presence of $G_{z,1}$, but spins in $z_3 < z < z_4$ in the presence of $G_{z,2}$.

5.1.4.3 Other Slice-Selective Pulses

Many slice-selective pulses in practical use yield better selection profiles than the popular sinc pulse. A simple example is the Gaussian pulse defined by

$$B_1^e(t) = Ae^{-a(t-\tau/2)^2} \tag{5.46}$$

which has reduced sidelobe amplitudes compared to the sinc pulse. Another more complicated example is the hyperbolic secant pulse in the general form

$$B_1^e(t) = B_1 \text{sech}(\beta t)^{1+i\mu} \tag{5.47}$$

This pulse is insensitive to B_1 inhomogeneities, often encountered in practice, and is particularly useful for slice-selective spin inversion. Detailed discussion of these and other selective pulses are beyond the scope of this book. The interested reader is referred to [19] for more information.

5.2   Spatial Information Encoding

After a signal has been activated by a selective or nonselective pulse, spatial information can be encoded into the signal during the free precession period. Since an
activated MR signal is in the form of a complex exponential, we have essentially
two ways to encode spatial information: *frequency encoding* and *phase encoding*.

5.2.1   Frequency Encoding

Frequency encoding, as the name implies, makes the oscillation frequency of
an activated MR signal linearly dependent on its spatial origin. The physical
principle used to realize this is rather simple. Consider first an idealized one-
dimensional object with spin distribution $\rho(x)$. If the magnetic field that the
object experiences after an excitation is the homogeneous B_0 field plus another
linear gradient field $(G_x x)$, the Larmor frequency at position x is

$$\omega(x) = \omega_0 + \gamma G_x x \tag{5.48}$$

Correspondingly, the FID signal generated locally from spins in an infinitesimal
interval dx at point x, with the omission of the transverse relaxation effect, is

$$dS(x,t) \propto \rho(x)dx e^{-i\gamma(B_0 + G_x x)t} \tag{5.49}$$

where the constant of proportionality is dependent on the flip angle (α), main
magnetic field strength (B_0), and so on. For notational convenience, we shall
neglect this scaling constant and rewrite Eq. (5.49) as

$$dS(x,t) = \rho(x)dx e^{-i\gamma(B_0 + G_x x)t} \tag{5.50}$$

The signal in Eq. (5.50) is said to be *frequency-encoded* because its oscillation frequency $\omega(x) = \gamma(B_0 + G_x x)$ is linearly related to the spatial location. For
the same reason, G_x is called a *frequency-encoding gradient*. The signal received
from the entire object in the presence of this gradient is

$$S(t) = \int_{\text{object}} dS(x,t) = \int_{-\infty}^{\infty} \rho(x)e^{-i\gamma(B_0 + G_x x)t} dx$$

$$= \left[\int_{-\infty}^{\infty} \rho(x)e^{-i\gamma G_x x t} dx \right] e^{-i\omega_0 t} \tag{5.51}$$

After demodulation (i.e., removal of the carrier signal $e^{-i\omega_0 t}$), we have

$$S(t) = \int_{-\infty}^{\infty} \rho(x)e^{-i\gamma G_x x t} dx \tag{5.52}$$

The effect of G_x on the frequency of the local MR signals is illustrated in Fig. 5.7. As can be seen from this example, the frequency-encoding gradient field, by assigning local signals to different frequencies, gradually pushes the local signals out of phase coherence. Therefore, the received frequency-encoded signal is expected to decay at a faster rate than its nonencoded counterpart.

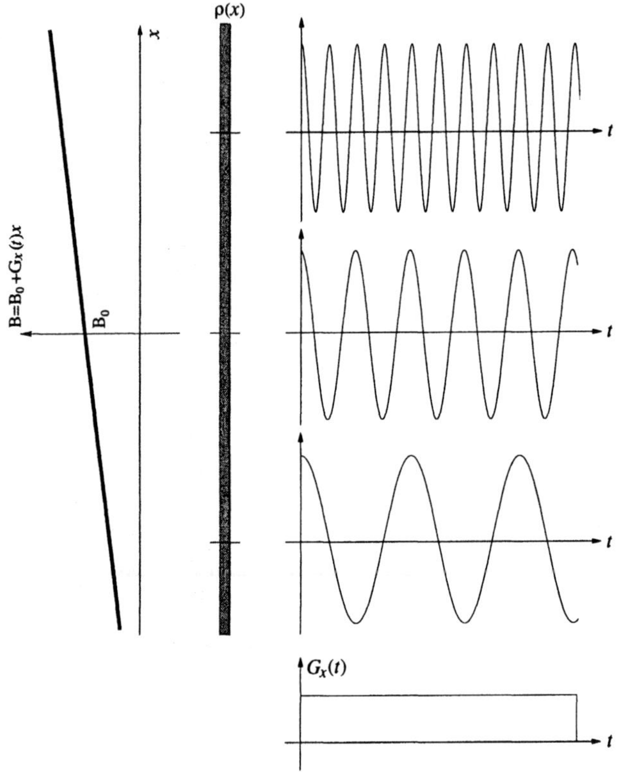

Figure 5.7   Localized signals from a hypothetical one-dimensional object in the presence of a frequency-encoding gradient.

This analysis can be generalized to the general case. Specifically, one can show that the received frequency-encoded FID signal after demodulation is, in general, given by

$$S(t) = \int_{\text{object}} \rho(\boldsymbol{r})e^{-i\gamma \boldsymbol{G}_{\text{fe}} \cdot \boldsymbol{r} t}d\boldsymbol{r} \tag{5.53}$$

where $\boldsymbol{G}_{\text{fe}}$ is the frequency-encoding gradient defined by

$$\boldsymbol{G}_{\text{fe}} = (G_x, G_y, G_z) \tag{5.54}$$

Similarly to Eq. (5.53), a general frequency-encoded echo signal can be expressed as

$$S(t) = \int_{\text{object}} \rho(\boldsymbol{r}) e^{-i\gamma \boldsymbol{G}_{\text{fe}} \cdot \boldsymbol{r}(t - T_{\text{E}})} d\boldsymbol{r} \tag{5.55}$$

An important question concerning Eqs. (5.53) and (5.55) is: Will each spatial point be assigned a unique frequency by turning on G_x, G_y, and G_z simultaneously? The answer to this question is *no*! To understand this point, let us examine the frequency distribution established by these gradients. Setting the Larmor frequency to be a constant yields

$$\gamma \boldsymbol{G}_{\text{fe}} \cdot \boldsymbol{r} = c \tag{5.56}$$

Clearly, in the two-dimensional case, Eq. (5.56) defines a family of isofrequency lines (depending on the value of c), all perpendicular to $\boldsymbol{G}_{\text{fe}}$, as illustrated in Fig. 5.8. In the three-dimensional case, Eq. (5.56) defines a family of isofrequency planes. Therefore, for a fixed frequency-encoded gradient vector $\boldsymbol{G}_{\text{fe}}$, spatial information is frequency-encoded only along the direction of $\boldsymbol{G}_{\text{fe}}$. In other words, only one-dimensional spatial localization along the gradient direction is achieved. For multidimensional localization, multiple encoded signals are necessary. Before discussing this topic, we introduce the concept of phase encoding.

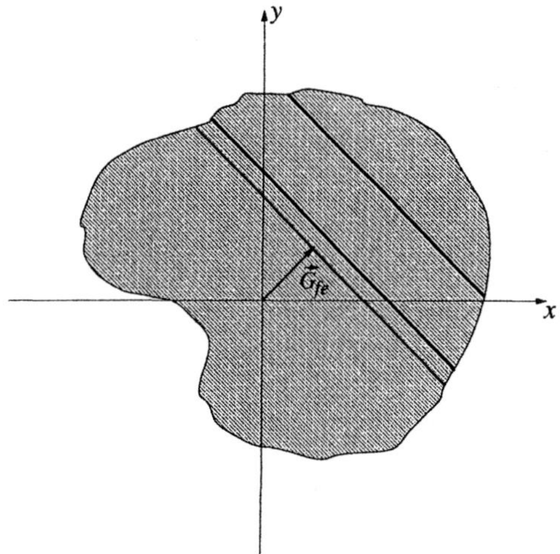

Figure 5.8   Iso-frequency lines established by the frequency-encoding gradient $\boldsymbol{G}_{\text{fe}}$.

5.2.2   Phase Encoding

With the principle of frequency encoding in hand, it is easy to understand phase encoding. To illustrate the idea, we again start with the one-dimensional case.

Imagine now that, after an RF pulse, we turn on a gradient G_x for a short interval T_{pe} and then turn it off. The local signal under the influence of this gradient is

$$dS(x, t) = \begin{cases} \rho(x)e^{-i\gamma(B_0 + G_x x)t} & 0 \leq t \leq T_{\mathrm{pe}} \\ \rho(x)e^{-i\gamma G_x x T_{\mathrm{pe}}}e^{-i\gamma B_0 t} & T_{\mathrm{pe}} \leq t \end{cases} \qquad (5.57)$$

It is evident that during the interval $0 \leq t \leq T_{\mathrm{pe}}$, the local signal is frequency-encoded. As a result of this frequency encoding, signals from different x-positions accumulate different phase angles after a time interval T_{pe}, as demonstrated in Fig. 5.9. Therefore, if we use the first time interval as a *preparatory period*, the signal collected afterward will bear an initial phase angle

$$\phi(x) = -\gamma G_x x T_{\mathrm{pe}} \qquad (5.58)$$

Since $\phi(x)$ is linearly related to the signal location x, we shall call the signal *phase-encoded*. For the same reason, G_x is referred to as the phase-encoding gradient and T_{pe} as the phase-encoding interval to emphasize their roles of imparting a position-dependent initial phase angle to the observed signal.

Phase encoding along an arbitrary direction can also be done for a multidimensional object by turning on G_x, G_y, and G_z simultaneously during the phase-encoding period. Similarly to Eq. (5.54), the phase-encoding gradient in this case is

$$\boldsymbol{G}_{\mathrm{pe}} = (G_x, G_y, G_z) \qquad 0 \leq t \leq T_{\mathrm{pe}} \qquad (5.59)$$

The initial phase angle is now given by

$$\phi(\boldsymbol{r}) = -\gamma \boldsymbol{G}_{\mathrm{pe}} \cdot \boldsymbol{r} T_{\mathrm{pe}} \qquad (5.60)$$

As in the case of frequency encoding, the received signal is the sum of all the local phase-encoded signals and is given by

$$\begin{aligned} S(t) &= \int_{\mathrm{object}} dS(\boldsymbol{r}, t) \\ &= \left[\int_{\mathrm{object}} \rho(\boldsymbol{r})e^{-i\gamma \boldsymbol{G}_{\mathrm{pe}} \cdot \boldsymbol{r} T_{\mathrm{pe}}} d\boldsymbol{r} \right] e^{-i\omega_0 t} \end{aligned} \qquad (5.61)$$

where the carrier signal $e^{-i\omega_0 t}$ will be removed after demodulation.

In summary, phase encoding is done by pre-frequency encoding the signal for a short time interval. As indicated by Eq. (5.61), a phase-encoded signal has the form of a nonencoded signal with a position-dependent initial phase angle. This phase angle can be adjusted with a variable phase-encoding gradient strength or phase-encoding interval. To gain a better understanding of both phase- and frequency-encoding schemes, we next look at them from a k-space perspective.

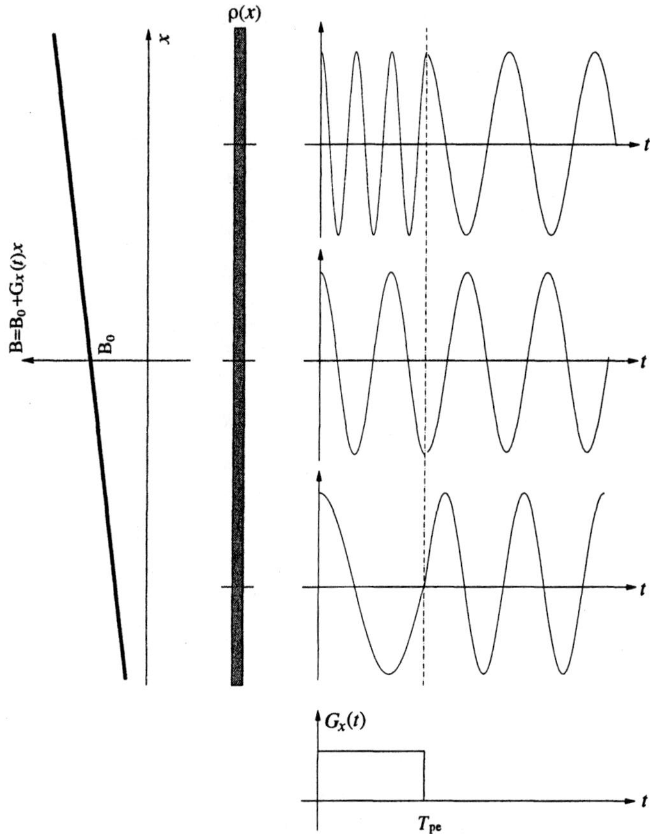

Figure 5.9 Phase-encoded signals from a one-dimensional object. Note that phase encoding is achieved by pre-frequency encoding the signals for a short period of time T_{pe}.

5.2.3   A k-Space Interpretation

This section establishes an important connection between spatial encoding (phase encoding and frequency encoding) and the Fourier transform. This connection enables us to describe complex imaging schemes clearly using the popular k-space notation.

5.2.3.1   Frequency-Encoded Signals

We first consider the frequency-encoded signal given in Eq. (5.52), from which
the following Fourier transform relationship is obtained:

$$S(k_x) = \int_{-\infty}^{\infty} \rho(x)e^{-i2\pi k_x x}dx \qquad (5.62)$$

by making a simple variable substitution,

$$k_x = \begin{cases} \gamma G_x t & \text{FID signals} \\ \gamma G_x(t - T_E) & \text{echo signals} \end{cases} \qquad (5.63)$$

It is clear that the role of the frequency-encoding gradient G_x is to map a time
signal to a k-space signal. In the extreme case that $G_x = 0$, this mapping is
trivial, since all the time data points are mapped to a single k-space data point
at $k_x = 0$. If $G_x \neq 0$, the activated time signal will be nontrivially mapped to
k-space. In other words, the frequency-encoding gradient uniquely encodes the
spatial information in the activated signal.

When multiple gradients are used for frequency encoding, the mapping relationship between t and k is given by

$$\boldsymbol{k} = \begin{cases} \gamma \boldsymbol{G}_{\text{fe}} t & \text{FID signals} \\ \gamma \boldsymbol{G}_{\text{fe}}(t - T_E) & \text{echo signals} \end{cases} \qquad (5.64)$$

and the corresponding k-space signal, according to Eq. (5.53), is

$$S(\boldsymbol{k}) = \int_{\text{object}} \rho(\boldsymbol{r})e^{-i2\pi \boldsymbol{k}\cdot\boldsymbol{r}}d\boldsymbol{r} \qquad (5.65)$$

Note that although the k-space signal in this case is in the form of a multidimensional Fourier transform, $S(\boldsymbol{k})$ is available only for a limited set of points in
k-space. The k-space coordinates of these points define the so-called *sampling
trajectory* of k-space. In the two-dimensional case, for example, the sampling
trajectory of an FID signal, according to Eq. (5.64), is defined by

$$\begin{cases} k_x = \gamma G_x t \\ k_y = \gamma G_y t \end{cases} \qquad (5.66)$$

or

$$\begin{cases} k_x = k \cos \phi \\ k_y = k \sin \phi \end{cases} \qquad (5.67)$$

where

$$k = \gamma G_{\text{fe}} t = \gamma t \sqrt{G_x^2 + G_y^2} \qquad (5.68)$$

and

$$\phi = \tan^{-1}\left(\frac{G_y}{G_x}\right) \qquad (5.69)$$

Equation (5.67) specifies a straight line originating from the k-space origin, as illustrated in Fig. 5.10a. The orientation of the line is adjustable by selecting different relative values for G_x and G_y. For an echo signal,

$$\begin{cases} k_x = \gamma G_x(t - T_E) \\ k_y = \gamma G_y(t - T_E) \end{cases} \tag{5.70}$$

which corresponds a straight line going through the k-space origin, as illustrated in Fig. 5.10b.

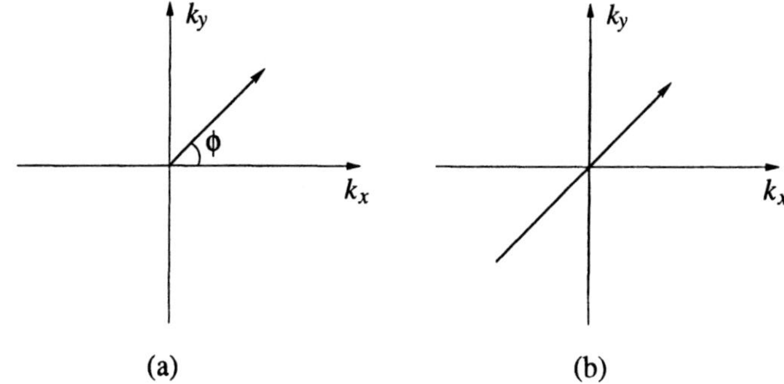

Figure 5.10 K-space sampling trajectories of (a) a frequency-encoded FID signal, and (b) a frequency-encoded echo signal.

The conclusion can be extended to three dimensions. Specifically, similarly to Eq. (5.67), we have

$$\begin{cases} k_x = k \sin\theta \cos\phi \\ k_y = k \sin\theta \sin\phi \\ k_z = k \cos\theta \end{cases} \tag{5.71}$$

where

$$k = \begin{cases} \gamma t \sqrt{G_x^2 + G_y^2 + G_z^2} & \text{FID signals} \\ \gamma(t - T_E)\sqrt{G_x^2 + G_y^2 + G_z^2} & \text{echo signals} \end{cases} \tag{5.72a}$$

$$\theta = \tan^{-1}\left(\frac{\sqrt{G_x^2 + G_y^2}}{G_z} \right) \tag{5.72b}$$

$$\phi = \tan^{-1}\left(\frac{G_y}{G_x} \right) \tag{5.72c}$$

Note that the k-space sampling trajectory of a frequency-encoded signal is a straight line only if constant gradients are used for frequency encoding. If G_{fe} is a function of time, the mapping relationship between t and k should be written as

$$k(t) = \gamma \int_0^t G_{\mathrm{fe}}(\tau)d\tau \qquad (5.73)$$

where the time origin corresponds to the instant when an RF excitation pulse is switched off. Therefore, a signal can traverse k-space linearly or nonlinearly depending on the waveform of the frequency-encoding gradient G_{fe}.

■ Example 5.2

This example calculates the k-space sampling trajectory in the presence of sinusoidal gradients, shown in Fig. 5.11.

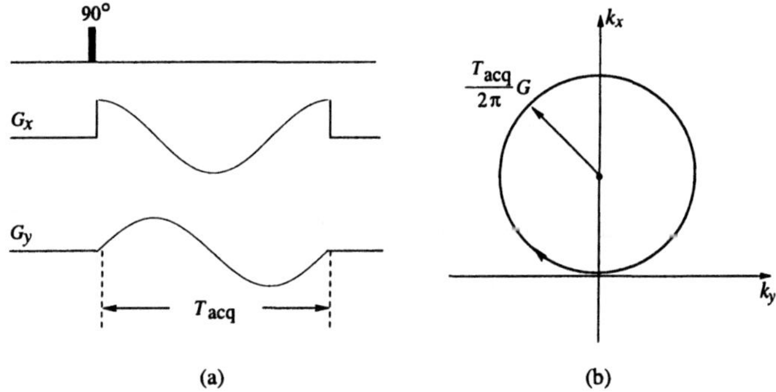

Figure 5.11 (a) A frequency-encoding scheme using a pair of sinusoidal gradients and (b) the corresponding k-space sampling trajectory.

According to Fig. 5.11a, we have

$$\begin{cases} G_x(t) = G\cos\left(\dfrac{2\pi t}{T_{\mathrm{acq}}}\right) \\[3mm] G_y(t) = G\sin\left(\dfrac{2\pi t}{T_{\mathrm{acq}}}\right) \end{cases} \qquad (5.74)$$

Substituting the above expressions into Eq. (5.73) yields

$$k_x(t) = \gamma \int_0^t G \cos\left(\frac{2\pi\tau}{T_{\mathrm{acq}}}\right) d\tau = \frac{T_{\mathrm{acq}}}{2\pi} G \sin\left(\frac{2\pi t}{T_{\mathrm{acq}}}\right) \tag{5.75a}$$

$$k_y(t) = \gamma \int_0^t G \sin\left(\frac{2\pi\tau}{T_{\mathrm{acq}}}\right) d\tau = \frac{T_{\mathrm{acq}}}{2\pi} G \left[1 - \cos\left(\frac{2\pi t}{T_{\mathrm{acq}}}\right)\right] \tag{5.75b}$$

for $0 \le t \le T_{\mathrm{acq}}$ It is easy to see that these equations describe a circular sampling trajectory, as shown in Fig. 5.11b.

■ Example 5.3

In this example, we examine the effect of a 180° pulse on k-space trajectories.

Recall from Eq. (3.101) that

$$M_{x'y'} \xrightarrow{\pi_\varphi} M^*_{x'y'} e^{-i2\varphi} \tag{5.76}$$

To highlight the k-dependence, we express the prepulse transverse magnetization as

$$M_{x'y'} = \rho(r)dr e^{-i2\pi k \cdot r} \tag{5.77}$$

Then, according to Eq. (5.76), the postpulse transverse magnetization is given by

$$M_{x'y'} = \rho(r)dr e^{i(2\pi k \cdot r - 2\varphi)} \tag{5.78}$$

It is evident from Eqs. (5.77) and (5.77) that

$$k \xrightarrow{\pi_\varphi} -k \tag{5.79}$$

In other words, a 180° pulse will swing the transverse magnetization to the opposite location in k-space.

One may notice from Eq. (5.78) that a 180° pulse will also introduce a phase shift (-2φ) to the received signal. This phase shift is related to the direction of the pulse. For example, the phase shift is 0 for a $180°_{x'}$ pulse and π for a $180°_{y'}$ pulse.

■ Example 5.4

This example examines the k-space sampling trajectories of a frequency-encoded FID signal, gradient-echo signal, and spin-echo signal generated by the excitation schemes shown in Fig. 5.12.

It is customary to set $t = 0$ to be the time instant when the $90°$ excitation pulse is applied. For the FID signal in Fig. 5.12a, we have

$$k_x = \gamma G_x t \qquad 0 \le t \le T_{\text{acq}} \tag{5.80}$$

Therefore, the sampling trajectory is a half-line along the k_x-axis, starting at $k_x = 0$ and ending at $k_x = \gamma G_x T_{\text{acq}}$.

For the gradient-echo signal in Fig. 5.12b, we have during the preparatory period that

$$k_x = -\gamma G_x t \qquad 0 \le t \le T_{\text{acq}}/2 \tag{5.81}$$

During the subsequent data acquisition period, we have

$$\begin{aligned}
k_x &= -\gamma G_x T_{\text{acq}}/2 + \gamma G_x \left(t - T_{\text{acq}}/2\right) \\
&= \gamma G_x \left(t - T_{\text{acq}}/2\right) \\
&= \gamma G_x (t - T_E) \qquad |t - T_E| \le T_{\text{acq}}/2
\end{aligned} \tag{5.82}$$

which corresponds to a symmetric line about the k-space origin, starting at $k_x = -\gamma G_x T_{\text{acq}}/2$ and ending at $k_x = \gamma G_x T_{\text{acq}}/2$.

For the spin-echo signal in Fig. 5.12c, k_x is given, during the preparatory period, by

$$k_x = \gamma G_x t \qquad 0 \le t \le T_{\text{acq}}/2 \tag{5.83}$$

At the end of the preparatory period, $k_x = \gamma G_x T_{\text{acq}}/2$, which stays the same until the $180°$ is applied. The $180°$ reverses the k_x value, giving

$$k_x = -\gamma G_x T_{\text{acq}}/2 \tag{5.84}$$

Consequently, during the data acquisition period, we have

$$\begin{aligned}
k_x &= -\gamma G_x T_{\text{acq}}/2 + \gamma G_x \left(t - T_{\text{acq}}/2\right) \\
&= \gamma G_x \left(t - T_{\text{acq}}/2\right) \\
&= \gamma G_x (t - T_E) \qquad |t - T_E| \le T_{\text{acq}}/2
\end{aligned} \tag{5.85}$$

which is the same as that of the gradient-echo signal. This example demonstrates that both gradient-echo signals and spin-echo signals can cover k-space symmetrically.

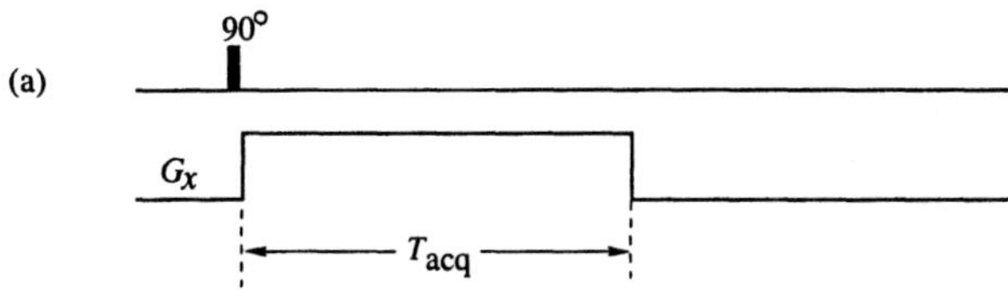

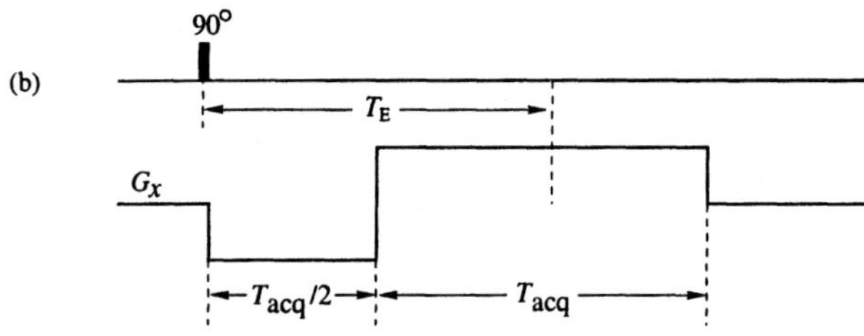

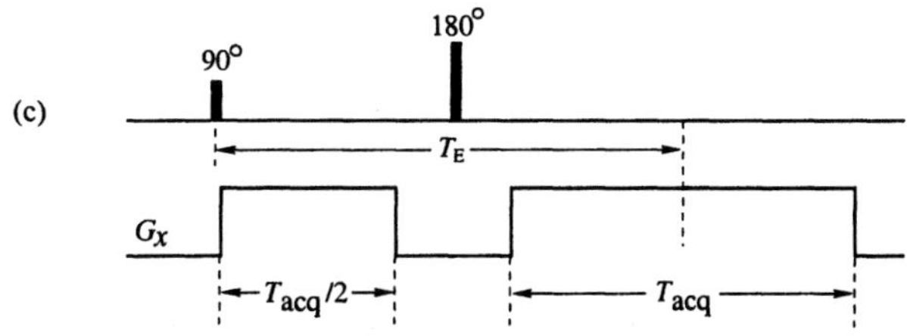

Figure 5.12 Excitation sequences for generating a frequency-encoded
(a) FID signal (b) gradient-echo signal, and (c) spin-echo signal.

5.2.3.2 Phase-Encoded Signals

As in frequency encoding, the effect of phase encoding can also be described by
the Fourier transform. Specifically, we can express the phase-encoded signal in
Eq. (5.61) as

$$S(k) = \int_{\text{object}} \rho(r)e^{-i2\pi k \cdot r}\,dr \tag{5.86}$$

by dropping the carrier signal $e^{-i\omega_0 t}$ and assuming

$$k = \gamma G_{\text{pe}}T_{\text{pe}} \tag{5.87}$$

Note that $S(k)$, as a function of k, has the same form for both frequency and phase
encodings, as shown in Eq. (5.86) and Eq. (5.65). However, a given time signal

is mapped to k-space differently by phase and frequency encoding. Specifically, k has a fixed value for a given G_{pe} and T_{pe} in phase encoding, while k is always a function of time in frequency encoding. Therefore, phase encoding influences only the starting point but not the shape and form of the k-space trajectory for an evolving transient MR signal.

In the general case in which G_{pe} is a function of time, k is given by

$$k = \gamma \int_0^{T_{pe}} G_{pe}(\tau)d\tau \tag{5.88}$$

Therefore, if the area under the gradient pulse remains the same, the form and shape of a phase-encoding gradient pulse are unimportant as far as k-space mapping is concerned. To better understand this point, consider the three gradient waveforms shown in Fig. 5.13. In the first case,

$$k_x = \gamma \left[\int_0^1 \tau d\tau + \int_1^2 d\tau + \int_2^3 (3 - \tau)d\tau \right] = 2\gamma \tag{5.89}$$

It is easy to show that $k_x = 2\gamma$ for both the second and third cases as well. Therefore, the three gradient waveforms have the same phase-encoding effect. Note that all three pulses have the same peak gradient value, but the trapezoidal and triangular pulses are smoother and longer than the rectangular pulse. During the phase-encoding period, k_x advances from $k_x = 0$ to $k_x = 2\gamma$ at different speeds for different gradient waveforms. Specifically, since

$$\frac{dk_x(t)}{dt} = \gamma G_x(t) \tag{5.90}$$

k_x traverses from the origin to the required phase-encoding value at a constant speed in the presence of a constant gradient but at variable speeds in all of the other cases.

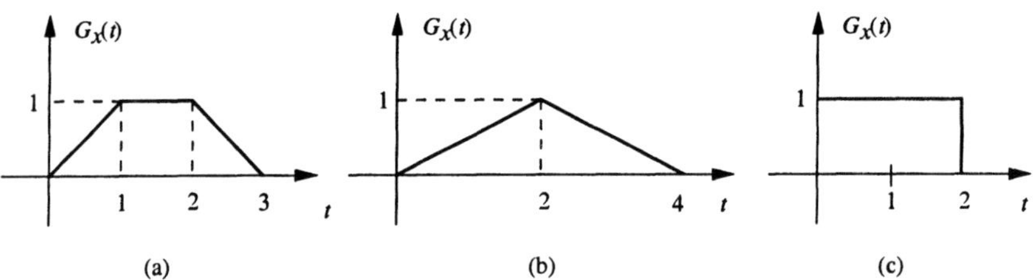

Figure 5.13 Three gradient pulses used for phase encoding.

5.3   Basic Imaging Methods

We discuss in this section how to use the signal localization principles described
in the preceding section for multidimensional imaging. Although the "ultimate"
goal of imaging is to recover the image function from the activated signal, here
we emphasize only the relationship between the measured data and the desired
image function. Therefore, the discussion in this section takes us only to the point
of arriving at an imaging equation. Chapter 6 explains how to recover the image
function from the measured data.

5.3.1   One-Dimensional Imaging

Given a three-dimensional object, one-dimensional imaging could mean two different things: (a) to obtain a one-dimensional projection image along a particular
direction, or (b) to obtain an image line. Both cases are concerned with resolving
spatial distribution along one direction, but the resulting image function can be
very different.

Consider the first case. For simplicity, we assume that the projection is taken
along the x-direction. Then, the desired image function $I(x)$ can be expressed as

$$I(x) = \int_{-\infty}^{\infty} \int_{-\infty}^{\infty} \rho(x, y, z)\,dy\,dz \tag{5.91}$$

A spin-echo imaging sequence for generating this image function is shown in
Fig. 5.14. In this sequence, the object is first excited with a hard pulse and then
a nonselective $180°$ refocusing pulse. The resulting spin-echo signal is acquired
in the presence of a frequency-encoding gradient G_x. Since all the pulses are
nonselective, the spin-echo signal can be expressed as

$$S(t) = \int_{-\infty}^{\infty} \int_{-\infty}^{\infty} \int_{-\infty}^{\infty} \rho(x, y, z)e^{-i\gamma G_x(t-T_E)}\,dx\,dy\,dz$$

$$= \int_{-\infty}^{\infty} I(x)e^{-i\gamma G_x(t-T_E)}\,dx \tag{5.92}$$

for $|t - T_E| < T_{\mathrm{acq}}/2$ Substituting $k_x = \gamma G_x(t - T_E)$ yields

$$S(k_x) = \int_{-\infty}^{\infty} I(x)e^{-i2\pi k_x x}\,dx \tag{5.93}$$

This is regarded as the one-dimensional imaging equation.

We next consider imaging a line in a three-dimensional object. Again, we
assume that a line along the x-direction is desired. The image function can be
expressed as

$$I(x) = \int_{y_0-\Delta y/2}^{y_0+\Delta y/2} \int_{z_0-\Delta z/2}^{z_0+\Delta z/2} \rho(x, y, z)\,dy\,dz \tag{5.94}$$

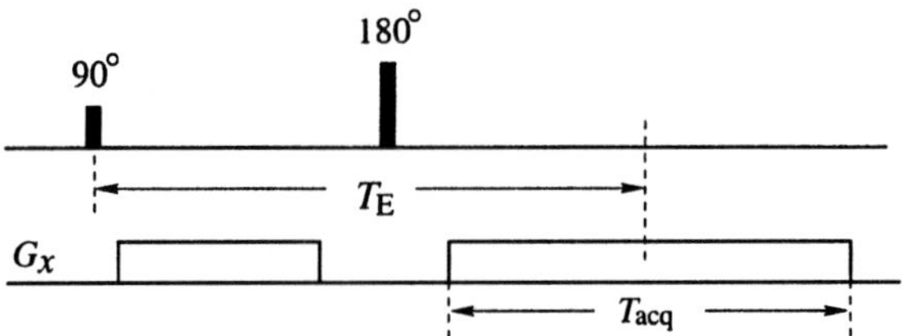

Figure 5.14 Pulse sequence to generate a spin-echo signal from which a projection image along the x-direction can be formed. Note that $G_y = G_z = 0$ in this excitation sequence.

where (y_0, z_0) specifies the line location and $(\Delta y, \Delta z)$ specifies the line widths. A typical excitation scheme for generating data necessary to form this line image is shown in Fig. 5.15, in which the first pulse selects a transverse plane while the second excites a coronal plane. The signal generated from the two selective pulses will be exclusively from the intersection—a line. To resolve spatial distribution along this line, a frequency-encoding gradient (G_x) is applied during the data acquisition.

$$S(t) = \int_{-\infty}^{\infty} \int_{y_0-\Delta y/2}^{y_0+\Delta y/2} \int_{z_0-\Delta z/2}^{z_0+\Delta z/2} \rho(x, y, z)e^{-i\gamma G_x(t-T_E)}\,dx\,dy\,dz$$

$$= \int_{-\infty}^{\infty} I(x)e^{-i\gamma G_x(t-T_E)}\,dx \tag{5.95}$$

for $|t - T_E| < T_{\text{acq}}/2$. Therefore, the measured signal is related to the desired image function in the same fashion as in the first case and can be put in the form of a one-dimensional Fourier transform.

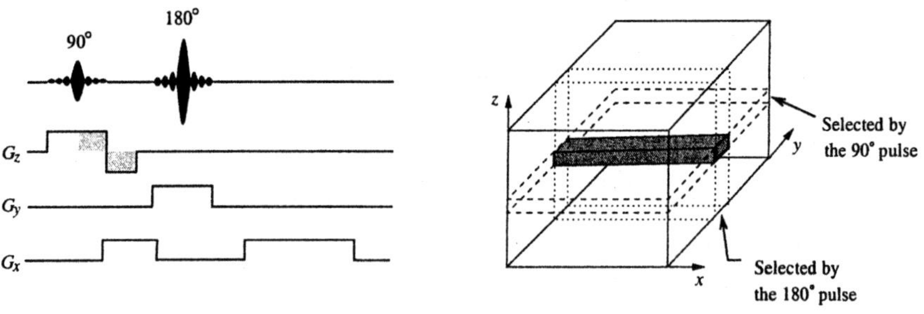

Figure 5.15 Line imaging: (a) pulse sequence and (b) effects of the selective pulses.

5.3.2 Two-Dimensional Imaging

As in one-dimensional imaging, we have the option of creating a two-dimensional image as either a projection or a slice of a three-dimensional object, depending on the applications. Although the outcome of the two imaging scenarios would be drastically different, the imaging principle is very similar, except that for generating each time signal one uses a hard pulse in the first case but a slice-selective soft pulse in the second. For the present discussion, therefore, we will ignore this subtle difference and focus on the key concept of encoding two-dimensional spatial information in the time signal. Denoting the desired image function by $I(x, y)$, it is easy to see that $I(x, y)$ is related to the underlying three-dimensional object function $\rho(x, y, z)$, in the projective imaging case, by

$$I(x, y) = \int_{-\infty}^{\infty} \rho(x, y, z) dz \tag{5.96}$$

and in the slice-selective imaging case, by

$$I(x, y) = \int_{z_0 - \Delta z/2}^{z_0 + \Delta z/2} \rho(x, y, z) dz \tag{5.97}$$

The basic imaging equation is the two-dimensional Fourier transform

$$S(k_x, k_y) = \int_{-\infty}^{\infty} \int_{-\infty}^{\infty} I(x, y) e^{-i2\pi(k_x x + k_y y)} dx dy \tag{5.98}$$

Therefore, a basic task of planar imaging is to generate sufficient data to cover k-space. A conventional strategy is to generate a set of "identical" signals $\{S_n(t)\}$ using repetitive excitations and then encode each properly so that k-space will be covered with multiple lines. Figure 5.16 shows a classical implementation of this strategy. As can be seen, this imaging sequence excites an object periodically with a pair of slice-selective $90°$ and $180°$ pulses, which generate a set of spin-echo signals. Spatial information is then encoded in the spin-echo signals by two-dimensional frequency-encoding.

Denote the encoding gradients in the nth excitation cycle by

$$\begin{cases} G_{n,x} = G \cos \phi_n \\ G_{n,y} = G \sin \phi_n \end{cases} \tag{5.99}$$

It is easy to show that the spin-echo signal is related to the desired image function by

$$S_n(t) = \int_{-\infty}^{\infty} \int_{-\infty}^{\infty} I(x, y) e^{-i\gamma G(t - T_E)(x \cos \phi_n + y \sin \phi_n)} dx dy \tag{5.100}$$

for $|t - T_E| < T_{\text{acq}}/2$, where $I(x, y)$ is defined in Eq. (5.97). Putting it in k-space notation immediately yields the generic imaging equation in Eq. (5.98).

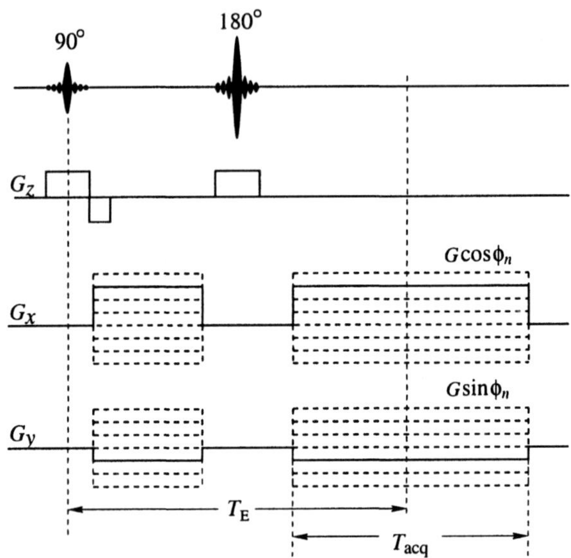

Figure 5.16 A two-dimensional imaging sequence. Note that it is customary to draw only one excitation period, in which the multiple values of G_x and G_y correspond to different excitation cycles. In the nth excitation cycle, $G_x = G\cos\phi_n$ and $G_y = G\sin\phi_n$ are applied during both intervals: $t_0 < t < t_0 + T_{\text{acq}}/2$ and $|t - T_E| < T_{\text{acq}}/2$.

We next analyze the k-space sampling pattern of this imaging scheme. Consider the signal generated in the nth excitation cycle. Following the same analysis used in Example 5.4, we have, in the interval between the 90° and 180° pulses,

$$\begin{cases} k_x = \gamma G(t - t_0)\cos\phi_n \\ k_y = \gamma G(t - t_0)\sin\phi_n \end{cases} \qquad t_0 < t < T_{\text{acq}}/2 + t_0 \qquad (5.101)$$

where t_0 and T_{acq} are defined in Fig. 5.16. Equation (5.101) indicates that k-space is traversed from the origin to point A as indicated in Fig. 5.17a, where

$$\boldsymbol{k}_{\text{A}} = \gamma G \frac{T_{\text{acq}}}{2}(\cos\phi_n, \sin\phi_n) \qquad (5.102)$$

The subsequent 180° pulse swings the trajectory to point B such that

$$\boldsymbol{k}_{\text{B}} = -\boldsymbol{k}_{\text{A}} \qquad (5.103)$$

During the subsequent data acquisition interval, we have

$$\begin{cases} k_x = \gamma G\cos\phi_n(t - T_E) \\ k_y = \gamma G\sin\phi_n(t - T_E) \end{cases} \qquad |t - T_E| < T_{\text{acq}}/2 \qquad (5.104)$$

which defines a radial line starting at k_B, going through the k-space origin, and ending at k_A. Since

$$\phi_n = \arctan\left(\frac{G_{n,y}}{G_{n,x}}\right) \tag{5.105}$$

one can easily change ϕ_n by adjusting the relative strengths of the frequency-encoding gradients. Therefore, by varying ϕ_n from one excitation cycle to another, k-space can be effectively covered. This method is sometimes referred to as the *Radon transform* (or *projection*) *imaging method*, since the radial k-space data are directly related to the projections of the desired image function.

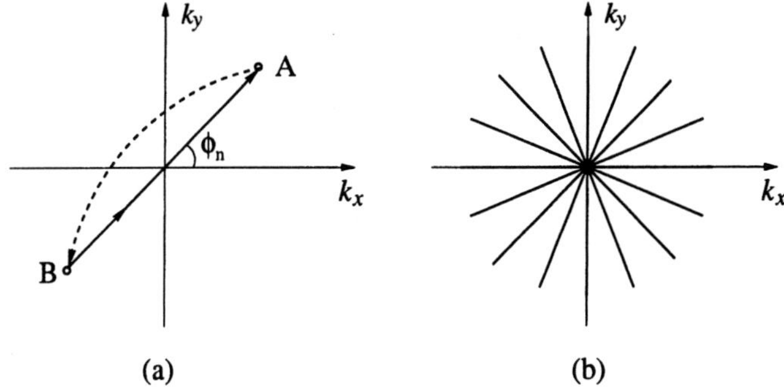

Figure 5.17 K-space coverage of the imaging sequence in Fig. 5.16: (a) k-space trajectory of a single excitation cycle, and (b) k-space coverage by a set of the frequency-encoded spin echoes.

To further illustrate the k-space coverage concept, let us analyze another basic imaging scheme shown in Fig. 5.18. This scheme uses the same excitation sequence as in Fig. 5.16a, but the signals generated are encoded differently. Specifically, each spin-echo signal is first phase-encoded along the y-direction and then acquired in the presence of a frequency-encoding gradient G_x.

To understand how k-space is traversed by this imaging scheme, consider the nth excitation. During the phase-encoding interval, we have

$$\begin{cases} k_x = \gamma G_x(t - t_0) \\ k_y = \gamma n \Delta G_y(t - t_0) \end{cases} \qquad t_0 < t < T_\mathrm{acq}/2 + t_0 \tag{5.106}$$

which represents a radial line from the origin to point A defined by

$$k_\mathrm{A} = (\gamma G_x T_\mathrm{pe}, \gamma n \Delta G_y T_\mathrm{pe}) \tag{5.107}$$

The subsequent $180°$ pulse swings the trajectory to point B, as shown in Fig. 5.19a,

$$k_\mathrm{B} = -k_\mathrm{A} \tag{5.108}$$

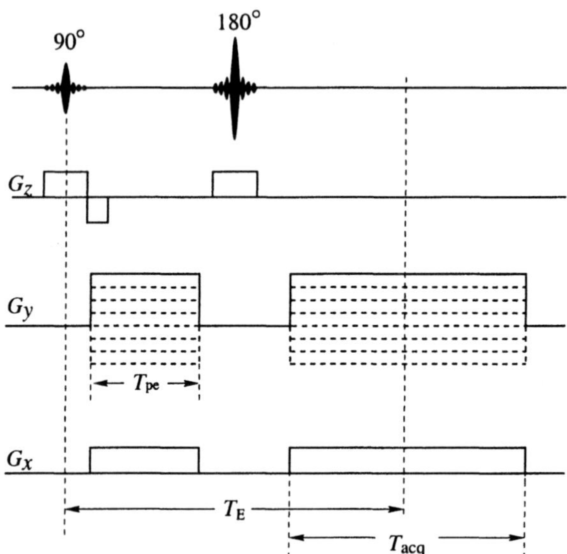

Figure 5.18　A two-dimensional imaging sequence with phase-encoding along the y-direction and frequency-encoding along the x-direction. Specifically, in the nth excitation cycle, $G_y = n\Delta G_y$ is applied during the interval $t_0 < t < t_0 + T_{\mathrm{pe}}$ to phase-encode the signal, which is then acquired in the presence of the frequency-encoding gradient G_x.

During the subsequent data acquisition interval, we have

$$\begin{cases} k_x = \gamma G(t - T_E) \\ k_y = \gamma n\Delta G_y T_{\mathrm{pe}} \end{cases} \qquad |t - T_E| < T_{\mathrm{acq}}/2 \qquad (5.109)$$

which is a horizontal line parallel to the k_x-axis, whose interception on k_y-axis is $\gamma n\Delta G_y T_{\mathrm{pe}}$. Therefore, by varying the phase-encoding strength, each line will assume different k_y locations resulting in the rectilinear sampling of k-space, as shown in Fig. 5.19b.

In the literature, this hybrid phase- and frequency-encoding scheme is known as the *phase-encoding method* because different time signals are phase-encoded using a variable gradient.[4] Note that symmetric coverage of k-space is provided by the use of spin echoes along the k_x-direction and by the use of both positive and negative phase-encoding gradients along the k_y-direction. However, spin echoes are not essential as far as k-space coverage is concerned. One can design an imaging sequence to give the same k-space coverage with gradient echoes. This is left to the reader.

---

[4]It is also possible to achieve the same phase-encoding effect by keeping the amplitude of the phase-encoding gradient constant but changing its duration from one excitation to another.

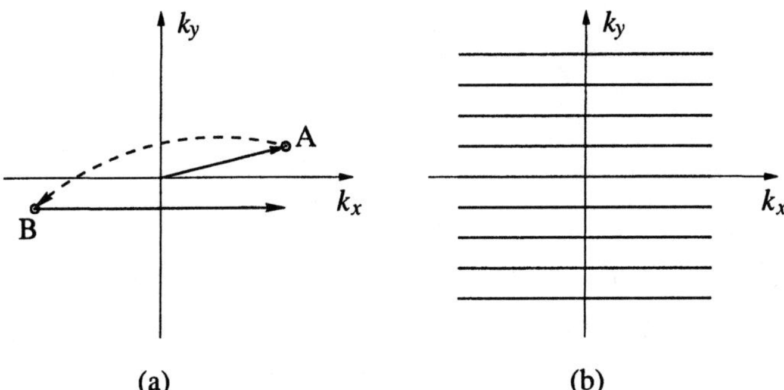

Figure 5.19 K-space coverage of the imaging sequence in Fig. 5.18. (a) k-space trajectory during a single excitation cycle, and (b) k-space coverage by a set of phase-encoded spin-echo signals.

5.3.3 Three-Dimensional Imaging

MR excitation is inherently a three-dimensional technique in the sense that signals generated by a short pulse will come from the entire object. In other words, it is easier to generate signals from the entire volume than from a limited region. The challenge in three-dimensional imaging lies in sorting out all the signal components from different spatial locations. There are many ways to accomplish this task. The simplest is perhaps the multislice imaging method, which uses slice-selective excitations for localization in the third dimension, leaving the other two to be done with encoding methods. This method generally produces a stack of two-dimensional images, each of which is acquired using the two-dimensional localization principles discussed in Section 5.3.2.

For true three-dimensional imaging, nonselective pulses are used for signal generation, and information along all three dimensions must be encoded into the activated signals. Because of the nature of MR signals, information along one dimension is naturally frequency-encoded, while information along the other two dimensions can be either phase- or frequency-encoded. Regardless of what the encoding scheme is, the general imaging equation is in the form of a three-dimensional Fourier transform:

$$S(k_x, k_y, k_z) = \int_{-\infty}^{\infty} \int_{-\infty}^{\infty} \int_{-\infty}^{\infty} I(x, y, z) e^{-i2\pi(k_x x + k_y y + k_z z)} dx\,dy\,dz \quad (5.110)$$

Different encoding schemes will only lead to different sampling patterns of the three-dimensional k-space. To demonstrate this point, consider the excitation sequence shown in Fig. 5.20, in which the x-direction is frequency-encoded while the y- and z-directions are phase-encoded. In this case, k-space is filled by rectilinear lines parallel to the k_x-axis as described by

$$\begin{cases} k_x = \gamma G_x(t - T_E) \\ k_y = \gamma G_y T_{\text{pe}} \\ k_z = \gamma G_z T_{\text{pe}} \end{cases} \qquad |t - T_E| < T_{\text{acq}}/2 \qquad (5.111)$$

where G_x is a constant, but $G_y = m\Delta G_y$ and $G_z = n\Delta G_z$.

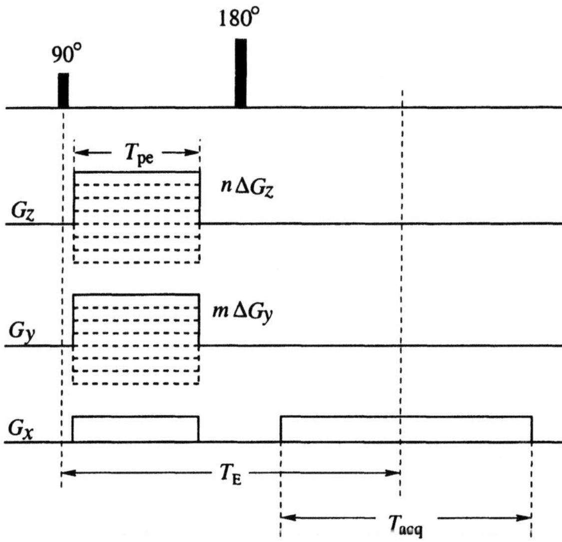

Figure 5.20   Three-dimensional phase-encoding imaging sequence.

As another example, a three-dimensional frequency-encoding imaging sequence is shown in Fig. 5.21. In contrast to the phase-encoding case, k-space is now filled with radial lines going through the origin. This can be understood by noting the following k-space sampling trajectory equation for each frequency-encoded signal:

$$\begin{cases} k_x = \gamma G_x(t - T_E) \\ k_y = \gamma G_y(t - T_E) \\ k_z = \gamma G_z(t - T_E) \end{cases} \qquad |t - T_E| < T_{\text{acq}}/2 \qquad (5.112)$$

where G_x, G_y, and G_z are selected according to the following formulas:

$$\begin{cases} G_x = G \sin\theta_n \cos\phi_m \\ G_y = G \sin\theta_n \sin\phi_m \\ G_z = G \cos\theta_n \end{cases} \qquad (5.113)$$

The foregoing discussion shows that the concept of three-dimensional imaging is not very different from that of two-dimensional imaging. However, three-dimensional imaging does present some unique practical problems because many more encodings are required to cover k-space. Chapter 8 discusses some of the practical imaging issues related to limited data acquisition time, resolution, and signal-to-noise ratio.

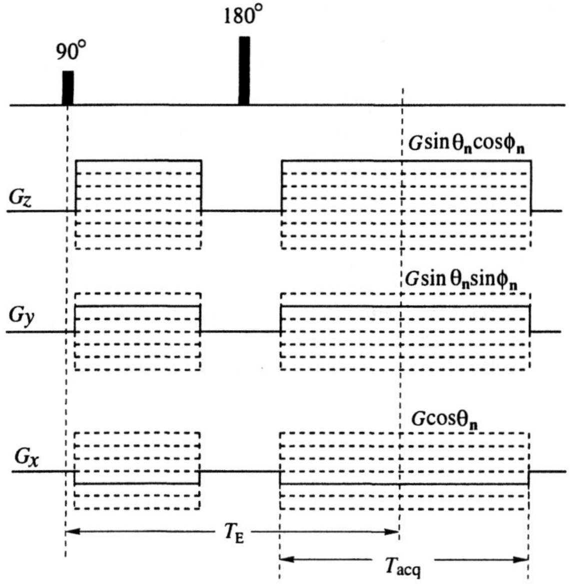

Figure 5.21   Three-dimensional frequency-encoding imaging sequence.

5.4   Sampling of k-Space

The discussion in Section 5.3 indicates that the key to multidimensional imaging lies in generating a sufficient number of signals to cover k-space. This section describes the sampling requirements of k-space signals. We first review the basic Shannon sampling theorem and then discuss its implications for selecting the data acquisition parameters.

5.4.1   The Sampling Theorem

Let us first review the definitions of some bandlimited signals.

Definition 5.1 *A time signal $g(t)$ is said to be time-limited if $g(t) = 0$ for $t > T$, where T is a finite number.*

Definition 5.2 *A time signal $g(t)$ is said to be (frequency) bandlimited if its frequency spectrum $\{\mathcal{F}g\}(f)$ is zero for $|f| > f_{\max}$, with $f_{\max}$ being the signal's frequency bandwidth.*

Definition 5.3 *A space signal $g(x)$ is said to be space-limited if $g(x) = 0$ for $|x| > W$.*

Definition 5.4 *A space signal $g(x)$ is said to be (frequency) bandlimited if its frequency spectrum $\{\mathcal{F}g\}(k)$ is zero for $|k| > k_{\max}$, with $k_{\max}$ being the signal's frequency bandwidth.*

We next describe the basic sampling theorem and some of its generalizations without proof. The reader interested in a thorough discussion of this topic is referred to [44, 45].

5.4.1.1 Uniform Sampling

The Shannon sampling theorem states that a bandlimited function can be reconstructed perfectly from its sampled values taken uniformly at an interval not exceeding the reciprocal of twice the signal bandwidth.

To be more specific, let $g(t)$ be bandlimited to $f_{\max}$. The sampling theorem requires that

$$\Delta t \le \frac{1}{2f_{\max}} \qquad \text{or} \qquad f_{\mathrm{s}} = \frac{1}{\Delta t} \ge 2f_{\max} \tag{5.114}$$

which is known as the *Nyquist sampling criterion*. The largest sampling interval permissible by the Nyquist criterion is $\Delta t = 1/(2f_{\max})$, which is called the *Nyquist interval*. Correspondingly, $f_{\mathrm{s}} = 2f_{\max}$ is called the *Nyquist frequency*, which is the minimum sampling rate required for exact recovery of $g(t)$.

Let $g(n\Delta t)$ be the sampled values taken from $g(t)$, with Δt satisfying the Nyquist criterion. Then, $g(t)$ can be reconstructed from $g(n\Delta t)$ using the following well-known interpolation formula:

$$g(t) = \sum_{n=-\infty}^{\infty} g(n\Delta t)\mathrm{sinc}[\pi f_{\mathrm{s}}(t - n\Delta t)] \tag{5.115}$$

which is illustrated in Fig. 5.22. It is also easy to show that Eq. (5.115) can be written in terms of the signal bandwidth as

$$g(t) = \frac{2f_{\max}}{f_{\mathrm{s}}} \sum_{n=-\infty}^{\infty} g(n\Delta t)\mathrm{sinc}[2\pi f_{\max}(t - n\Delta t)] \tag{5.116}$$

5.4.1.2 Interlaced Sampling

Interlaced sampling is a special case of nonuniform sampling, which finds useful application in echo-planar imaging discussed in Chapter 9. As shown in Fig. 5.23, interlaced sampling satisfies the Nyquist criterion in the average sense

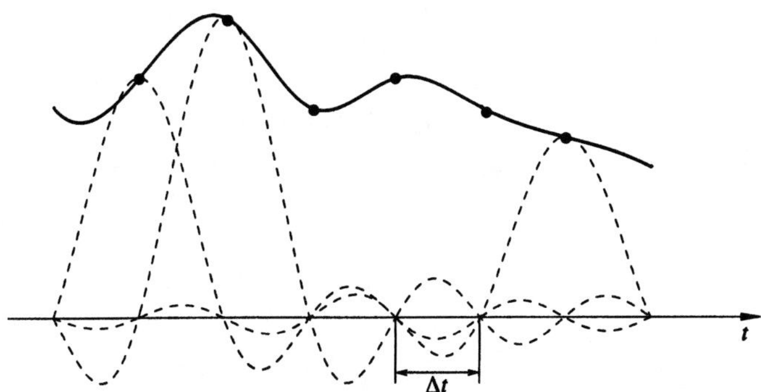

Figure 5.22   Illustration of the recovery of a continuous function from its samples by a summation of weighted sinc functions.

if $\Delta t \leq 1/f_{\max}$. It has been shown [44] that $g(t)$ can be recovered from this set of nonuniformly sampled values using the following interpolation formula:

$$g(t) = \sum_{n=-\infty}^{\infty} [g(n\Delta t)h(t - n\Delta t) + g(n\Delta t + \delta)h(-t + n\Delta t + \delta)] \quad (5.117)$$

where the interpolation kernel function $h(t)$ is given by

$$h(t) = \frac{\cos(2\pi f_{\max}t - \pi\delta f_{\max}) - \cos(\pi\delta f_{\max})}{2\pi f_{\max}t \sin(\pi\delta f_{\max})} \quad (5.118)$$

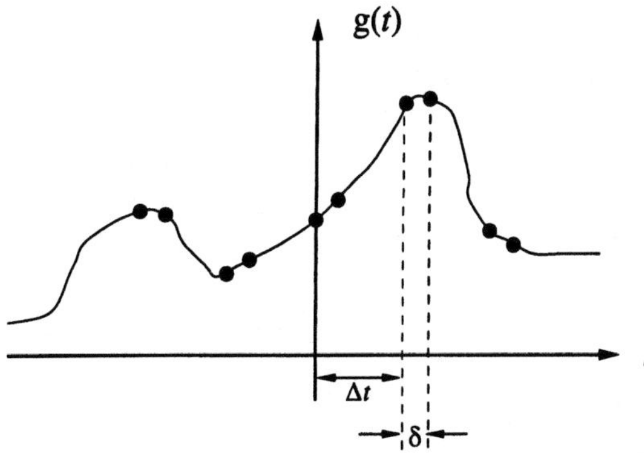

Figure 5.23   An example of interlaced sampling.

5.4.1.3   Sampling of Bandlimited Periodic Functions

It is well known that periodic functions (satisfying the Dirichlet conditions) can be expressed in terms of the Fourier series. If a periodic function is also bandlimited, the Fourier series will have only a finite number of terms. We summarize the result regarding the sampling of these functions here because it is useful for describing polar sampling of k-space.

Consider the following finite Fourier series:

$$g(t) = \sum_{n=-N}^{N} c_n e^{-i2\pi nt/T} \tag{5.119}$$

Clearly, $g(t)$ is periodic in t with period T and bandlimited to N/T. Since $g(t)$ is uniquely specified by the $2N + 1$ coefficients, it is expected that $2N + 1$ samples taken within a single period would suffice to uniquely reconstruct $g(t)$. Therefore, the Nyquist sampling criterion in this case can be stated as

$$\Delta t \leq \frac{T}{2N + 1} \tag{5.120}$$

Assume that $N_s \geq 2N + 1$ samples are taken from $g(t)$ in interval $\Delta t = T/N_s$. It has been shown that $g(t)$ can be reconstructed from this set of samples using the following interpolation formula:

$$g(t) = \sum_{n=0}^{N_s-1} g(n\Delta t) \frac{\sin\left[\frac{\pi}{T}(2N + 1)(t - n\Delta t)\right]}{N_s \sin\left[\frac{\pi}{T}(t - n\Delta t)\right]} \tag{5.121}$$

Detailed derivation of Eq. (5.121) can be found in [45, 252].

5.4.2   Sampling Requirements of k-Space Signals

Sampling of k-space is a multidimensional sampling problem. In practice, however, one treats sampling along each dimension separately, thus reducing it to a one-dimensional sampling problem. The resulting sampling pattern is not optimal; nonetheless, it guarantees "perfect" reconstruction of the underlying continuous k-space signal. We therefore adopt this conventional treatment to determine the sampling requirements on the MRI data acquisition parameters for two popular imaging schemes: rectilinear sampling and polar sampling. Here, we consider only two-dimensional imaging, since the treatment can be easily extended to higher-dimensional cases if necessary.

We first consider the rectilinear sampling case. Assume that the object being imaged is bounded by a rectangle of widths W_x and W_y, as shown in Fig. 5.24. Then, according to the sampling theorem we have

$$\Delta k_x \leq \frac{1}{W_x} \quad \text{and} \quad \Delta k_y \leq \frac{1}{W_y} \tag{5.122}$$

We further assume that frequency encoding is used along the x-direction and phase encoding is used along the y-direction. Then,

$$\begin{cases} \Delta k_x = \gamma |G_x| \Delta t \\ \Delta k_y = \gamma \Delta G_y T_{\text{pe}} \end{cases} \tag{5.123}$$

where

$$\begin{aligned} G_x &: & \text{frequency-encoding gradient} \\ \Delta t &: & \text{readout sampling time interval} \\ \Delta G_y &: & \text{phase-encoding gradient step size} \\ T_{\text{pe}} &: & \text{phase-encoding interval} \end{aligned}$$

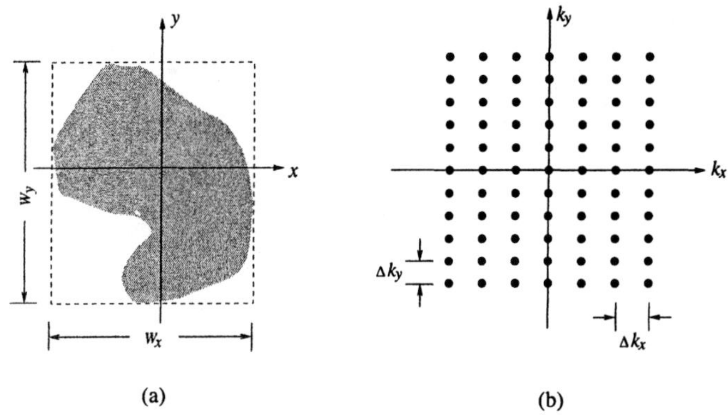

Figure 5.24   Illustration of (a) an object bounded by a rectangle of widths W_x and W_y, and (b) rectilinear sampling of k-space.

Substituting Eq. (5.123) into Eq. (5.122), we immediately obtain the following requirements on the data acquisition parameters:

$$\begin{cases} \Delta t \leq \dfrac{2\pi}{\gamma |G_x| W_x} \\ \Delta G_y \leq \dfrac{2\pi}{\gamma T_{\text{pe}} W_y} \end{cases} \tag{5.124}$$

We next consider the polar sampling case. In this imaging scheme, there are two essential data acquisition parameters: Δk and $\Delta \phi$. To obtain the requirements on these parameters, the following two standard assumptions are made:

(a) Space-limitedness (Fig. 5.25a):

$$\rho(x, y) = 0 \quad \text{for} \quad \sqrt{x^2 + y^2} \geq R_x \tag{5.125}$$

(b) Frequency-limitedness (Fig. 5.25b):

$$S(k_x, k_y) = \mathcal{F}\rho = 0 \quad \text{for} \quad \sqrt{k_x^2 + k_y^2} \geq R_k \tag{5.126}$$

The first assumption is valid because practical object functions are space limited. The second assumption is only an approximation since a function cannot be both space- and frequency-limited at the same time. This assumption is, however, necessary to enable us to derive a minimum sampling requirement along the ϕ-direction.

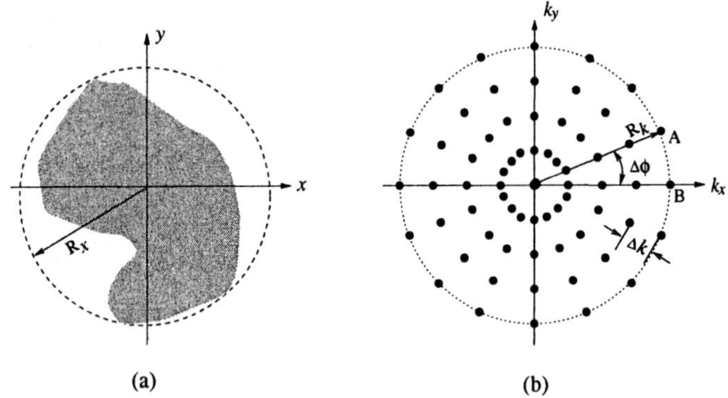

Figure 5.25   Illustration of (a) an object bounded by a circle of radius R_x and (b) polar sampling of k-space.

With assumption (a), the sampling requirement along the k-direction for each ϕ can be found easily. Specifically, it is easy to show that

$$\Delta k = \gamma G \Delta t \leq \frac{1}{2R_x} \tag{5.127}$$

or

$$\Delta t \leq \frac{\pi}{\gamma G R_x} \tag{5.128}$$

where $G = \sqrt{G_x^2 + G_y^2}$.

Determining the minimum sampling requirement along the ϕ-direction is more complicated than determining it along the k-direction. Because $S_p(k, \phi)$ is periodic in ϕ for a given k, we can express it in terms of the Fourier series as

$$S_p(k, \phi) = \sum_{n=-\infty}^{\infty} c_n(k) e^{-in\phi} \tag{5.129}$$

where

$$c_n(k) = \frac{1}{2\pi} \int_{-\pi}^{\pi} S_p(k, \phi) e^{in\phi} d\phi \tag{5.130}$$

The largest angular sampling interval $\Delta\phi$ allowed for $S_p(k, \phi)$ is determined by the number of significant terms in the Fourier series in Eq. (5.129). For a circularly symmetric object, $S_p(k, \phi)$ is a constant over ϕ and the series will have only a dc term. In general, the number of significant terms increases with $|k|$. A well-known result concerning this problem is derived in [231], which states that $S_p(k, \phi)$ is bandlimited to $R_x 2\pi|k| + 1$ with respect to ϕ. In other words, the Fourier series coefficients $c_n(k)$ in Eq. (5.129) are not significant for $|n| > [R_x 2\pi|k|] + 1$, where the brackets represent rounding $R_x 2\pi|k|$ to the next higher integer. Based on the assumption of frequency-limitedness stated in Eq. (5.126), c_n can be ignored for any measured k values if $|n| > [2\pi R_x R_k] + 1$. Therefore, according to the results concerning sampling of bandlimited periodic functions presented in Section 5.4.1, the angular sampling interval that satisfies the Nyquist criterion for all of the sampled k values is given by

$$\Delta\phi \leq \frac{2\pi}{2([2\pi R_x R_k] + 1) + 1} \tag{5.131}$$

A more insightful relationship can be derived based on Eq. (5.131), which directly relates the number of radial lines (or projections), denoted by N_ϕ, to the number of samples per line, denoted by N_k. More specifically, taking into account the fact that data at $n\Delta\phi$ and $n\Delta\phi + \pi$ are collected simultaneously, we can express N_ϕ as

$$N_\phi = \frac{\pi}{\Delta\phi} \geq [2\pi R_x R_k] + 1.5 \tag{5.132}$$

Replacing R_x and R_k with

$$R_x = \frac{1}{2\Delta k} \tag{5.133}$$

and

$$R_k = \frac{N_k}{2}\Delta k \tag{5.134}$$

we immediately get

$$\frac{N_\phi}{N_k} \approx \frac{\pi}{2} \tag{5.135}$$

Equation (5.135) indicates that the number of projections required is roughly the same as the number of samples per projection.

Interestingly, the result in Eq. (5.135) can also be obtained by setting the worst-case azimuthal resolution and the radial resolution to be approximately the same. Inspection of Fig. 5.25 indicates that the worst-case azimuthal resolution is given by

$$\overline{AB} = \Delta\phi R_k = \frac{\pi}{N_\phi}\frac{N_k}{2}\Delta k \tag{5.136}$$

Setting $\overline{AB} \approx \Delta k$ immediately yields Eq. (5.135).

Exercises

5.1 Selection of an envelope function for an RF pulse has nothing to do with the B_0 field strength. True or false? Why?

5.2 Why do we need stronger frequency-encoding gradients for imaging at higher fields?

5.3 Phase-encoded spin-echo signals should decay faster than nonencoded spin-echo signals. True or false? Why?

5.4 What is the cross-talk artifact in slice-selective excitations? How can it be reduced?

5.5 In slice-selective excitation, how is the width of a selected slice related to the strength of the slice-selection gradient? Assume that G_z is the desired gradient strength. What is the consequence if the gradient system malfunctions such that the effective gradient the object sees is

(a) $G_{\text{eff}} = 0$

(b) $G_{\text{eff}} = G_z/2$

(c) $G_{\text{eff}} = 2G_z$

5.6 Assume that in the presence of a z-gradient (G_z) only, a given slice-selective pulse $B_1(t)$ excites a slice defined by $z = z_0$ of width Δz such that $\gamma G_z z_0 = f_0$. Which slice will $B_1(t)$ excite if G_x, G_y, and G_z are turned on simultaneously during the excitation?

(a) Derive the equation describing the new slice selected.

(b) Calculate the new slice thickness in terms of Δz_0.

5.7 Slice-selective excitation is made possible through the use of an inhomogeneous magnetic field. No matter what kind of field distribution we have, a frequency-selective pulse will always excite spins on a plane of a certain orientation and thickness. True or false? If your answer is "false," give an example showing that a nonplanar slice is selected by an RF pulse.

5.8 Phase encoding of spatial information is achieved by assigning different initial phase angles to local NMR signals. True or false?

5.9 Explain why a frequency-encoded signal decays faster than its nonencoded counterpart.

5.10 Why do we need to use multiple phase-encoding gradient values but only one frequency-encoding gradient value in the conventional phase-encoding imaging excitation sequence? Discuss whether the same thing could be accomplished with a single phase-encoding gradient value but with a variable gradient duration.

5.11 Echo signals (spin echoes or gradient echoes) are often used in MRI primarily because:

(a) They are useful for symmetric k-space sampling.

(b) They are always available.

(c) They are easier to generate than FID signals.

(d) None of the above.

Select all the answers that apply.

5.12 For the excitation sequence shown in (a), the FID signals generated are mapped to k-space as shown in (b). Discuss how to modify this excitation sequence so that the FID signals will generate the k-space coverage shown in (c).

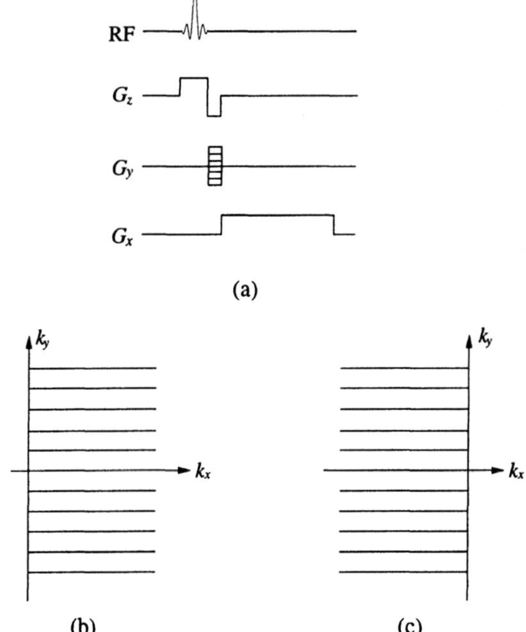

5.13 For the following three excitation schemes,

(a) Find the mathematical expression for the activated signal.

(b) Assuming that the signals are sampled with the same time interval Δt, sketch how the sampled data are mapped into k-space for each case.

Scheme 1:

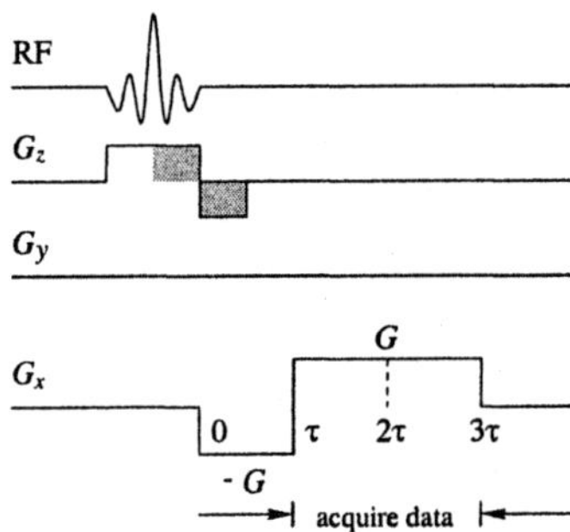

Scheme 2:

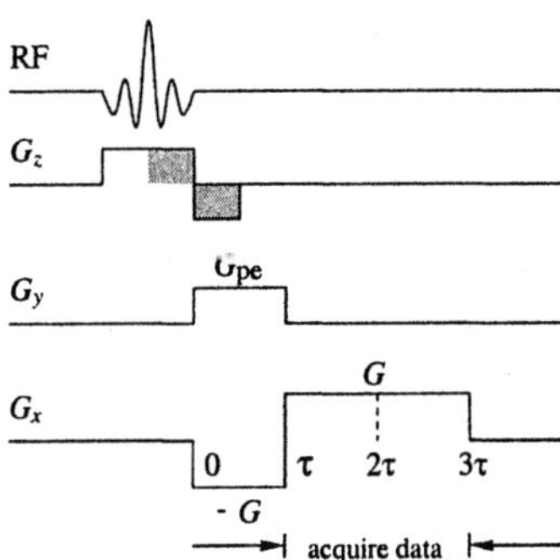

Scheme 3:

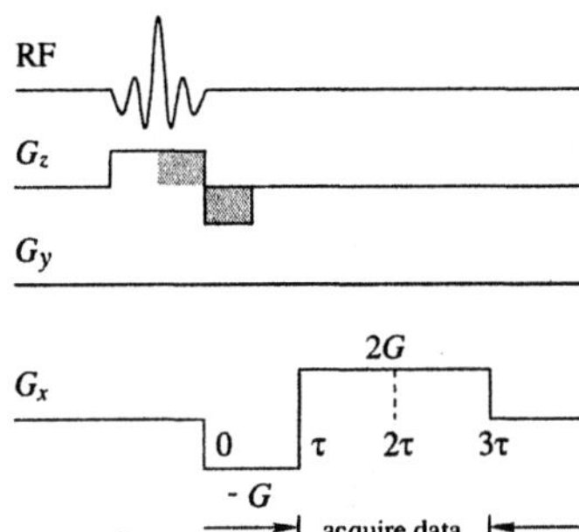

5.14 Draw a gradient-echo imaging sequence with rectilinear sampling of k-space.

5.15 Draw a gradient-echo imaging sequence with radial sampling of k-space.

5.16 An MRI system is equipped with a gradient system that can provide variable G_x and G_y gradients. Design a spin-echo imaging sequence that gives the k-space sampling trajectories shown below. Sketch the pulse sequence and specify the necessary gradient functions.

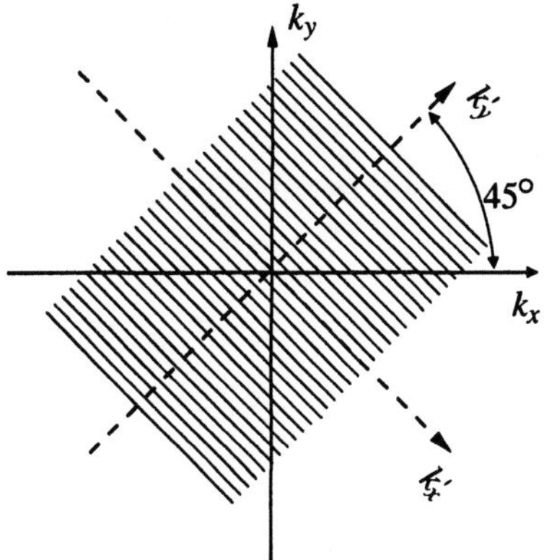

5.17 Design an excitation sequence to generate the concentric k-space coverage shown below, assuming each circle of data is from one excitation. Let $S_n(t)$ be the time signal generated by the nth excitation. Mark the k-space locations of the sampled data points $S_n(m\Delta t)$.

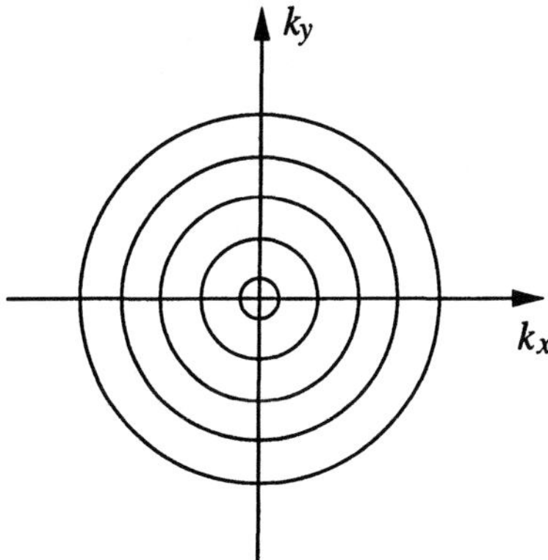

5.18 Design an excitation sequence that generates data mapped to the following elliptical k-space trajectory.

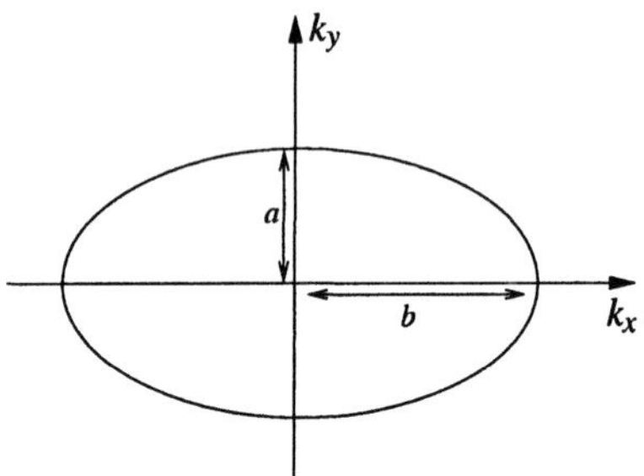

5.19   For the excitation sequences given below:

    (a)   Derive an expression for the FID signal.

    (b)   Map the time signal to k-space and sketch the sampling trajectory.

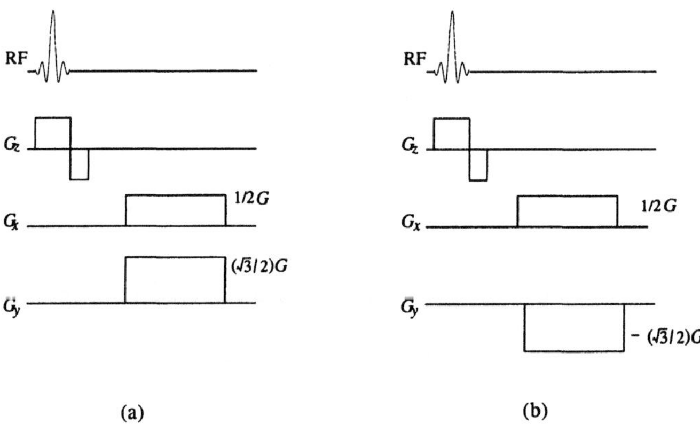

                    (a)   (b)

5.20   For a given object function $\rho(x, y)$, the frequency-encoded signal measured in the presence of a gradient G_x is $S_1(t)$, and its largest time interval permissible by the sampling theorem is Δt. Assume that a new signal $S_2(t)$ is measured in the presence of a frequency-encoding gradient twice the strength of G_x.

    (a)   How is the new measured signal $S_2(t)$ related to $S_1(t)$?

    (b)   What is the largest sampling interval allowed for $S_2(t)$?

    (c)   If the inverse Fourier transform (with respect to t) of $S_1(t)$ and $S_2(t)$ is $\tilde{\rho}_1(x)$ and $\tilde{\rho}_2(x)$, respectively, how is $\tilde{\rho}_1(x)$ related to $\tilde{\rho}_2(x)$ and to $\rho(x, y)$?

5.21 Determine the frequency bandwidth of the following signals:

(a) $\sin(10\pi t + 45°) + e^{i2.5\pi t}$

(b) $\mathrm{sinc}(\pi t)$

(c) $\mathrm{sinc}^2(\pi t)$

(d) $\mathrm{sinc}(\pi t) + \mathrm{sinc}^2(\pi t)$

(e) $\mathrm{sinc}(\pi t)\cos(100\pi t)$

5.22 Let $g(t)$ be a signal with Nyquist frequency f_s. Determine the Nyquist frequency for each of the following signals:

(a) $g(t) + g(t - 3)$

(b) $\dfrac{dg(t)}{dt}$

(c) $g^2(t)$

(d) $g(t)\cos f_s t$

5.23 Show that if $g(t)$ is bandlimited to $f_{\max}$, then

$$g(t) = g(t) * 2f_{\max}\mathrm{sinc}(2\pi f_{\max}t)$$

5.24 Derive Eq. (5.116) from Eq. (5.115).

Chapter 6

Image Reconstruction

One picture is worth a thousand words.

Old folk saying

Image synthesis (or reconstruction) is an important topic of tomographic imaging because spatial information is encoded into the measured data during the data acquisition step. Depending on how spatial information is encoded into the measured data, the image reconstruction technique necessary can vary considerably. In this chapter, we single out two fundamental image reconstruction problems for detailed discussion: (a) reconstruction from Fourier transform samples, and (b) reconstruction from Radon transform samples. Many practical MRI data acquisition schemes lend themselves naturally to one of these two reconstruction problems. For example, if k-space is sampled rectilinearly as shown in Fig. 6.1a, we directly have the first reconstruction problem; if k-space is sampled radially as shown in Fig. 6.1b, we have the second reconstruction problem. For other k-space coverage, signal interpolation is often used to regrid the measured data into one of these two "standard" formats so that a basic reconstruction algorithm can be applied.

This chapter is organized as follows. First, some general issues in image reconstruction are discussed. Then, the theory and algorithms of Fourier reconstruction are described. Finally, image reconstruction from Radon transform data is discussed, starting with a detailed description of the inverse Radon transform, which is followed by an exposition of various practical algorithms. Advanced topics of image reconstruction are presented in Chapter 10.

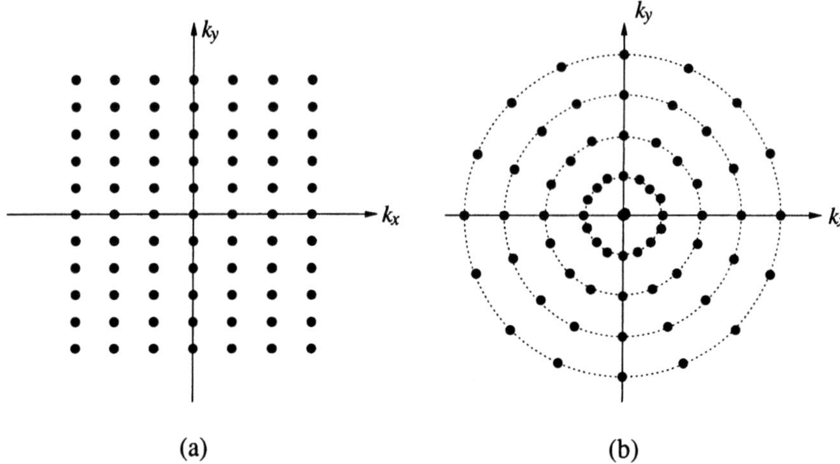

Figure 6.1 Two basic k-space coverage used in MRI experiments.

6.1 General Issues of Image Reconstruction

We may formally state the image reconstruction problem as finding an image function I that is consistent with the measured signal S according to a known imaging equation:

$$S = \mathcal{T}\{\mathcal{I}\} \tag{6.1}$$

where $\mathcal{T}$ is usually an integral transformation operator. In MRI, $\mathcal{T}$ represents any of the spatial information encoding schemes. Equation (6.1) is often referred to as the data-consistency constraint, and any function satisfying this constraint is called a *feasible reconstruction*. A more formal definition of feasible reconstruction is as follows.

Definition 6.1 *An arbitrary function is a feasible reconstruction if a physical object built based on this function will produce the measured data with the same experimental procedure.*

The data-consistency constraint is important because image reconstruction does no more than convert information in the measured data into an image format. A violation of the data-consistency constraint can mean that this conversion step is not faithful, and a loss of valid information or a gain of spurious information may result. Nevertheless, it should not be taken for granted that any image reconstruction technique satisfies the data-consistency constraint. In practice, data consistency can be sacrificed in a controlled way in exchange for other more desirable image properties. For example, in the windowed Fourier reconstruction technique described later, the data-consistency constraint is purposely violated to reduce the Gibbs ringing artifact described in Chapter 8.

Theoretically, if $\mathcal{T}$ is invertible, a data-consistent I can be obtained from the inverse transform such that

$$I = \mathcal{T}^{-1}\{S\} \tag{6.2}$$

However, in real life $\mathcal{T}^{-1}\{S\}$ cannot be computed because the data space is only partially sampled. Therefore, instead of directly implementing the inversion formula, one focuses on finding an image function that satisfies the data-consistency constraint either by an approximate implementation of the inverse transform or by methods that may have nothing to do with it. Some general issues with such an image reconstruction procedure are *existence*, *uniqueness*, and *stability*.

It is easy to understand that, given a set of measured data, an image function I that is consistent with the data always exists since the data are generated from a physical object. Whether such an image function is unique depends on how the data space is sampled. If finite sampling is used, as is always the case in practice, there are many feasible image functions for the given measured data. In this case, some optimality criterion has to be applied to select an image from the many feasible ones, a topic discussed further in later sections. Stability of an image reconstruction technique is related to how perturbations in the data domain are translated to possible image errors. More specifically, if the data are perturbed by ΔS and, as a consequence, the image function is in error by ΔI, then

$$S + \Delta S = \mathcal{T}\{I + \Delta I\} \tag{6.3}$$

An important practical question is: will ΔI be small for a small ΔS? The answer is not necessarily yes. For example, for Fourier imaging, $\mathcal{T}$ is the Fourier transform operator. According to the well-known Riemann–Lebesgue lemma, we can add a frequency component of arbitrarily large amplitude to the image function without greatly perturbing the k-space data. For example, let

$$\Delta I = A \sin(2\pi k_0 x) \tag{6.4}$$

Then, we have (see Problem 6.1)

$$\lim_{k_0 \to \infty} \Delta S = \lim_{k_0 \to \infty} \int_{-W_x/2}^{W_x/2} \Delta I(x) e^{-i2\pi kx} dx = 0 \tag{6.5}$$

where W_x is the size of the object. Equations (6.4) and (6.5) imply that ΔS can be made negligible while ΔI is arbitrarily large. An operator with this property is called *ill-conditioned*. Because most imaging operators are ill-conditioned in nature and do not have a unique solution owing to finite sampling, the reconstruction problem is considered to be an *ill-posed* problem. Consequently, obtaining the exact true image function is theoretically impossible, which caused some doubts about the practical usefulness of tomographic imaging in the early days. However, as we will find out later, if we pick the image function "appropriately," an acceptable image can be obtained with a known deviation from the true image function. This deviation can be fully characterized by a point spread function if the imaging process is linear, and it can be made negligible under certain circumstances. The rest of the chapter takes up the specifics of various image reconstruction algorithms.

6.2 Reconstruction from Fourier Transform Samples

6.2.1 Problem Formulation

The problem of reconstructing a function from its Fourier transform samples can be formulated as follows:

$$\text{Given} \quad S(k_n) = \int I(r)e^{-i2\pi k_n \cdot r}\,dr \quad k_n \in \mathcal{D} \quad (6.6)$$

$$\text{determine} \quad I(r)$$

where $\mathcal{D}$ contains the set of k-space points at which measured data are collected.

This problem occurs in many scientific disciplines and was studied long before the birth of MRI. It is now widely known that given a set of uniformly sampled Fourier transform samples, the discrete Fourier transform (DFT) is the computational tool to use for image reconstruction. This section discusses the theoretical basis and limitations of the DFT image reconstruction technique.

6.2.2 Basic Theory

To simplify our presentation, we consider only the one-dimensional case here. This simplification is acceptable owing to the separability of the multidimensional Fourier transform discussed in Section 2.5.

In the one-dimensional case, Eq. (6.6) can be written as

$$S(k_n) = \int_{-\infty}^{\infty} I(x)e^{-i2\pi k_n x}\,dx \quad (6.7)$$

Furthermore, assume that k-space is uniformly sampled such that

$$\mathcal{D} = \{k_n = n\Delta k, n = \ldots, -2, -1, 0, 1, 2, \ldots\} \quad (6.8)$$

The imaging equation becomes

$$S[n] = S(n\Delta k) = \int_{-\infty}^{\infty} I(x)e^{-i2\pi n\Delta k x}\,dx \quad (6.9)$$

An important formula governing how to reconstruct $I(x)$ from $S(n\Delta k)$ is

$$\sum_{n=-\infty}^{\infty} S[n]e^{i2\pi n\Delta kx} = \frac{1}{\Delta k}\sum_{n=-\infty}^{\infty} I\left(x - \frac{n}{\Delta k}\right) \qquad (6.10)$$

The left-hand side of Eq. (6.10) can be viewed as a Fourier series, with Δk being the fundamental frequency and $S[n]$ being the series coefficient of the nth harmonic. The right-hand side is a periodic extension of $I(x)$ with period $1/\Delta k$. Equation (6.10) can be proven as follows.

First, the following equality (commonly known as the *Poisson formula*) holds in a distribution sense (see Example 2.7):

$$\sum_{n=-\infty}^{\infty} e^{i2\pi n\Delta kx} = \frac{1}{\Delta k}\sum_{n=-\infty}^{\infty} \delta\left(x - \frac{n}{\Delta k}\right) \qquad (6.11)$$

Next, based on the definition we have

$$\sum_{n=-\infty}^{\infty} S[n]e^{i2\pi n\Delta kx} = \sum_{n=-\infty}^{\infty}\left[\int_{-\infty}^{\infty} I(\hat{x})e^{-i2\pi n\Delta k\hat{x}}\,d\hat{x}\right]e^{i2\pi n\Delta kx}$$

$$= \sum_{n=-\infty}^{\infty}\int_{-\infty}^{\infty} I(\hat{x})e^{i2\pi n\Delta k(x-\hat{x})}\,d\hat{x}$$

$$= \int_{-\infty}^{\infty} I(\hat{x})\sum_{n=-\infty}^{\infty} e^{i2\pi n\Delta k(x-\hat{x})}\,d\hat{x}$$

$$= \int_{-\infty}^{\infty} I(\hat{x})\frac{1}{\Delta k}\sum_{n=-\infty}^{\infty} \delta\left(x - \hat{x} - \frac{n}{\Delta k}\right)d\hat{x}$$

$$= \frac{1}{\Delta k}\sum_{n=-\infty}^{\infty}\int_{-\infty}^{\infty} I(\hat{x})\delta\left(x - \hat{x} - \frac{n}{\Delta k}\right)d\hat{x}$$

$$= \frac{1}{\Delta k}\sum_{n=-\infty}^{\infty} I\left(x - \frac{n}{\Delta k}\right)$$

which proves the result in Eq. (6.10).

■ **Example 6.1**

This example examines the periodic extension of a support-limited function and its Fourier series representation.

Consider $I(x) = \Lambda(x)$ shown in Fig. 6.2a. We construct

$$\tilde{I}_1(x) = \sum_{n=-\infty}^{\infty} \Lambda(x - 2n)$$

and

$$\tilde{I}_2(x) = \sum_{n=-\infty}^{\infty} \Lambda(x - 3n)$$

Clearly, $\tilde{I}_1(x)$ and $\tilde{I}_2(x)$ are periodic extensions of $I(x)$ with period 2 and 3, respectively, as can be seen from Figs. 6.2b and 6.2c. To calculate their Fourier series representations, we need to know the Fourier transform of $\Lambda(x)$. From Example 2.4, we have

$$\mathcal{F}\Lambda(k) = \mathrm{sinc}^2(\pi k)$$

The fundamental frequencies of $\tilde{I}_1(x)$ and $\tilde{I}_2(x)$ are $\Delta k = \frac{1}{2}$ and $\frac{1}{3}$, respectively. Therefore,

$$\tilde{I}_1(x) = \frac{1}{2} \sum_{n=-\infty}^{\infty} \mathrm{sinc}^2(n\pi/2) e^{in\pi x}$$

and

$$\tilde{I}_1(x) = \frac{1}{3} \sum_{n=-\infty}^{\infty} \mathrm{sinc}^2(n\pi/3) e^{i2n\pi x/3}$$

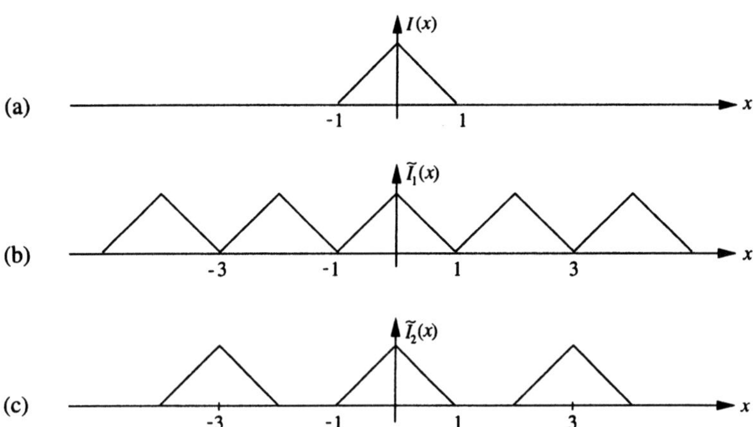

Figure 6.2   Illustration of $\Lambda(x)$ and its periodic extensions.

In the remainder of this section, we derive the Fourier reconstruction formulas based on Eq. (6.10). For clarity, we first discuss the infinite sampling case and then extend the result to the practical case of finite sampling.

6.2.2.1 Infinite Sampling

In this hypothetical case of infinite sampling, $S(k)$ is available at $k \in \mathcal{D}$, where

$$\mathcal{D} = \{n\Delta k, -\infty < n < \infty\} \tag{6.12}$$

Therefore, there is sufficient information to define the Fourier series in Eq. (6.10). The question now is if $I(x)$ can be recovered from its periodic extension as defined in Eq. (6.10). The answer is yes provided that Δk satisfies the Nyquist sampling criterion discussed in Section 5.4. To illustrate this point, we first make use of the fact that any practical $I(x)$ is a support-limited function. That is, there exists a finite W_x such that

$$I(x) = 0, \qquad |x| > W_x/2 \tag{6.13}$$

where the region defined by $|x| < W_x/2$ is referred to as the *field of view* (FOV) in the MRI literature.

If the relationship

$$W_x < \frac{1}{\Delta k} \qquad \text{or} \qquad \Delta k < \frac{1}{W_x} \tag{6.14}$$

holds, then there is no overlap among the various periodic replicas $I(x - n/\Delta k)$ for different n. Hence, one can obtain $I(x)$ from the Fourier series as formed in Eq. (6.10) by chunking out any period. More specifically,

$$I(x) = \Delta k \Pi \left(\frac{x}{\Delta k}\right) \sum_{n=-\infty}^{\infty} S[n] e^{i2\pi n \Delta k x} \tag{6.15}$$

In practice, $I(x)$ is evaluated only within the FOV; the scoping function, $\Pi(x/\Delta k)$, is often dropped from Eq. (6.15) for notational convenience. Therefore, the reconstruction formula is simply written as

$$I(x) = \Delta k \sum_{n=-\infty}^{\infty} S[n] e^{i2\pi n \Delta k x} \qquad |x| < \frac{1}{\Delta k} \tag{6.16}$$

This convention will be followed in the rest of the book whenever it is not necessary to make the distinction between the support-limited image function and the corresponding Fourier series representation.

6.2.2.2 Finite Sampling

In many practical situations, only a finite number of k-space points are collected. Following convention, we assume that $S(k)$ is known for $k \in \mathcal{D}$, where

$$\mathcal{D} = \{n\Delta k, -N/2 \le n < N/2\} \tag{6.17}$$

This set of data is not sufficient to define the Fourier series as required by the reconstruction formula in Eq. (6.16). As a result, the feasible reconstruction is not unique.

Remark 6.1 *If $I(x)$ is a feasible reconstruction, then $\hat{I}(x) = I(x) + e^{i2\pi m\Delta k x}$ is also a feasible reconstruction for any $|m| > N/2$*

Remark 6.2 *$I(x)$ given in Eq. (6.16) is a feasible reconstruction, if the unmeasured coefficients take finite arbitrary values. In other words,*

$$I(x) = \Delta k \sum_{n=-N/2}^{N/2-1} S[n]e^{i2\pi n\Delta k x} + \sum_{n<-N/2; n\ge N/2} c_n e^{i2\pi n\Delta k x} \tag{6.18}$$

is a feasible reconstruction for arbitrary (finite) c_n.

An important question regarding image reconstruction from finite Fourier transform samples is: what values should we assign to the c_n? Clearly, the answer is application-dependent. In practice, the c_n is often selected based on the minimum-norm constraint.[1] As a result, the unmeasured Fourier series coefficients are all forced to be zero because, according to the Parseval theorem,

$$\int_{-\frac{\Delta k}{2}}^{\frac{\Delta k}{2}} |I(x)|^2 dx = \Delta k^2 \sum_{n=-N/2}^{N/2-1} |S[n]|^2 + \sum_{n<-N/2; n\ge N/2} |c_n|^2 \tag{6.19}$$

which reaches the minimum when $c_n = 0$. Therefore, the minimum-norm, feasible reconstruction is in the form of a truncated Fourier series:

$$I(x) = \Delta k \sum_{n=-N/2}^{N/2-1} S[n]e^{i2\pi n\Delta k x} \qquad |x| < \frac{1}{\Delta k} \tag{6.20}$$

Equation (6.20) is popularly known as the *Fourier reconstruction formula*.

Clearly, the Fourier reconstruction is not identical to the true image function. In fact, as a result of the series truncation, the inherent data continuity of $S(k)$ is violated,[2] leading to the well-known *Gibbs ringing artifact*, further characterized

---

[1] Reconstruction using other constraints is discussed in Chapter 10.

[2] Note that $S(k)$ is an analytic function from the discussion in Section 2.5.

in Chapter 8. A simple way to cope with this problem is to multiply the data with a window (or filter) function w_n that decays smoothly to zero at $n = \pm N/2$. A variety of such filter functions are available. The most popular one is perhaps the Hamming window function[3] defined in Section 2.3. After a filter function is selected, the windowed Fourier (series) reconstruction is then given by

$$I(x) = \Delta k \sum_{n=-N/2}^{N/2-1} S[n] w_n e^{i2\pi n \Delta k x} \qquad |x| < \frac{1}{\Delta k} \qquad (6.21)$$

Note that the windowed Fourier reconstruction is not data-consistent since

$$\int_{-\Delta k/2}^{\Delta k/2} I(x) e^{-i2\pi n \Delta k x} dx = w_n S[n] \qquad (6.22)$$

One will see from Chapter 8 that this violation of data consistency manifests itself as a loss of spatial resolution. For this reason, it is commonly said that windowed Fourier reconstruction reduces Gibbs ringing at the expense of spatial resolution (rather than data consistency).

6.2.3   Computational Algorithms

We now discuss the formation of a digital image from the continuous image function given in Eq. (6.20) or Eq. (6.21) through use of the fast Fourier transform (FFT) algorithm. Note that in spite of the discreteness of the measured data, the reconstructed image is a continuous function of space. Discretization of the image function is necessitated by numerical computation and display.

6.2.3.1   DFT and FFT

Given a finite-duration sequence d_n, $n = 0, 1, \ldots, N - 1$, its discrete Fourier transform (DFT) is another N-point sequence defined by

$$D_m = \sum_{n=0}^{N-1} d_n e^{-i2\pi mn/N} \qquad m = 0, 1, \ldots, N - 1 \qquad (6.23)$$

Given D_m, we can recover d_n exactly using the following formula:

$$d_n = \frac{1}{N} \sum_{n=0}^{N-1} D_m e^{i2\pi mn/N} \qquad n = 0, 1, \ldots, N - 1 \qquad (6.24)$$

---

[3] The Hamming window function needed here can be expressed as:

$$w_n = 0.54 + 0.46 \cos(2\pi n/N) \qquad \text{for } -N/2 \leq n < N/2$$

Equations (6.23) and (6.24) are often referred to as the *forward* and *inverse* transforms, respectively. Note that as defined here, d_n and D_m are periodic sequences of period N. Therefore, for a finite-duration sequence, its DFT representation automatically performs a periodic extension on d_n.

Direct evaluation of the DFT is time-consuming. Inspection of Eqs. (6.23) and (6.24) reveals that direct calculation of D_m or d_n requires N^2 multiplications and $N(N-1)$ additions, assuming that $e^{-i2\pi mn/N}$ is precalculated. In practice, the DFT is computed using a so-called fast Fourier transform (FFT) algorithm. The existence of an FFT algorithm became generally known only in the mid-1960s through the landmark work of Cooley and Tukey [126]. In retrospect, we now know that efficient algorithms for computing DFT had been independently discovered many times in history, starting with Gauss in 1805.

The fundamental principle underlying all FFT algorithms is that of decomposing the computation of the DFT of a sequence of length N into successively shorter DFTs. To illustrate this principle, we consider the special case of N being an integer power of 2. That is, $N = 2^r$ for an integer r. Since N is an even integer, we can split d_n into two $N/2$-point sequences consisting of the even-indexed points and odd-indexed points in d_n, respectively, such that

$$D_m = \sum_{n \text{ even}} d_n e^{-i2\pi mn/N} + \sum_{n \text{ odd}} d_n e^{-i2\pi mn/N} \tag{6.25}$$

Simple variable substitution yields

$$D_m = \sum_{p=0}^{N/2-1} d_{2p} e^{-i2\pi m2p/N} + \sum_{p=0}^{N/2-1} d_{2p+1} e^{-i2\pi m(2p+1)/N}$$

$$= \sum_{p=0}^{N/2-1} d_{2p} e^{-i2\pi mp/(N/2)} + e^{-i2\pi m/N} \sum_{p=0}^{N/2-1} d_{2p+1} e^{-i2\pi mp/(N/2)}$$

$$= G_m + e^{-i2\pi m/N} H_m \tag{6.26}$$

This decomposition is the core of the so-called *decimation-in-time radix-2 FFT algorithm*. Each sum in the decomposition can be recognized as an $N/2$-point DFT. Although the index m ranges over N values for D_m, G_m and H_m need only be computed for m between 0 and $N/2 - 1$ because they are each periodic in m with period $N/2$. With $N = 2^r$ the decomposition can be applied to the evaluation of G_m and H_m by breaking each down to two $N/4$-point DFTs, and the process continues until only two-point DFTs remain. The whole process requires $\log_2 N$ steps of decomposition. Since calculations at each step involve N multiplications and N additions, the whole process requires a total of $N \log_2 N$ multiplications and $N \log_2 N$ additions. Therefore, this algorithm offers tremendous savings in computational time over the straightforward method. For example, with $N = 1024$, $N^2 = 1,048,576$, $N \log_2 N = 10,240$, and the time-saving factor is $1,048,576/10,240 = 102.4$.

6.2.3.2 Direct FFT Reconstruction

To convert $I(x)$ given in Eq. (6.20) or Eq. (6.21) to a digital image, the sampling interval (or digital pixel size) has to satisfy the Nyquist criterion to avoid loss of image information. Since $I(x)$ is a frequency bandlimited function (because of finite sampling) in the sense that $\mathcal{F}\{I\}(k) = 0$ for $|k| > (N/2)\Delta k$, $I(x)$ can be uniquely recovered from $I[m] = I(m\Delta x)$ as long as $\Delta x \leq 1/(N\Delta k)$ according to the Nyquist criterion. Therefore, the largest acceptable pixel size for $I(x)$ is

$$\Delta x = \frac{1}{N\Delta k} \tag{6.27}$$

which is called the *Fourier pixel size*. At this pixel size, exactly N pixels are available within the FOV. Namely,

$$\frac{\text{FOV}}{\Delta x} = \frac{1/\Delta k}{1/N\Delta k} = N \tag{6.28}$$

The N pixels are determined by

$$I[m] = \Delta k \sum_{n=-N/2}^{N/2-1} S[n]e^{i2\pi nm/N} \qquad -N/2 \leq m < N/2 \tag{6.29}$$

Equation (6.29) is called the *direct DFT (or FFT) reconstruction*, which generates N pixels by directly applying the inverse FFT to an N-point measured data sequence.

Inspection of Eq. (6.29) reveals that given a data set $\{S[n]\}$, one can calculate $\{I[m]\}$ without knowing the precise value of Δk. Therefore, one can always treat $\Delta k = 1$ and, consequently, $\Delta x = 1/N$. With these normalized values for Δk and Δx, Eq. (6.29) can be rewritten as

$$I[m] = \sum_{n=-N/2}^{N/2-1} S[n]e^{i2\pi nm/N} \qquad -N/2 \leq m < N/2 \tag{6.30}$$

Another subtle point worth noting is that the standard FFT subroutine is rewritten according to the DFT sum as defined in Eqs. (6.23) and (6.24). To use such a routine to evaluate Eq. (6.30), some pre- and post-processing is needed. More specifically, let $\hat{m} = m + N/2$ and $\hat{n} = n + N/2$. Then $\hat{m}$ and $\hat{n}$ will each have values ranging from 0 to $N - 1$, and Eq. (6.30) can be converted to the standard DFT format as follows.

$$
\begin{aligned}
I[m] &= \sum_{\hat{n}=0}^{N-1} S[\hat{n} - N/2]e^{i2\pi(\hat{n}-N/2)m/N} \\
&= e^{-im\pi} \sum_{\hat{n}=0}^{N-1} S[\hat{n} - N/2]e^{i2\pi\hat{n}(\hat{m}-N/2)/N} \\
&= e^{-im\pi} \sum_{\hat{n}=0}^{N-1} S[\hat{n} - N/2]e^{-i\hat{n}\pi}e^{i2\pi\hat{n}\hat{m}/N} \\
&= (-1)^m \sum_{\hat{n}=0}^{N-1} (-1)^{\hat{n}} S[\hat{n} - N/2]e^{i2\pi\hat{n}\hat{m}/N}
\end{aligned}
\tag{6.31}
$$

or

$$
I[m - N/2] = (-1)^m \sum_{n=0}^{N-1} (-1)^n S[n - N/2]e^{i2\pi nm/N}
\tag{6.32}
$$

Equation (6.32) suggests that we first reverse the sign of the alternate elements in S_n, then feed it to an FFT routine, and finally change the sign of the alternate elements of the output sequence. This processing scheme is schematically shown in Fig. 6.3.

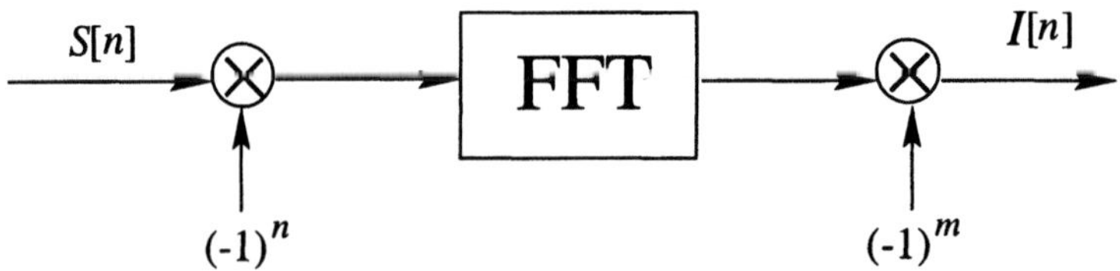

Figure 6.3 Schematic diagram of direct FFT reconstruction from symmetric k-space data.

6.2.3.3 Zero-Filled FFT Reconstruction

Zero-filled FFT reconstruction differs from direct FFT reconstruction in that the data sequence is padded with zeros at one or both ends before the FFT algorithm is applied. Zero-padding is used for two main reasons. First, if N is not an integer power of 2, padding the data set with zeros will bring its length to the next power of two so that the radix-2 FFT algorithm can be used. For example, with $N = 96$, padding 32 zeros to the data sequence will bring its length to $128 = 2^7$. Second, and perhaps more frequently used, zero-padding increases the digital resolution of the resulting image, thus generating the so-called digital zooming or interpolation effect.

To understand the interpolation effect, let us suppose that $\hat{N} > N$ pixels are desired from $I(x)$ with pixel size $\Delta\hat{x} = 1/(\hat{N}\Delta k) = 1/\hat{N}$ with $\Delta k = 1$. Based on Eq. (6.20), this set of pixel values is given by

$$I[m] = \sum_{n=-N/2}^{N/2-1} S[n]e^{i2\pi nm/\hat{N}} \qquad -\hat{N}/2 \le m < \hat{N}/2 \qquad (6.33)$$

These pixels cannot be directly evaluated by the FFT algorithm because $\{I[m]\}$ and $\{S[n]\}$ have different lengths. To get around this problem, $\{S[n]\}$ is expanded to $\hat{N}$ points by adding $\hat{N} - N$ zeros. Specifically, let

$$\hat{S}[n] = \begin{cases} S[n] & -N/2 \le n \le N/2 - 1 \\ 0 & -\hat{N}/2 \le n < -N/2,\ N/2 \le n < \hat{N}/2 \end{cases} \qquad (6.34)$$

Equation (6.33) can then be written as

$$I[m] = \sum_{n=-\hat{N}/2}^{\hat{N}/2-1} \hat{S}[n]e^{i2\pi nm/\hat{N}} \qquad -\hat{N}/2 \le m < \hat{N}/2 \qquad (6.35)$$

which can now be evaluated directly by an $\hat{N}$-point FFT.

Note that Eq. (6.34) suggests that zeros be padded at both ends of the data sequence. It is sometimes more convenient to pad all the zeros at one end of the data sequence. The resulting FFT reconstruction will have a linear phase shift, which is inconsequential when only the magnitude image is desired.

The zooming effect of zero-filling can sometimes make the image look "better," but no information is gained by zero-filling the data sequence. By the same token, zero-filling does not violate the data-consistency constraint and thus will not introduce additional image artifacts, although some existing image artifacts may appear more obvious in the zero-padded FFT reconstruction.

6.3   Reconstruction from Radon Transform Samples

6.3.1   Problem Formulation

Image reconstruction from Radon transform samples is commonly known as image reconstruction from projections. Let $P(p, \mu)$ denote the measured projection profiles. This problem can be formulated in general as follows:

$$\text{Given} \qquad P(p, \mu) = \mathcal{R}\{I\} = \int_{\mathbb{R}^n} I(r)\delta(p - \mu \cdot r)dr \qquad (6.36)$$

$$\text{determine} \qquad I(r)$$

where $(p, \mu) \in \mathcal{D}$ with $\mathcal{D}$ containing the set of Radon-space points at which measured data are collected.

Although MRI does not collect Radon transform data per se, these techniques are useful for image reconstruction from radially sampled k-space data. In the following discussion, we assume that the "measured" data are directly from the Radon space. As in the Fourier transform case, if the Radon space is fully sampled, $I(r)$ can be uniquely determined from the inverse Radon transform formula. In practice, the Radon space is partially sampled, leading to an underdetermined problem. Consequently, the feasible reconstruction is not unique. Various reconstruction techniques discussed in this section represent different ways to select a reconstruction from the many feasible ones.

6.3.2 The Inverse Radon Transform

Before describing the practical reconstruction algorithms, we discuss the inverse Radon transform in order to gain some theoretical insight. Let us start with the multidimensional inverse Fourier transform in vector form

$$I(r) = \int_{\mathbb{R}^n} S(k)e^{i2\pi k \cdot r}dk \tag{6.37}$$

In spherical (or hyperspherical) polar coordinates (see Section 2.6 for definitions), Eq. (6.37) becomes

$$I(r) = \int_{|\mu|=1} \int_0^\infty S_p(k\mu)e^{i2\pi k\mu \cdot r}k^{n-1}dkd\mu \tag{6.38}$$

Extending the lower limit of the inner integral from 0 to $-\infty$ by multiplying the integrand with a unit step function $u(k)$ yields

$$I(r) = \int_{|\mu|=1} \int_{-\infty}^\infty S_p(k\mu)k^{n-1}u(k)e^{i2\pi k\mu \cdot r}dkd\mu \tag{6.39}$$

The inner integral can now be recognized as a one-dimensional inverse Fourier transform along the k-axis. Therefore, Eq. (6.39) can be rewritten as

$$I(r) = \int_{|\mu|=1} \mathcal{F}_k^{-1}\{S_p(k\mu)k^{n-1}u(k)\}(\mu \cdot r)d\mu \tag{6.40}$$

where $\mathcal{F}_k^{-1}$ denotes taking the inverse Fourier transform along the k-axis.

Based on the projection-slice theorem and the derivative property of the

Fourier transform, we have

$$\mathcal{F}_k^{-1}\{S_p(k\mu)k^{n-1}u(k)\}$$

$$= \frac{1}{(i2\pi)^{n-1}}\mathcal{F}_k^{-1}\{S_p(k\mu)(i2\pi k)^{n-1}\} * \mathcal{F}_k^{-1}\{u(k)\}$$

$$= \frac{1}{(i2\pi)^{n-1}}\frac{\partial^{n-1}P(p,\mu)}{\partial p^{n-1}} * \left[\frac{1}{2}\delta(p) - \frac{1}{i2\pi p}\right] \tag{6.41}$$

$$= \frac{1}{(i2\pi)^{n-1}}\left[\frac{1}{2}\frac{\partial^{n-1}P(p,\mu)}{\partial p^{n-1}} - \frac{1}{i2\pi}\frac{\partial^{n-1}P(p,\mu)}{\partial p^{n-1}} * \frac{1}{p}\right]$$

Substituting this result into Eq. (6.40), we immediately obtain the following general inversion formula:

$$I(r) = \frac{1}{2(i2\pi)^{n-1}}\int_{|\mu|=1}\frac{\partial^{n-1}P(p,\mu)}{\partial p^{n-1}}\bigg|_{p=\mu\cdot r}d\mu$$

$$- \frac{1}{(i2\pi)^n}\int_{|\mu|=1}\int_{-\infty}^{\infty}\frac{\partial^{n-1}P(p,\mu)/\partial p^{n-1}}{\mu\cdot r - p}dpd\mu \tag{6.42}$$

The two terms in Eq. (6.42) have the following interesting properties:

(a)

$$\frac{1}{2(i2\pi)^{n-1}}\int_{|\mu|=1}\frac{\partial^{n-1}P(p,\mu)}{\partial p^{n-1}}\bigg|_{p=\mu\cdot r}d\mu = 0 \qquad n \text{ even} \tag{6.43}$$

(b)

$$-\frac{1}{(i2\pi)^n}\int_{|\mu|=1}\int_{-\infty}^{\infty}\frac{\partial^{n-1}P(p,\mu)/\partial p^{n-1}}{\mu\cdot r - p}dpd\mu = 0 \qquad n \text{ odd} \tag{6.44}$$

Proof of these identities can be found in the Appendix of this chapter.

The above properties result in the following well-known inversion formulas. For functions of odd dimensions,

$$I(r) = \frac{1}{2(i2\pi)^{n-1}}\int_{|\mu|=1}\frac{\partial^{n-1}P(p,\mu)}{\partial p^{n-1}}\bigg|_{p=\mu\cdot r}d\mu \tag{6.45}$$

For functions of even dimensions,

$$I(r) = -\frac{1}{(i2\pi)^n}\int_{|\mu|=1}\int_{-\infty}^{\infty}\frac{\partial^{n-1}P(p,\mu)/\partial p^{n-1}}{\mu\cdot r - p}dpd\mu \tag{6.46}$$

Two special cases of practical interest are $n = 2$ and $n = 3$. For $n = 2$, we have

$$I(x,y) = \frac{1}{2\pi^2}\int_0^\pi\int_{-\infty}^{\infty}\frac{\partial P(p,\phi)/\partial p}{x\cos\phi + y\sin\phi - p}dpd\phi \tag{6.47}$$

and for $n = 3$,

$$I(x, y, z) = -\frac{1}{8\pi^2} \int_0^{2\pi} \int_0^{\pi} \frac{\partial^2 P(p, \boldsymbol{\mu}_3)}{\partial p^2}\bigg|_{p=\boldsymbol{\mu}_3 \cdot \boldsymbol{r}} \sin\theta\, d\theta\, d\phi \qquad (6.48)$$

where $\boldsymbol{\mu}_3 = (\sin\theta\cos\phi, \sin\theta\sin\phi, \cos\theta)$. Equation (6.48) can be equivalently written as [16]

$$I(x, y, z) = -\frac{1}{8\pi^2} \left(\frac{\partial^2}{\partial x^2} + \frac{\partial^2}{\partial y^2} + \frac{\partial^2}{\partial z^2} \right) \int_0^{2\pi} \int_0^{\pi} P(\boldsymbol{\mu}_3 \cdot \boldsymbol{r}, \boldsymbol{\mu}_3) \sin\theta\, d\theta\, d\phi$$

$$(6.49)$$

For $n > 2$, the inverse Radon transform can also be carried out in a multistage fashion. Specifically, according to Eq. (2.120), we have

$$\mathcal{R}_n^{-1} = \mathcal{R}_m^{-1} \mathcal{R}_{n-m+1}^{-1} \qquad (6.50)$$

As an example, $\mathcal{R}_3^{-1} = \mathcal{R}_2^{-1} \mathcal{R}_2^{-1}$, which means three-dimensional inverse transforms can be implemented as two-dimensional inverse transforms carried out in two stages.

6.3.3　Backprojection

This section defines the backprojection operator that is used in several reconstruction algorithms. Let $P(p, \boldsymbol{\mu})$ be a projection profile from the Radon transform of an arbitrary function. The backprojection operator $\mathcal{B}$ is defined by

$$\mathcal{B}\{P(p, \boldsymbol{\mu})\} = P(\boldsymbol{\mu} \cdot \boldsymbol{r}, \boldsymbol{\mu}) \qquad (6.51)$$

The term *backprojection* comes from fact that mapping $P(p, \boldsymbol{\mu})$ to $P(\boldsymbol{\mu} \cdot \boldsymbol{r}, \boldsymbol{\mu})$ is to *backproject* the value of $P(p_0, \boldsymbol{\mu})$ along the integration path of the Radon transform, as illustrated in Fig. 6.4.

With the general definition in Eq. (6.51), it is easy to define the backprojection operator in two and three dimensions. Specifically, in two dimensions

$$\mathcal{B}_2\{P(p, \phi)\} = P(x\cos\phi + y\sin\phi, \phi) \qquad (6.52)$$

and in three dimensions

$$\mathcal{B}_3\{P(p, \theta, \phi)\} = P(x\sin\theta\cos\phi + y\sin\theta\sin\phi + z\cos\theta, \theta, \phi) \qquad (6.53)$$

The backprojection operator maps a one-dimensional profile to a multidimensional function with constant values along a line (plane or hyperplane) defined by $\boldsymbol{\mu} \cdot \boldsymbol{r} = p$. This property can better be seen from the following example.

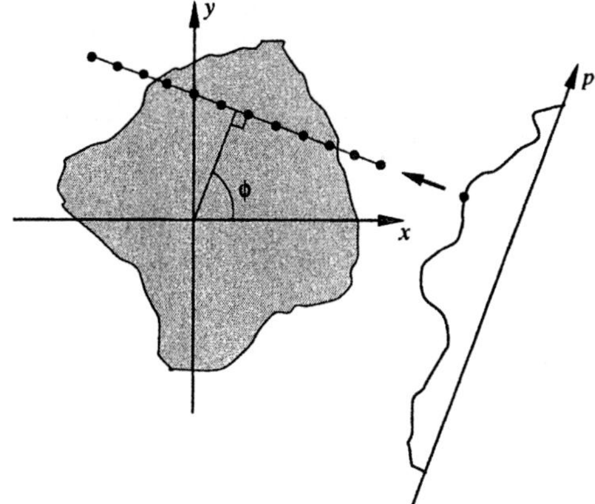

Figure 6.4   Illustration of backprojecting the value of a point in a projection profile to the pixels along a particular line.

■ **Example 6.2**

Consider two projection profiles $P(p, 0°) = \Pi(p/a)$ and $P(p, 45°) = \Pi(p/a)$. We calculate their corresponding backprojections.

According to Eq. (6.52), we have for the first case

$$\mathcal{B}_2\{P(p, 0°)\} = \Pi[(x\cos 0° + y\sin 0°)/a] = \Pi(x/a)$$

and for the second case

$$\mathcal{B}_2\{P(p, 45°)\} = \Pi[(x\cos 45° + y\sin 45°)/a] = \Pi[(x + y)/(\sqrt{2}a)]$$

$\mathcal{B}_2\{P(p, 0°)\}$ and $\mathcal{B}_2\{P(p, 45°)\}$ are illustrated in Fig. 6.5.

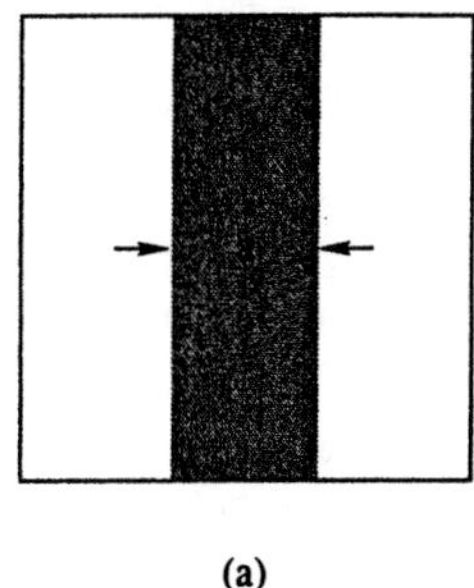

(a)

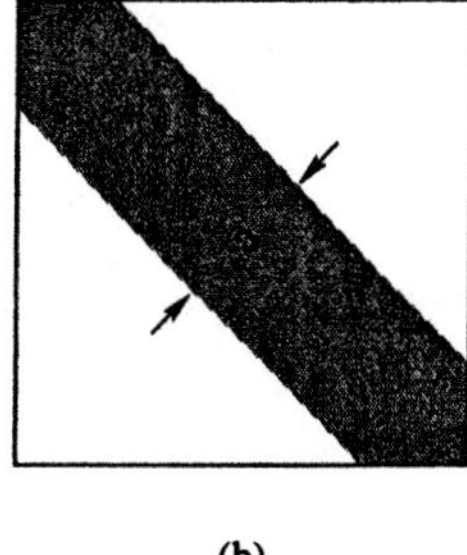

(b)

Figure 6.5   Illustration of $\mathcal{B}_2\{P(p, 0°)\}$ and $\mathcal{B}_2\{P(p, 45°)\}$ discussed in Example 6.2.

6.3.4   Practical Reconstruction Algorithms

We now discuss some popular algorithms used for image reconstruction from
Radon transform samples. We begin with the backprojection reconstruction and
filtered/convolution backprojection methods, which are directly motivated from
the inverse Radon transform. We then discuss two methods known as direct
Fourier reconstruction and algebraic reconstruction, which are not based on the
inverse Radon transform.

6.3.4.1   Direct Backprojection Method

The easiest, but somewhat crude, way of implementing the inverse Radon transform formula is to directly backproject the measured projections, as illustrated in
Fig. 6.6. The general backprojection reconstruction formula is

$$I(r) = c \int_{|\mu|=1} \mathcal{B}\{P(p,\mu)\} d\mu \tag{6.54}$$

where the measured projection profiles are first backprojected and then integrated
over the unit sphere. Clearly, the scaling constant c in Eq. (6.54) is unimportant
as far as image quality is concerned. In practice, c is set to $1/2$ in two dimensions
and to $1/(2\pi)$ in three dimensions so that the point spread functions associated
with backprojection reconstruction become $1/\sqrt{x^2 + y^2}$ and $1/\sqrt{x^2 + y^2 + z^2}$,
respectively. This topic is discussed in Section 8.1.3.

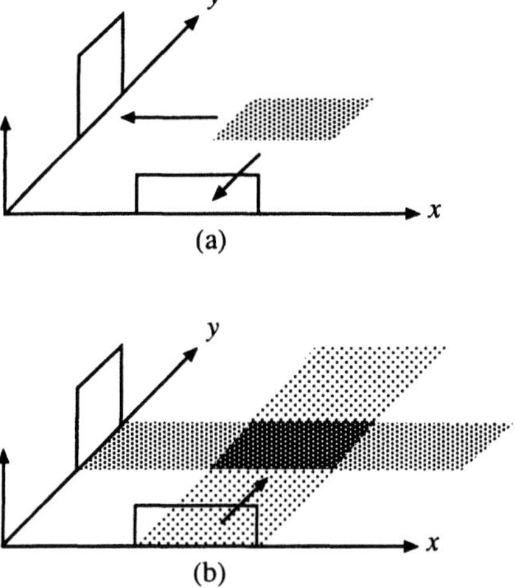

Figure 6.6   (a) Two projection profiles from a rectangular object. (b)
Backprojection reconstruction.

Based on the definition of the backprojection operator in Eq. (6.52), the backprojection reconstruction formula can be written explicitly in two dimensions as

$$I(x,y) = \frac{1}{2} \int_0^{2\pi} P(x\cos\phi + y\sin\phi, \phi)d\phi \tag{6.55}$$

or

$$I(x,y) = \int_0^{\pi} P(x\cos\phi + y\sin\phi, \phi)d\phi \tag{6.56}$$

noting that $P(p,\phi) = P(-p, \phi + \pi)$. Similarly, in three dimensions, we have

$$I(x,y,z) = \frac{1}{2\pi} \int_0^{2\pi} \int_0^{\pi} P(x\sin\theta\cos\phi + y\sin\theta\sin\phi + z\cos\theta, \theta, \phi)\sin\theta d\theta d\phi \tag{6.57}$$

In practice, the measured projections are discretized both angularly and radially. So, the above reconstruction formulas are implemented in discrete forms. In two dimensions, we may assume that $P(p,\phi)$ is available at the following points

$$p = n_p\Delta p \qquad n_p = -N_p/2, \ldots, N_p/2 - 1 \tag{6.58a}$$
$$\phi = n_\phi\Delta\phi \qquad n_\phi = 0, 1, \ldots, N_\phi - 1 \tag{6.58b}$$

Then,

$$I(x,y) = \Delta\phi \sum_{n_\phi=0}^{N_\phi-1} P(p_n, n_\phi\Delta\phi) \tag{6.59}$$

where it is understood that prior to the summation p_n is replaced by

$$p_n = x\cos n_\phi\Delta\phi + y\sin n_\phi\Delta\phi \tag{6.60}$$

In three dimensions, we may assume that $P(p, \phi, \theta)$ is available for

$$p = n_p\Delta p \qquad n_p = -N_p/2, \ldots, N_p/2 - 1 \tag{6.61a}$$
$$\theta = n_\theta\Delta\theta \qquad n_\theta = 0, 1, \ldots, N_\theta - 1 \tag{6.61b}$$
$$\phi = n_\phi\Delta\phi \qquad n_\phi = 0, 1, \ldots, N_\phi - 1 \tag{6.61c}$$

Then,

$$I(x,y,z) = \frac{\Delta\phi\Delta\theta}{2\pi} \sum_{n_\phi=0}^{N_\phi-1} \sum_{n_\theta=0}^{N_\theta-1} P(p_n, n_\theta\Delta\theta, n_\phi\Delta\phi)\sin n_\theta \tag{6.62}$$

where

$$p_n = x\sin n_\theta\Delta\theta\cos n_\phi\Delta\phi + y\sin n_\theta\Delta\theta\sin n_\phi\Delta\phi + z\cos n_\theta\Delta\theta \tag{6.63}$$

When $I(x, y)$ or $I(x, y, z)$ is evaluated on the rectangular grid points, say $(x, y) = (n_x \Delta x, n_y \Delta y)$ or $(x, y, z) = (n_x \Delta x, n_y \Delta y, n_z \Delta z)$, it is necessary to perform one-dimensional signal interpolation along the p-axis on the measured projection profiles. Why do we need signal interpolation? This is because p_n as determined by Eqs. (6.60) and (6.63) may not fall exactly on the sampling points along the p-axis. In other words, $p_n \neq n_p \Delta p$, for $-N_p/2 \leq n_p < N_p/2$.

A variety of signal interpolation schemes can be used to solve this problem. The most efficient one is the *nearest-neighbor* interpolator, which determines the value of $P(p_n, \mu)$ as follows:

$$P(p_n, \mu) = P(m\Delta p, \mu) \tag{6.64}$$

where

$$m = \arg \min |p_n - m\Delta p| \tag{6.65}$$

Higher-order interpolators are often more accurate but computationally less efficient. For example, in the linear interpolation method, we select m such that $m\Delta p \leq p_n < (m + 1)\Delta p$ and estimate $P(p_n, \mu)$ by

$$\frac{(m + 1)\Delta p - p_n}{\Delta p} P(m\Delta p, \mu) + \frac{p_n - m\Delta p}{\Delta p} P[(m + 1)\Delta p, \mu] \tag{6.66}$$

A notable limitation of the backprojection method is that it produces blurred images as discussed in Chapter 8 and illustrated in Fig. 6.7. This problem can be overcome using the filtered backprojection reconstruction method discussed in Section 6.3.4.2.

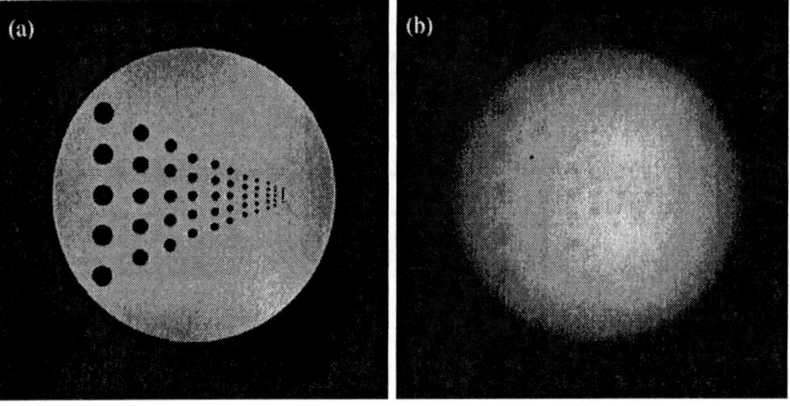

Figure 6.7   Reconstruction of a phantom image: (a) The "gold" standard, and (b) backprojection reconstruction with 256 projections uniformly covering ϕ from 0 to π.

6.3.4.2   Filtered Backprojection Reconstruction

Filtered backprojection reconstruction is a direct implementation of the inverse Radon transform formula. It differs from direct backprojection reconstruction only in that measured projections are filtered before they are backprojected.

Let $P(p, \mu)$ be the measured projections of $I(r)$, and let $S_p(k\mu)$ be the Fourier transform of $I(r)$ in the polar form. Filtered backprojection reconstruction is expressed in general as

$$I(r) = \int_{|\mu|=1} \mathcal{B}\{\bar{P}(p, \mu)\}d\mu \tag{6.67}$$

where the filtered projections $\bar{P}(p, \mu)$ are given, according to Eq. (6.39), by

$$\bar{P}(p, \mu) = \int_{-\infty}^{\infty} S_p(k\mu)k^{n-1}u(k)e^{i2\pi kp}dk \tag{6.68}$$

There are many ways to implement filtered backprojection reconstruction based on variants of Eq. (6.68). In two dimensions, for example, it is more convenient to write the filtered backprojection reconstruction as

$$I(x, y) = \int_0^\pi \mathcal{B}_2\{\bar{P}(p, \phi)\}d\phi \tag{6.69}$$

where

$$\bar{P}(p, \phi) = \int_{-\infty}^{\infty} S_p(k, \phi)|k|e^{i2\pi kp}dk \tag{6.70}$$

or

$$\bar{P}(p, \phi) = \frac{1}{2\pi^2}\frac{\partial P(p, \phi)}{\partial p} * \frac{1}{p} \tag{6.71}$$

Similarly, in three dimensions, we have[4]

$$I(x, y, z) = \int_0^\pi \int_0^\pi \mathcal{B}_3\{\bar{P}(p, \theta, \phi)\} \sin\theta d\theta d\phi \tag{6.72}$$

where

$$\bar{P}(p, \theta, \phi) = \int_{-\infty}^{\infty} S_p(k, \theta, \phi)k^2 e^{i2\pi kp}dk \tag{6.73}$$

or based on Eq. (6.48)

$$\bar{P}(p, \theta, \phi) = -\frac{1}{4\pi^2}\frac{\partial^2 P(p, \theta, \phi)}{\partial p^2} \tag{6.74}$$

---

[4]The three-dimensional Radon inversion formula can be written as

$$I(x, y, z) = \int_0^\pi \int_0^\pi \int_{-\infty}^{\infty} S_p(k, \theta, \phi)k^2 e^{i2\pi kp} \sin\theta dk d\theta d\phi$$

noting that $S_p(k, \theta, \phi) = S_k(-k, \theta + \pi, \pi - \phi)$, for $k \geq 0$ and $0 \leq \theta, \phi \leq \pi$.

Equations (6.70) and (6.73) are k-space implementations of the filter operation, whereas Eqs. (6.71) and (6.74) are Radon-space implementations. If data are directly measured in k-space, as is the case with MRI, it is often more convenient to implement Eqs. (6.70) and (6.73). Based on the preceding discussion, we may rewrite the filtered projections in general as

$$\bar{P}(p, \mu) = \mathcal{F}_k^{-1}\{S_p(k, \mu)H(k)\} \tag{6.75}$$

where $H(k)$ is a one-dimensional filter function. In two dimensions, the "ideal" filter function, according to the inverse Radon transform formula, is given by

$$H(k) = |k| \tag{6.76}$$

Because this filter amplifies high-frequency noise, an approximate filter function is generally used in practice. Specifically, to limit the unbounded nature of the $|k|$ filter in the high-frequency range, we can multiply it with a bandlimiting function such as the rectangular window function $\Pi(k/W_k)$, where W_k is the desired frequency band. This gives rise to the well-known Ram–Lak filter proposed by Ramachandran and Lakshminarayanan. This function is also referred to as the "M" filter because its shape resembles the character "M". A list of commonly used filter functions are as follows:

- Ram–Lak filter:

$$H(k) = |k|\Pi\left(\frac{k}{W_k}\right) \tag{6.77}$$

- Shepp–Logan filter:

$$H(k) = |k|\text{sinc}\left(\frac{\pi k}{W_k}\right)\Pi\left(\frac{k}{W_k}\right) \tag{6.78}$$

- Low-pass cosine filter:

$$H(k) = |k|\cos\left(\frac{\pi k}{W_k}\right)\Pi\left(\frac{k}{W_k}\right) \tag{6.79}$$

- Generalized Hamming filter:

$$H(k) = |k|\left[0.54 + 0.46\cos\left(\frac{2\pi k}{W_k}\right)\right]\Pi\left(\frac{k}{W_k}\right) \tag{6.80}$$

These filter functions are graphically shown in Fig. 6.8.

In higher dimensions, the ideal filter function required by the inverse Radon transform is different from the $|k|$ filter. For example, in three dimensions, we have

$$H(k) = k^2 \tag{6.81}$$

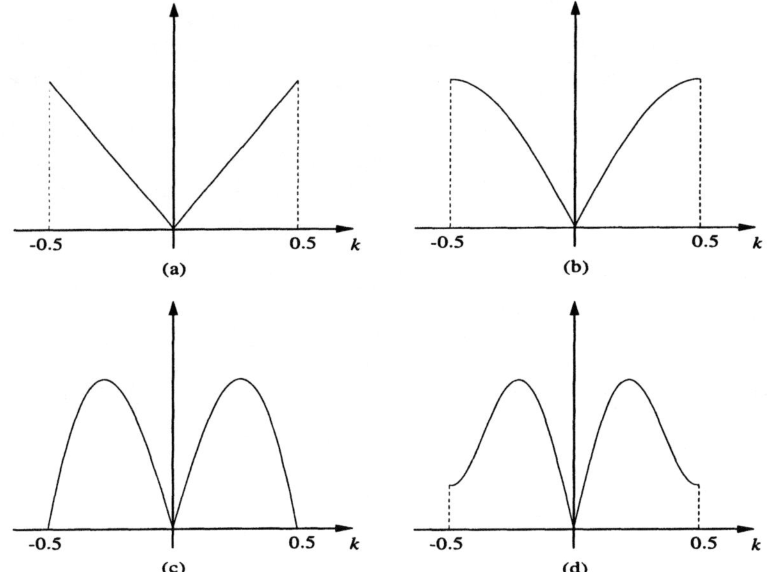

Figure 6.8 Filter functions for two-dimensional filtered backprojection reconstruction: (a) Ram-Lak filter, (b) Shepp-Logan filter, (c) Low-pass cosine filter, and (d) Generalized Hamming filter. Note the desired frequency band W_k is normalized to 1.

This filter can be modified to reduce its noise sensitivity in the same way as is done to the $|k|$ filter. Two examples of filtered backprojection reconstruction are shown in Fig. 6.9 to illustrate the effect of different filter functions on filtered backprojection reconstruction. As can be seen from this example, different filters result in noticeably different reconstructions.

6.3.4.3   Direct Fourier Reconstruction

As discussed in Sections 6.3.4.1 and 6.3.4.2, direct and filtered backprojection reconstructions are approximate implementations of the inverse Radon transform. In this and the following subsections, we briefly describe two reconstruction methods that bypass the inverse Radon transform: the direct Fourier reconstruction method and the algebraic reconstruction method.

The direct Fourier reconstruction method consists of three major steps:

(a) Conversion of the projection data to Fourier data by one-dimensional Fourier transformation of each projection (projection-slice theorem)

(b) Conversion of Fourier data on a polar grid to a rectangular grid (signal interpolation)

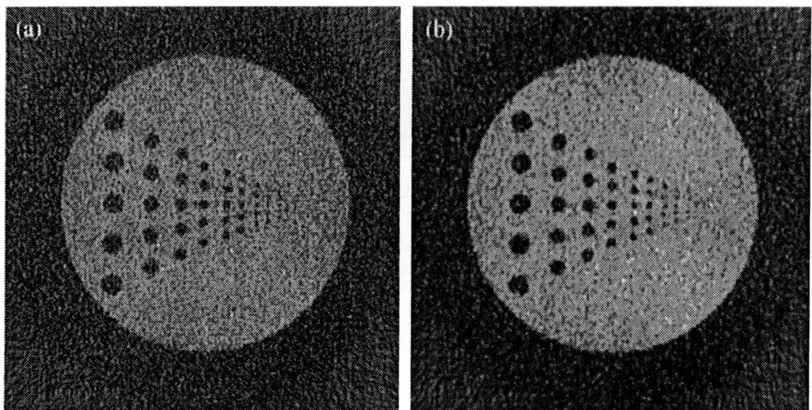

Figure 6.9 Filtered backprojection reconstructions of a phantom image using (a) the Ram-Lak filter, and (b) the low-pass cosine filter. Note that image (b) is less noisy than (a) because the low-pass cosine filter suppresses some of the high-frequency noise.

(c) The standard Fourier reconstruction

The first step is not necessary when Fourier data are directly measured, as is the case in MRI. The last step detailed in Section 6.2 is straightforward. Hence, the key step with direct Fourier reconstruction is the conversion of polar-raster data to rectangular raster data. Detailed discussion of this signal interpolation problem and available algorithms is beyond the scope of this text. The interested reader is referred to [168, 200, 212, 230, 250, 251] for more details. An important point to bear in mind here is that the rectangular-raster data generated by signal interpolation often contain errors. Particularly, because k-space is sparsely sampled in the high-frequency range with polar sampling, the interpolation step is prone to aliasing effects. These errors can create noticeable image artifacts when the signal interpolator is not properly chosen.

6.3.4.4 Algebraic Reconstruction Techniques

Algebraic reconstruction techniques (ART), as the name implies, formulate the image reconstruction problem as one of solving a set of algebraic equations [143, 158]. Although ART is not widely used in MRI, some understanding of the underlying principle is useful.

To illustrate the concept, let us focus on the two-dimensional case. ART parameterizes the desired image function $I(x, y)$ in terms of a finite set of known basis functions $\varphi_\ell(x, y)$ such that

$$I(x, y) = \sum_{\ell=1}^{L} c_\ell \Phi_\ell(x, y) \tag{6.82}$$

where c_ℓ are the model coefficients (parameters). With this model, the data-consistency constraint can be expressed as

$$P(p_m, \phi_n) = \sum_{\ell=1}^{L} c_\ell \mathcal{R}\left\{\Phi_\ell(x, y)\right\}(p_m, \phi_n) \tag{6.83}$$

where $0 \leq m < N_p$, and $0 \leq n < N_\phi$ assuming that there are N_ϕ projections, each with N_p samples in the measured data set. It is evident from Eq. (6.83) that the c_ℓ can be determined uniquely by the data-consistency constraint alone if the following two conditions are met:

(a)   The basis functions are well-chosen (or linearly independent).

(b)   The total number of model parameters L is not greater than the total number of data points $N = N_p \times N_\phi$.

A particular set of the basis functions corresponds to $\Phi_\ell(x, y)$ being the indicator function of the ℓth pixel. That is

$$\Phi_\ell(x, y) = \begin{cases} 1 & (x, y) \in \ell\text{th pixel pixel region} \\ 0 & \text{otherwise} \end{cases} \tag{6.84}$$

In this case, c_ℓ becomes the desired image pixel value. This model arises when we discretize the image function $I(x, y)$ on an $N_x \times N_y = L$ grid and assume that $I(x, y)$ is a constant within each pixel. Putting Eq. (6.82) in matrix form yields

$$\mathbf{W}c = d \tag{6.85}$$

where d is an N-element vector containing all the measured data $P(p_m, \phi_n)$ and $\mathbf{W}$ is an $N \times L$ matrix containing the weighting coefficients. When N and L are small, we can use conventional linear system solvers to find the solution to Eq. (6.85). However, in practice L may be as large as 65,000 (for a 256×256 image). Assume that 128 projections are taken, each with 512 data points. Then $N = 65,000$, and $\mathbf{W}$ becomes a square matrix of size $65,536 \times 65,536$. Solving such a linear system directly is highly undesirable even if possible. In practice, Eq. (6.85) is solved iteratively. One popular iterative method was first proposed by Kaczmarz [172] and later elucidated by Tanabe [254]. In this algorithm, one first makes an initial guess at the solution c_0. This initial guess is projected onto the hyperplane represented by the first equation, $w_1 \cdot c = d_1$, of Eq. (6.85) giving c_1. After c_1 has been obtained, we take its projection[5] onto the hyperplane

---

[5]Note the difference between the projection of a vector onto a plane and the projection of an object function defined by the Radon transform.

represented by the second equation $w_2 \cdot c = d_2$, which gives c_2. This process is repeated with the third hyperplane and so on, until we get c_N, the projection onto the last hyperplane. One now iterates by again projecting c_N on the first hyperplane. This process continues until all the N hyperplanes have been cycled through, resulting in I_{2N}. The next iteration starts by projecting I_{2N} onto the first hyperplane again, and so on. The projection onto the jth hyperplane from that on the $(j-1)$th hyperplane is given by

$$c_j = c_{j-1} - \frac{c_{j-1} \cdot w_j - d_j}{w_j \cdot w_j} w_j \tag{6.86}$$

It has been shown that the iteration in Eq. (6.86) converges to the right solution of the linear system if a unique solution exists. If the solution is not unique (e.g., in the underdetermined case when $N < L$), the algorithm converges to one of the feasible solutions that is closest to the initial guess, c_0. On the other hand, if the linear system is overdetermined, no unique solution exists. The algorithm in this case will not converge to a single point; rather, it will oscillate in the neighborhood of the region of the intersection of the hyperplanes. The convergence rate of the algorithm depends on both the initial guess and the orthogonality of the hyperplanes. In the ideal case that the hyperplanes are mutually orthogonal, one iteration of the algorithm through all the hyperplanes is enough. On the other hand, if the angles between the hyperplanes are very small, the convergence of the algorithm can be very slow. This algorithm is illustrated in Fig. 6.10, where only two variables are considered.

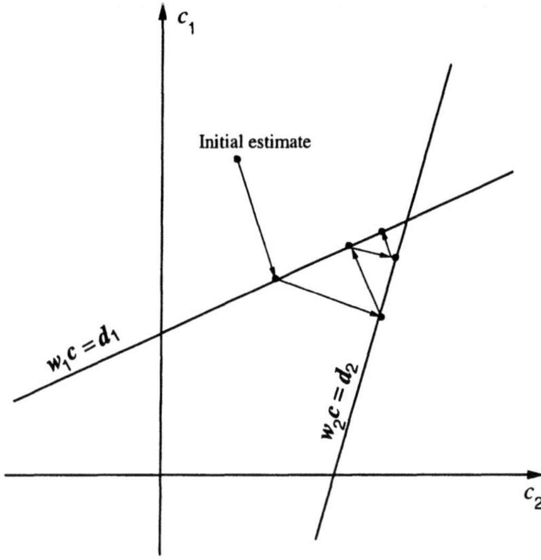

Figure 6.10   Illustration of the Kaczmarz algorithm for the case of two variables.

6.4 Appendix

This appendix presents a proof of the results stated in Eqs. (6.43) and (6.44). Let $f(\mu)$ and $g(\mu)$ represent the integrands in the two equations. Namely,

$$f(\mu) = \left. \frac{\partial^{n-1}\mathcal{R}\{I\}(p,\mu)}{\partial p^{n-1}} \right|_{p=\mu\cdot r} \tag{6.87}$$

and

$$g(\mu) = \int_{-\infty}^{\infty} \frac{\frac{\partial^{n-1}\mathcal{R}\{I\}(p,\mu)}{\partial p^{n-1}}}{\mu\cdot r - p}\, dp \tag{6.88}$$

We then have

$$\begin{aligned}
f(-\mu) &= \left. \frac{\partial^{n-1}\mathcal{R}\{I\}(p,-\mu)}{\partial p^{n-1}} \right|_{p=-\mu\cdot r} \\[2mm]
&= \left. \frac{\partial^{n-1}\mathcal{R}\{I\}(-p,\mu)}{\partial p^{n-1}} \right|_{p=-\mu\cdot r} \\[2mm]
&= (-1)^{n-1} \left. \frac{\partial^{n-1}\mathcal{R}\{I\}(-p,\mu)}{\partial(-p)^{n-1}} \right|_{p=-\mu\cdot r} \\[2mm]
&= (-1)^{n-1} \left. \frac{\partial^{n-1}\mathcal{R}\{I\}(p,\mu)}{\partial p^{n-1}} \right|_{p=\mu\cdot r} \\[2mm]
&= (-1)^{n-1} f(\mu)
\end{aligned} \tag{6.89}$$

and, similarly,

$$\begin{aligned}
g(-\mu) &= \int_{-\infty}^{\infty} \frac{\frac{\partial^{n-1}\mathcal{R}\{I\}(p,-\mu)}{\partial p^{n-1}}}{-\mu\cdot r - p}\, dp \\[2mm]
&= \int_{-\infty}^{\infty} \frac{\frac{\partial^{n-1}\mathcal{R}\{I\}(-p,\mu)}{\partial p^{n-1}}}{-\mu\cdot r - p}\, dp \\[2mm]
&= (-1)^{n-1} \int_{-\infty}^{\infty} \frac{\frac{\partial^{n-1}\mathcal{R}\{I\}(\hat{p},\mu)}{\partial \hat{p}^{n-1}}}{-\mu\cdot r + \hat{p}}\, d\hat{p} \\[2mm]
&= (-1)^{n} \int_{-\infty}^{\infty} \frac{\frac{\partial^{n-1}\mathcal{R}\{I\}(\hat{p},\mu)}{\partial \hat{p}^{n-1}}}{\mu\cdot r - \hat{p}}\, d\hat{p} \\[2mm]
&= (-1)^{n} g(\mu)
\end{aligned} \tag{6.90}$$

where symmetry relation $\mathcal{R}\{I\}(p,\mu) = \mathcal{R}\{I\}(-p,-\mu)$ is used. Equations (6.89) and (6.90) suggest that $f(\mu)$ is an even function for odd n but an odd function for even n; on the other hand, $g(\mu)$ is an odd function for odd n but an even function for even n. The results in Eqs. (6.43) and (6.44) are now evident, noting that $f(\mu)$ and $g(\mu)$ are integrated over the unit (hyper)sphere.

Exercises

6.1 Show that if W_x is a finite number, then

$$\lim_{k_0 \to \infty} \int_{-W_x/2}^{W_x/2} A \sin(2\pi k_0 x) e^{-i2\pi k x} dx = 0$$

6.2 Let

$$S[n] = \int_{-\infty}^{\infty} I(x) e^{-i2\pi n \Delta k x} dx$$

and

$$\epsilon^2 = \int_{-1/\Delta k}^{1/\Delta k} \left| I(x) - \Delta k \sum_{n=-N/2}^{N/2-1} S[n] w_n e^{i2\pi n \Delta k x} \right|^2 dx$$

Assume that $I(x) = 0$ for $|x| > W_x/2$ and $\Delta k \leq 1/W_x$. Show that ϵ is minimized when w_n is a rectangular window function. That is,

$$w_n = \begin{cases} 1 & -N/2 \leq n < N/2 \\ 0 & \text{otherwise} \end{cases}$$

6.3 Let $I(x)$ be the trapezoidal pulse defined in Problem 2.21.

(a) Construct and sketch a periodic extension of $I(x)$ with period $3b$.

(b) Find the Fourier series expansion for the resulting periodic function.

6.4 Let $I(x) = \Lambda(x)$ and $\tilde{I}(x) = \sum_{n=-\infty}^{\infty} I(x + n)$.

(a) Sketch $\tilde{I}(x)$.

(b) Is $\tilde{I}(x)$ a periodic function of period $1, 2, \cdots$?

(c) Find the Fourier series representation for $\tilde{I}(x)$.

6.5 Show that the Fourier reconstruction is always data-consistent regardless of the sampling interval Δk and the number of data points available. In other words, let

$$\hat{I}(x) = \Delta k \Pi\left(\frac{x}{\Delta k}\right) \sum_{m=-N/2}^{N/2-1} S(m\Delta k) e^{i2\pi m \Delta k x}$$

Then

$$\mathcal{F}\{\hat{I}\}(m\Delta k) = S(m\Delta k) \qquad \text{for } -N/2 \leq n < N/2 \text{ and } \forall \Delta k$$

holds for any $\Delta k > 0$.

6.6 Let $I(x)$ be a feasible reconstruction consistent with the measured data $S(n\Delta k)$, $-N/2 \leq n < N/2$. Show that $\hat{I}(x) = I(x) + e^{i2\pi m \Delta k x}$ is also a feasible reconstruction for any $|m| > N/2$.

6.7 Prove the relation in Eq. (6.19).

6.8 Assume that a k-space data set $S[m, n]$ yields the image in (a) after a two-dimensional FFT.

(a) Discuss how to modify $S[m, n]$ to generate the image in (b) with the same processing.

(b) Let $\hat{S}[m, n]$ be the k-space data for image (b). How can $S[m, n]$ be restored from $\hat{S}[m, n]$?

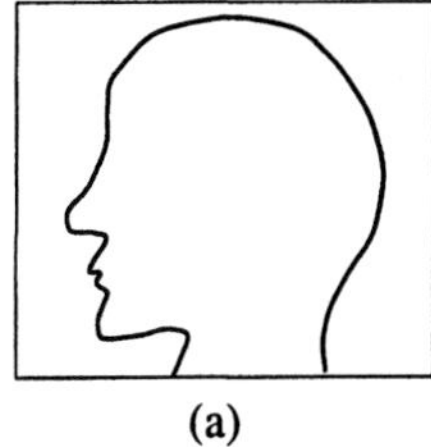

(a)

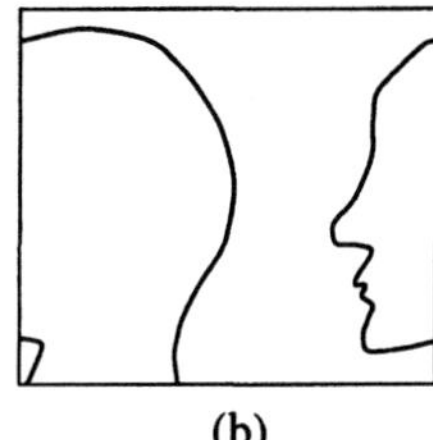

(b)

6.9 Prove the following equality:

$$\int_0^{2\pi} \int_0^{\infty} S_p(k, \phi) e^{i2\pi k(x \cos \phi + y \sin \phi)} k\, dk\, d\phi$$
$$= \int_0^{\pi} \int_{-\infty}^{\infty} S_p(k, \phi) e^{i2\pi k(x \cos \phi + y \sin \phi)} |k|\, dk\, d\phi$$

6.10 Show that Eqs. (6.48) and (6.49) are equivalent.

6.11 Discuss whether the images reconstructed using the following techniques are data-consistent:

(a) Direct backprojection method

(b) Filtered backprojection method

(c) Direct Fourier reconstruction method

(d) Algebraic reconstruction method

6.12 A rectangular object function is defined by

$$I(x, y) = \begin{cases} A & |x| < a \text{ and } |y| < a \\ 0 & \text{otherwise} \end{cases}$$

where $a < 1$ assuming FOV $= 1$.

(a) Sketch the object function.

(b) Calculate and plot the projection for $\phi = 0°$.

(c) Calculate and plot the corresponding filtered projection defined by the inverse Radon transform formula.

(d) Calculate and sketch the backprojection images from the projections obtained in (b) and (c), respectively.

6.13 Let

$$\begin{cases} 0.6c_1 + 0.4c_2 = 10 \\ 0.3c_1 + 0.7c_2 = 5 \end{cases}$$

represent two discretized Radon transform equations.

(a) Find the "true" image pixel values (c_1, c_2) defined by the two equations.

(b) Calculate the reconstructed pixel values after two iterations of the Karczmarz algorithm with initial guess $c_0 = (0, 0)$.

Chapter 7

Image Contrast

Be different in order to be seen.

Common sense

We have discussed so far how to generate an MR image from an object, starting from signal generation, through spatial information encoding, to image reconstruction. This chapter focuses on the end result—the image. Specifically, we examine how image contrast can be adjusted in several basic imaging schemes.

7.1   Introduction

Image contrast is an important imaging parameter because the human visual system is not good at judging absolute illuminance values. A well-known example is shown in Fig. 7.1, where the two smaller squares in the middle have equal intensity but the one on the right appears brighter.

Although image contrast perception depends on a number of factors, technically, image contrast is defined in terms of differences in image intensity. Specifically, let I_A and I_B be the image intensity of tissues A and B, and C_{AB} be their contrast index. We have

$$C_{AB} = \frac{|I_A - I_B|}{I_{ref}}$$

(7.1)

where I_{ref} is a normalizing reference value. It is apparent from Eq. (7.1) that to enhance image contrast, one should maximize the differences in image intensity among different tissues.

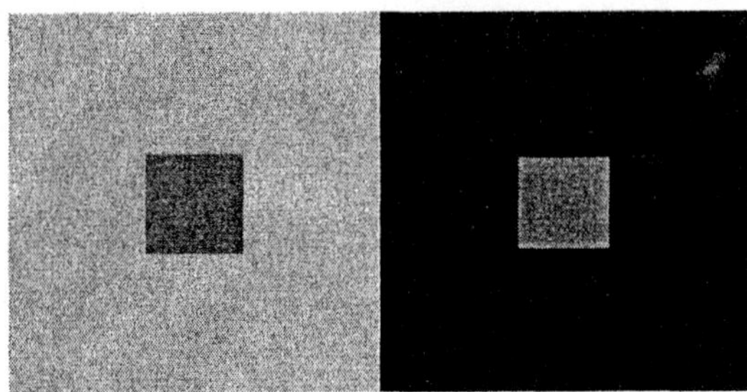

Figure 7.1 Visual illusion: small squares in the middle have equal intensity but do not appear equally bright.

In MRI, image intensity I is a multiparameter function of spin density ρ, relaxation times T_1, T_2, and T_2^*, diffusion coefficients D, and so on. We may, therefore, express the image contrast as

$$C_{\mathrm{AB}} = f(\rho, T_1, T_2, T_2^*, D, \ldots) \tag{7.2}$$

where the exact functional form of "f" is dependent on the data acquisition protocol. If the data acquisition parameters are chosen such that the T_1 effect is dominant, then

$$C_{\mathrm{AB}} \approx f(T_1) \tag{7.3}$$

and the resulting image is said to carry T_1 *contrast* or a T_1 *weighting*. Similarly, we have *spin density contrast* if

$$C_{\mathrm{AB}} \approx f(\rho) \tag{7.4}$$

and T_2 *contrast* if

$$C_{\mathrm{AB}} \approx f(T_2) \tag{7.5}$$

7.2 Saturation–Recovery Sequence

The basic saturation–recovery sequence consists of a string of equally spaced 90° pulses as illustrated in Fig. 7.2. The time interval between two successive 90° pulses is called the *repetition time* (T_{R}). For brevity, we may write this sequence as

$$(90° - T_{\mathrm{R}})_N \tag{7.6}$$

where N is the number of times that the 90° pulse is applied.

To analyze the image contrast behavior of this sequence, it is necessary to derive an expression for the signal in terms of the sequence parameters. Let $M_{z'}^{(n)}(0_-)$ and $M_{z'}^{(n)}(0_+)$ represent the longitudinal magnetization before and

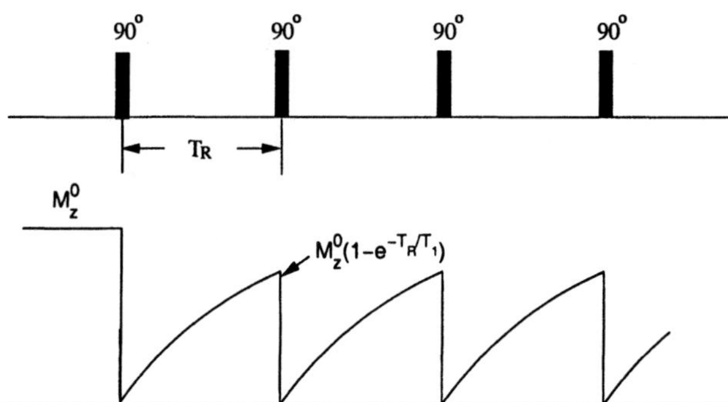

Figure 7.2   Basic saturation–recovery pulse sequence and the relaxation curve for the longitudinal magnetization.

after the nth 90°-pulse, and similarly, $M_{x'y'}^{(n)}(0_-)$ and $M_{x'y'}^{(n)}(0_+)$ denote the pre- and postpulse transverse magnetization. We have, as the initial condition, that

$$\begin{cases} M_{z'}^{(1)}(0_-) = M_z^0 \\ M_{z'}^{(1)}(0_+) = 0 \end{cases} \tag{7.7}$$

Based on the relaxation equation in Eq. (3.122), we obtain

$$M_{z'}^{(n)}(0_-) = M_z^0\left(1 - e^{-T_R/T_1}\right) + M_{z'}^{(n-1)}(0_+)e^{-T_R/T_1} \qquad n > 1 \tag{7.8}$$

For this excitation sequence, it is usually assumed that

$$M_{z'}^{(n)}(0_+) = 0 \qquad n \geq 1 \tag{7.9}$$

which is known as the *saturation condition*. This condition is met if

$$T_R \gg T_2 \tag{7.10}$$

The saturation condition means that the decay of the transverse magnetization resulting from a 90° pulse is complete before the next pulse is applied.[1]

---

[1] If T_R is less than $3T_2$, the residual $M_{x'y'}$ component is significant and will be converted to $M_{z'}$ by a 90° pulse. The effect of a 90° pulse on the residual $M_{x'y'}$ component depends on its location at the time of the pulse. For example, if $M_{x'y'}$ is perpendicular to the $\vec{B}_1$ field, it will be flipped onto the z-axis. On the other hand, if $M_{x'y'}$ is parallel to the $\vec{B}_1$ field, it will not be affected. For this reason, it is imperative that the transverse magnetization be completely dispersed (especially in the case of $T_R < 4T_2$) using, for example, a spoiler gradient if necessary before the next 90° pulse is applied.

With the result in Eq. (7.9), Eq. (7.8) can be written as

$$M_{z'}^{(n)}(0_-) = M_z^0 \left(1 - e^{-T_R/T_1}\right) \qquad n \geq 2 \qquad (7.11)$$

Equation (7.11) indicates that the spin system reaches a "steady state" by the time the second 90° pulse is applied. For this reason, the first 90° pulse is sometimes called the *preparatory pulse* and the corresponding signal is discarded.

From Eq. (7.11), we obtain

$$M_{x'y'}^{(n)}(0_+) = M_z^0 \left(1 - e^{-T_R/T_1}\right) \qquad n > 1 \qquad (7.12)$$

and correspondingly, the amplitude of the FID signal is

$$A_f \propto M_z^0 \left(1 - e^{-T_R/T_1}\right) \propto \rho \left(1 - e^{-T_R/T_1}\right) \qquad (7.13)$$

One can see from Eq. (7.13) that the FID signal bears a characteristic T_1-weighting factor, $(1 - e^{-T_R/T_1})$. Since this T_1-weighting factor is not affected by the subsequent steps in spatial information encoding and image reconstruction, the resulting image intensity will be similarly T_1-weighted as

$$I(r) = C\rho(r) \left[1 - e^{-T_R/T_1(r)}\right] \qquad (7.14)$$

where C is a scaling constant dependent on the encoding and image reconstruction methods used. Equation (7.14) indicates that a saturation–recovery sequence is capable of generating an image with either spin-density-weighted contrast or T_1-weighted contrast. Specifically, if a long T_R is used,

$$(1 - e^{-T_R/T_1}) \rightarrow 1 \qquad (7.15)$$

and the tissue contrast will come primarily from the difference in spin density. On the other hand, if a short T_R is used, the image will be T_1-weighted, and the tissue contrast will be due mainly to the difference in the tissue T_1 value. For biological samples, a T_R of less than 500 ms is considered to be short and a T_R greater than 1500 ms is considered to be long for sequences of this type.

■ Example 7.1

Assume that we have a sample consisting of two tissues with uniform spin density but different T_1 relaxation times $T_{1,A}$ and $T_{1,B}$. In this example, we calculate the optimal T_R value of a saturation–recovery sequence so that maximum T_1 contrast is achieved.

According to Eq. (7.14), we have

$$\begin{cases} I_A \propto \rho_A \left(1 - e^{-T_R/T_{1,A}}\right) \\ I_B \propto \rho_B \left(1 - e^{-T_R/T_{1,B}}\right) \end{cases} \tag{7.16}$$

and

$$\mathcal{C}_{AB} \propto |I_A - I_B| = C \left(e^{-T_R/T_{1,B}} - e^{-T_R/T_{1,A}}\right) \tag{7.17}$$

for $\rho_A = \rho_B$. The optimal value for T_R satisfies the following equation:

$$\frac{\partial \mathcal{C}_{AB}}{\partial T_R} = C \left(\frac{1}{T_{1,A}} e^{-T_R/T_{1,A}} - \frac{1}{T_{1,B}} e^{-T_R/T_{1,B}}\right) = 0 \tag{7.18}$$

whose solution is

$$T_R^o = \frac{\ln\left(\frac{T_{1,A}}{T_{1,B}}\right)}{\frac{1}{T_{1,B}} - \frac{1}{T_{1,A}}} \tag{7.19}$$

Following the same procedure, one can readily work out a solution for the more general case with $\rho_A \neq \rho_B$. This is left for the reader.

7.3   Inversion–Recovery Sequence

Inversion recovery is another popular T_1-weighted imaging sequence. As illustrated in Fig. 7.3, this sequence begins with a preparatory 180° pulse (or inversion pulse). In abbreviated form, it is written as

$$(180° - T_I - 90° - T_D)_N \tag{7.20}$$

where T_I is called the inversion time and T_D the recovery (or delay) time.

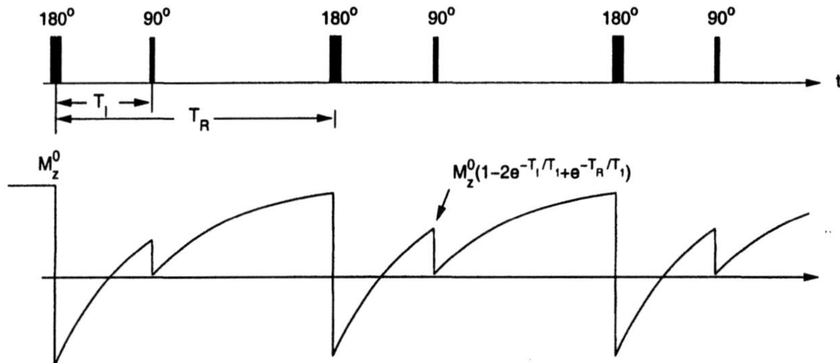

Figure 7.3   The basic inversion–recovery pulse sequence and the time evolution of $M_{z'}$.

The image intensity as a function of the T_1 relaxation time and the pulse timing parameters can be shown to be (see Example 7.2)

$$I(\boldsymbol{r}) \propto \rho(\boldsymbol{r}) \left[1 - 2e^{-T_\mathrm{I}/T_1(\boldsymbol{r})} + e^{-T_\mathrm{R}/T_1(\boldsymbol{r})} \right] \tag{7.21}$$

In contrast to the saturation–recovery sequence, we can now adjust two sequence parameters, T_I and T_R, for optimal T_1 contrast. Specifically, by properly choosing T_I we can make some tissue components to have negative or even zero intensities. For example, if we set T_I to the following value

$$T_\mathrm{I} = [\ln 2 - \ln(1 + e^{-T_\mathrm{R}/T_1^0})]T_1^0 \tag{7.22}$$

we have

$$1 - 2e^{-T_\mathrm{I}/T_1^0} + e^{-T_\mathrm{R}/T_1^0} = 0 \tag{7.23}$$

Then, any tissue components with $T_1 = T_1^0$ will contribute no signal in the final image. This is known as the *signal-nulling effect*.

Because of this property, the inversion–recovery sequence can generate greater T_1 contrast than the saturation–recovery sequence and is more useful for differentiation of tissues having similar spin density and T_2 values but slightly different T_1 values.

■ **Example 7.2**

In this example, we derive the expression in Eq. (7.21). As in the saturation–recovery sequence, the z magnetization in this sequence reaches a steady state prepulse value after the first 90° pulse. Therefore, to derive the signal expression in Eq. (7.21), we need only to calculate the z magnetization before the second 90° pulse.

Referring to Fig. 7.3, $M_{z'} = M_z^0$ at $t = 0$. After the first 180° pulse,

$$M_{z'} = -M_z^0$$

Based on the relaxation equation in Eq. (3.122), the longitudinal magnetization at $t = T_\mathrm{I}$ is given by

$$M_{z'} = M_z^0 \left(1 - 2e^{-T_\mathrm{I}/T_1} \right)$$

which is subsequently flipped onto the transverse plane by the 90° pulse applied at $t = T_\mathrm{I}$. At $t = T_\mathrm{R}$, the longitudinal magnetization regains the following value:

$$M_{z'} = M_z^0 \left(1 - e^{-(T_\mathrm{R} - T_\mathrm{I})/T_1} \right)$$

After the second $180°$,

$$M_{z'} = -M_z^0 \left(1 - e^{-(T_R - T_1)/T_1}\right)$$

Finally, applying the relaxation equation again, we have, immediately before the second $90°$ pulse, that

$$M_{z'} = M_z^0 \left(1 - e^{-T_1/T_1}\right) - M_z^0 \left(1 - e^{-(T_R - T_1)/T_1}\right) e^{-T_1/T_1}$$

$$= M_z^0 \left(1 - 2e^{-T_1/T_1} + e^{-T_R/T_1}\right)$$

The signal expression in Eq. (7.21) results immediately.

7.4   Basic Spin-Echo Imaging

The plain saturation–recovery and inversion–recovery sequences, as described in Sections 7.3 and 7.2, generate T_1-weighted FID signals. For symmetric coverage of k-space, echo signals are often used. In this section, we discuss the incorporation of spin echoes into these imaging sequences and the resulting image contrast.

We first study the saturation–recovery spin-echo sequence shown in Fig. 7.4. As in the plain saturation–recovery sequence, the z magnetization before a $90°$ pulse reaches a steady state after the first pulse, whose value is

$$M_{z'}(0_-) = M_z^0 \left(1 - 2e^{-(T_R - T_E/2)/T_1} + e^{-T_R/T_1}\right) \tag{7.24}$$

Therefore, the amplitude of the spin-echo signal is

$$A_E = M_z^0 \left(1 - 2e^{-(T_R - T_E/2)/T_1} + e^{-T_R/T_1}\right) e^{-T_E/T_2} \tag{7.25}$$

In practice, $T_E \ll T_R$ and Eq. (7.25) can be simplified to

$$A_E = M_z^0 \left(1 - e^{-T_R/T_1}\right) e^{-T_E/T_2} \tag{7.26}$$

The signal expression in Eq. (7.26) indicates that the image intensity of the saturation–recovery spin-echo sequence carries a T_1-weighting, T_2-weighting, and spin-density-weighting simultaneously, in general. However, we can selectively emphasize one of contrast mechanisms by properly choosing the sequence parameters T_R and T_E. For instance, if a short T_E is used, the term e^{-T_E/T_2} approaches 1 and the T_2-weighting factor can then be ignored. Effects of different sequence parameter values on image contrast for this excitation scheme is summarized in Table 7.1.

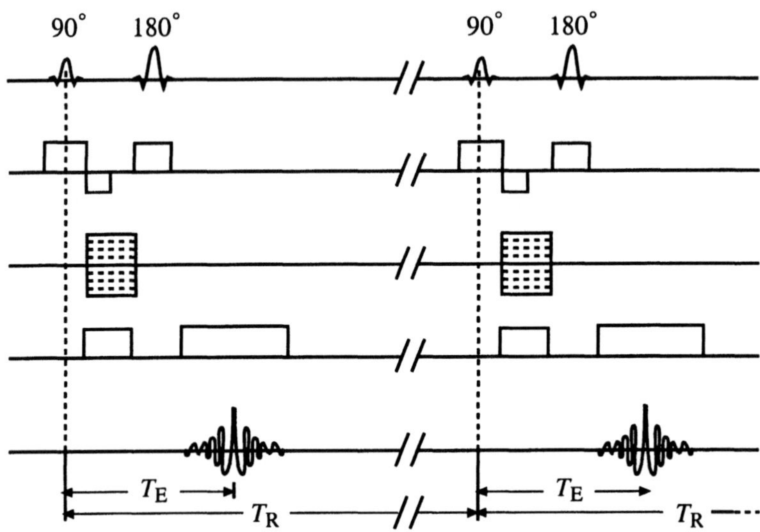

Figure 7.4 Saturation–recovery spin-echo imaging sequence.

Table 7.1 Image Contrast of a Saturation–Recovery SE Sequence

Contrast	T_E	T_R
T_1-weighting	short	appropriate
T_2-weighting	appropriate	long
ρ-weighting	short	long

We now extend the discussion to the inversion–recovery spin-echo sequence shown in Fig. 7.5. Correspondingly to Eq. (7.25), one can derive for the inversion–recovery sequence that

$$A_E = M_z^0 \left(1 - 2e^{-T_1/T_1} + 2e^{-(T_R - T_E/2)/T_1} - e^{-T_R/T_1}\right) e^{-T_E/T_2} \qquad (7.27)$$

Again, invoking the practical assumption that $T_E \ll T_R$, we have the following better known formula:

$$A_E = M_z^0 \left(1 - 2e^{-T_1/T_1} + e^{-T_R/T_1}\right) e^{-T_E/T_2} \qquad (7.28)$$

which indicates that this sequence can generate T_1-, T_2-, and spin-density-weighted contrast as the saturation–recovery spin-echo sequence does.

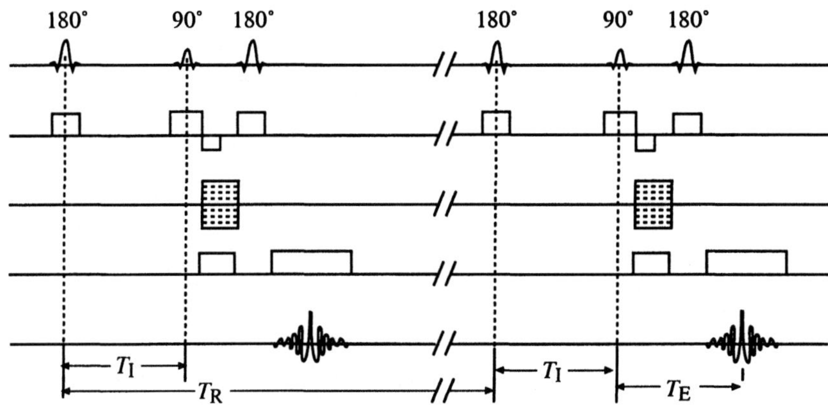

Figure 7.5 Inversion–recovery spin-echo imaging sequence.

7.5 Basic Gradient-Echo Imaging

The basic idea of gradient-echo imaging is to replace the 180° rephasing RF
pulses in a spin-echo imaging sequence by gradient rephasing pulses, as shown
in Fig. 7.6. With this replacement, it becomes efficient to use smaller flip-angle
excitations for fast imaging, a topic discussed in Chapter 9.

Gradient-echo imaging sequences show a wide range of variations as compared to spin-echo imaging sequences, and, as a result, the image contrast mechanism is also significantly richer. Specifically, gradient-echo imaging sequences
can generate images with T_1-, T_1/T_2-, T_2-, T_2^*-, and spin-density-weighted contrast with a proper selection of the T_R, T_E, and the flip angle. In this section, we
illustrate this concept by going through one specific example. More in-depth discussion of other gradient-echo imaging methods, in the context of fast imaging,
and their contrast behavior can be found in Chapter 9.

Consider the gradient-echo sequence in Fig. 7.6. We assume that $T_R \gg T_2$
such that

$$M_{x'y'}^{(n)}(0_-) = 0 \tag{7.29}$$

Equation (7.29) means that the transverse magnetization from the preceding excitation pulse is totally dephased.

Invoking the relaxation equation in Eq. (3.122), we obtain

$$M_{z'}^{(n)}(0_-) = M_z^0(1 - e^{-T_R/T_1}) + M_{z'}^{(n-1)}(0_+)e^{-T_R/T_1} \tag{7.30}$$

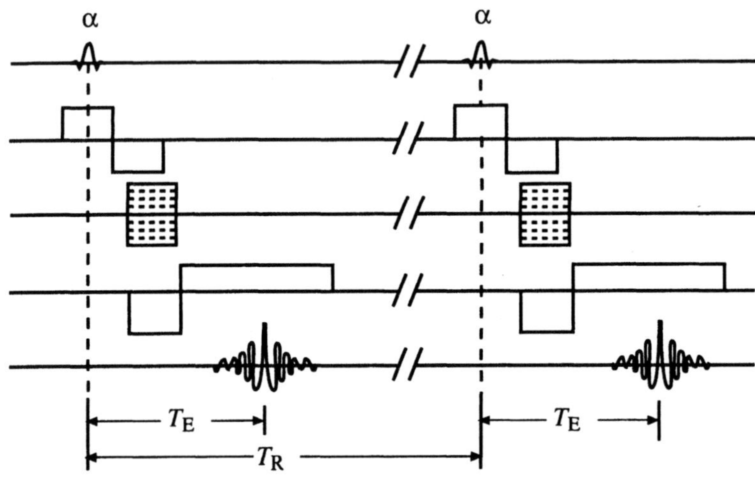

Figure 7.6   A generic gradient-echo imaging sequence.

where $M_{z'}^{(n)}(0_-)$ and $M_{z'}^{(n-1)}(0_+)$ represent the z magnetization before the nth pulse and after the $(n-1)$th pulse, respectively. Making use of the fact that

$$M_{z'}^{(n)}(0_+) = M_{z'}^{(n)}(0_-)\cos\alpha \tag{7.31}$$

Equation (7.30) can be rewritten as

$$M_{z'}^{(n)}(0_-) = M_z^0(1 - e^{-T_R/T_1}) + M_{z'}^{(n-1)}(0_-)\cos\alpha\, e^{-T_R/T_1} \tag{7.32}$$

Under the dynamic equilibrium condition that

$$M_{z'}^{(n)}(0_-) = M_{z'}^{(n-1)}(0_-) = M_{z'}^{ss}(0_-) \tag{7.33}$$

we have

$$M_{z'}^{ss}(0_-) = \frac{M_z^0(1 - e^{-T_R/T_1})}{1 - \cos\alpha\, e^{-T_R/T_1}} \tag{7.34}$$

Consequently, the postpulse transverse magnetization is

$$M_{x'y'}^{ss}(t) = \frac{M_z^0(1 - e^{-T_R/T_1})}{1 - \cos\alpha\, e^{-T_R/T_1}}\sin\alpha\, e^{-t/T_2^*} \tag{7.35}$$

and the echo amplitude is

$$A_E = \frac{M_z^0(1 - e^{-T_R/T_1})}{1 - \cos\alpha\, e^{-T_R/T_1}}\sin\alpha\, e^{-T_E/T_2^*} \tag{7.36}$$

Equation (7.36) clearly shows that the image intensity from this gradient-echo sequence carries both T_1- and T_2^*-weightings. The T_2^*-weighting factor is characteristic of a gradient-echo sequence, and it is controllable by adjusting the echo time T_E. This is similar to the way the T_2 contrast is adjusted in a spin-echo imaging sequence. Unlike the case of a spin-echo sequence, however, the T_1 contrast in the gradient-echo sequence is dependent mainly on the flip angle α instead of the repetition time T_R. Specifically, when α is small, $\cos\alpha \approx 1$ and the T_1-weighting factor is eliminated. As the flip angle is increased, the T_1-weighting factor becomes more significant, and it can be further regulated by selecting different repetition time.

7.6   Discussion

There are three primary types of contrast in MR imaging: *spin density contrast*, T_1 *contrast*, and T_2 *contrast*. Spin density contrast is linearly proportional to the tissue spin density differences, whereas T_1 and T_2 contrasts have an exponential dependence on the tissue T_1 and T_2 values. Normal soft tissues usually have a small variation in spin density but have quite different T_1 values. Therefore, T_1-weighted imaging is an effective method to obtain images of a good anatomical definition. Many disease states are characterized by a change of the tissue T_2 value, and T_2-weighted imaging is a sensitive method for disease detection.

For a given imaging sequence, all three types of contrast can contribute to the tissue contrast, but usually only one is emphasized. For example, in spin-echo imaging, one can eliminate the T_1 and T_2 factors with a large T_R and a small T_E. The resulting image will be spin-density-weighted. In practice, the minimum value of T_E possible is often limited by system hardware performance, and the maximum value of T_R is constrained by imaging time and practical considerations.

Although a large intensity difference is an important factor for good tissue visibility, there are also many other contributing factors, such as image pixel size and noise. Discussion of these topics is beyond the scope of this text.

To illustrate the concept of tissue contrast as a function of data acquisition parameters, three set of head images are shown in Figs. 7.7, 7.8, and 7.9. The images in Figs. 7.7 and 7.8 were acquired using a saturation–recovery spin-echo sequence with different T_1- and T_2-weightings. One can appreciate the change in image appearance due to different acquisition parameters by noting the typical brain tissue parameters listed in Table 7.2.

Figure 7.9. shows a set of brain images acquired using a gradient-echo sequence with different flip angles. As can be seen, at small flip angles, the images show mainly the proton density distribution, with cerebrospinal fluid having the highest intensity, followed by gray and white matters. At larger flip angles, the images become T_1-weighted.

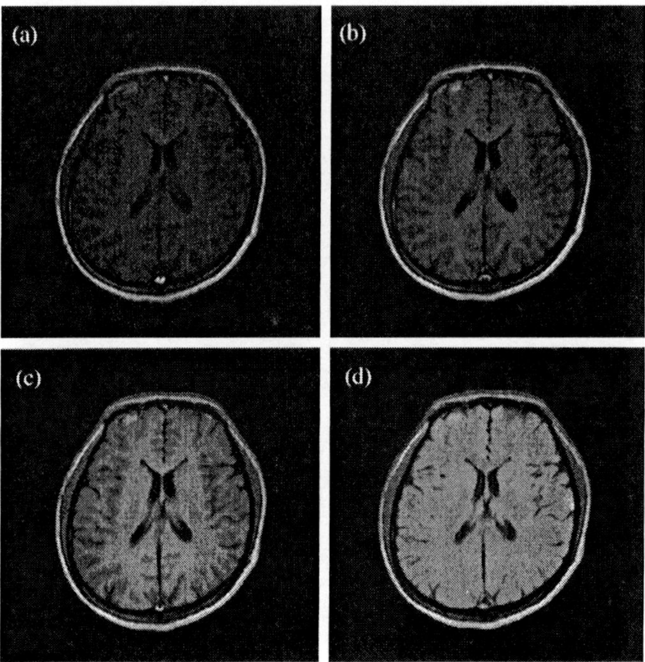

Figure 7.7 T_1-weighted head images obtained using a saturation–recovery SE sequence with different T_Rs: (a) $T_R = 250$ ms, (b) $T_R = 500$ ms, (c) $T_R = 1000$ ms, and (d) $T_R = 2000$ ms. The shorter T_R images are heavily T_1-weighted, while the long T_R image is more proton-density-weighted.

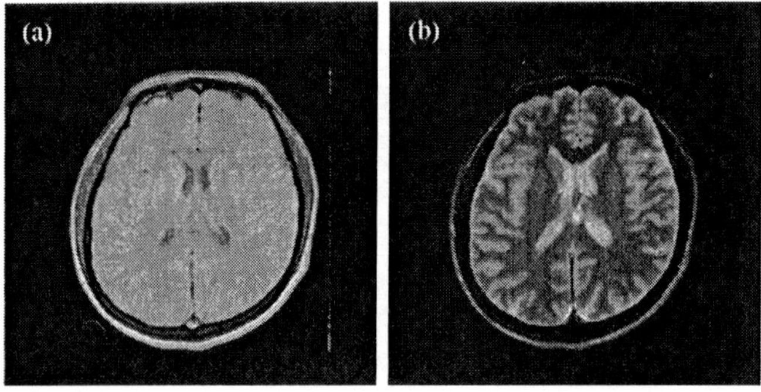

Figure 7.8 T_2-weighted head images obtained using the same sequence as in Fig. 7.7. Two different echo times were used: (a) $T_E = 20$ ms and (b) $T_E = 80$ ms, with the same $T_R = 2000$ ms. Image (a) is heavily proton-density-weighted, while image (b) is T_2-weighted.

Table 7.2   Typical Brain Tissue Parameters Measured at 1.5 T

Tissue	T_1 (ms)	T_2 (ms)	Relative ρ
White matter	510	67	0.61
Gray matter	760	77	0.69
Cerebrospinal fluid	2650	280	1.00

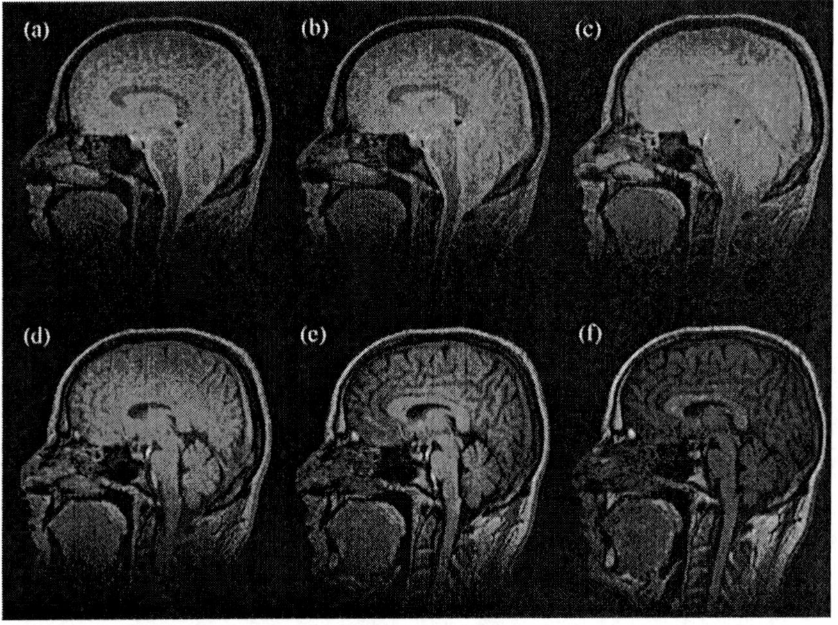

Figure 7.9   Brain images acquired using a gradient-echo sequence ($T_R = 25$ ms, $T_E = 4.75$ ms) with different flip angles: (a) $\alpha = 2°$, (b) $\alpha = 5°$, (c) $\alpha = 10°$, (d) $\alpha = 20°$, (e) $\alpha = 40°$, and (f) $\alpha = 60°$. Note that at small flip angles, the images show the characteristics of proton-density-weighting, whereas at larger flip angles, the T_1-weighting becomes dominant. Each of these images is acquired from a three-dimensional data set with $N_x = 512$, $N_y = 512$, $N_z = 80$, $\text{FOV}_x = 256$ mm, $\text{FOV}_y = 256$ mm, and $\text{FOV}_z = 160$ mm. The image in (a) was obtained by averaging two slices to improve the signal-to-noise ratio.

Exercises

7.1 Design a two-dimensional imaging pulse sequence that can be used to generate a T_1 map from a slice of an object and outline the signal processing steps required.

7.2 Design a two-dimensional imaging pulse sequence that can be used to generate a T_2 map from a slice of an object and outline the signal processing steps required.

7.3 Why is the data acquisition time for T_2-weighted imaging longer than that for T_1-weighted imaging?

7.4 A saturation–recovery spin-echo sequence can generate different kinds of image contrast. To generate a spin-density-weighted image, both the T_1-weighting and T_2-weighting factors are virtually eliminated. But for a T_1-weighted or T_2-weighted image, the spin density-weighting remains. True or false? Why?

7.5 Assume the following object with $\rho_A = 1$, $T_{1,A} = 1000$ ms, $T_{2,A} = 50$ ms, $\rho_B = 1$, $T_{1,B} = 500$ ms and $T_{2,B} = 100$ ms. Three images were obtained using a saturation–recovery spin-echo sequence, with $I_A = I_B$ for image 1, $I_A = 2I_B$ for image 2, and $I_A = 0.5I_B$ for image 3.

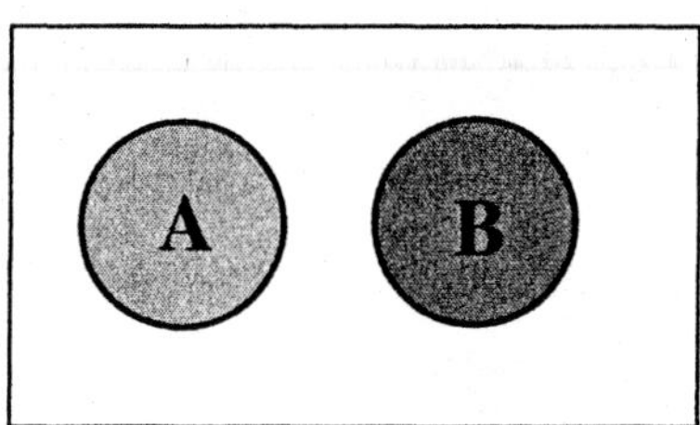

(a) For each case, determine if the image is ρ-weighted, T_1-weighted, or T_2-weighted.

(b) Determine the T_R and T_E values used to obtain each image, assuming that the contrast difference results from only one of three contrast mechanisms.

7.6 Derive the expression in Eq. (7.24).

7.7 Derive the expression in Eq. (7.27).

7.8 Discuss why image contrast is determined primarily by central k-space data.

7.9 The signal-nulling property of the inversion–recovery sequence can be exploited for fat suppression. The T_1 value of fat at 1.5 T is roughly 260 ms. If $T_R = 100$ ms, what is the value of T_I that will cause the M_z-component of fat to be zero at the times that the 90° pulses are applied?

Chapter 8

Image Resolution, Noise, and Artifacts

Nothing is invented and perfected at the same time.

Latin Proverb

This chapter further examines image characteristics with respect to various data acquisition and processing schemes. We focus specifically on issues related to image resolution, signal-to-noise ratio, and systematic image artifacts. The primary goal is to familiarize the reader with some commonly encountered image errors and to provide some insight into how to reduce them when appropriate.

8.1 Resolution Limitations

In any practical MRI experiment, the resultant image is never identical to the true image desired. This section discusses image errors due to limited resolution. However, instead of describing all the practical resolution-limiting factors, we focus on describing a useful point spread function (PSF) concept and show how to use it to analyze resolution limitation in several practical imaging schemes.

8.1.1 Point Spread Function

Consider an idealized object consisting of a single point. It is likely that the image we obtain from it is a blurred point. Nevertheless, we are still able to identify it as a point. Now, we add another point to the object. If the two points are farther apart, we will see two blurred points. However, as the two points are moving closer to each other, the image looks less like two points. In fact, the two points will merge together to become a single blob when their separation is below a certain threshold. We call this threshold value the resolution limit of the imaging system. Formally stated, *the spatial resolution of an imaging system is the smallest separation δx of two point sources necessary for them to remain resolvable in the resultant image.* In order to arrive at a more quantitative definition of resolution, we next introduce the point spread function concept.

We first define what is called a linear imaging process. Assume that for a given imaging system, object $I_1(x)$ produces image $\hat{I}_1(x)$, and object $I_2(x)$ produces image $\hat{I}_2(x)$. We then construct a composite object as

$$I_3(x) = aI_1(x) + bI_2(x) \tag{8.1}$$

for arbitrary constants a and b. If the image resulting from $I_3(x)$ is described by

$$\hat{I}_3(x) = a\hat{I}_1(x) + b\hat{I}_2(x) \tag{8.2}$$

this imaging system is a linear system. For such a system, an elegant relationship exists between an arbitrary object function $I(x)$ and its image $\hat{I}(x)$ (see Problem 8.2). That is,

$$\hat{I}(x) = I(x) * h(x) \tag{8.3}$$

where the convolution kernel function $h(x)$ is known as the point spread function since $\hat{I}(x) = h(x)$ for $I(x) = \delta(x)$.

It is clear from Eq. (8.3) that the image from an imaging system is an exact representation of the underlying object function only if the point spread function is a δ-function. If $h(x)$ deviates from a δ-function, $\hat{I}(x)$ will be a blurred version of $I(x)$. The amount of blurring introduced to $\hat{I}(x)$ by an imperfect $h(x)$ can be quantified by the width of $h(x)$. To illustrate this point, consider a simple case in which $h(x)$ is a boxcar function. As shown in Fig. 8.1, the two sources are resolvable in the resultant image only when the separation between them is larger than the width of the boxcar function. Therefore, based on the observation, we can state that the resolution limit of an imaging system is the width of its point spread function.

When $h(x)$ is not a boxcar function, its width definition is not unique. Two practical definitions are as follows:

Definition 8.1 *The effective width W_h of $h(x)$ is the full width at the half maximum of $h(x)$.*

Definition 8.2 *The effective width W_h of $h(x)$ is the width of an approximating boxcar function that has the same height and area as $h(x)$; or, more precisely,*

$$W_h = \frac{1}{h(0)} \int_{-\infty}^{\infty} h(x)dx \tag{8.4}$$

where it is assumed that $h(0)$ is the maximum point of $h(x)$.

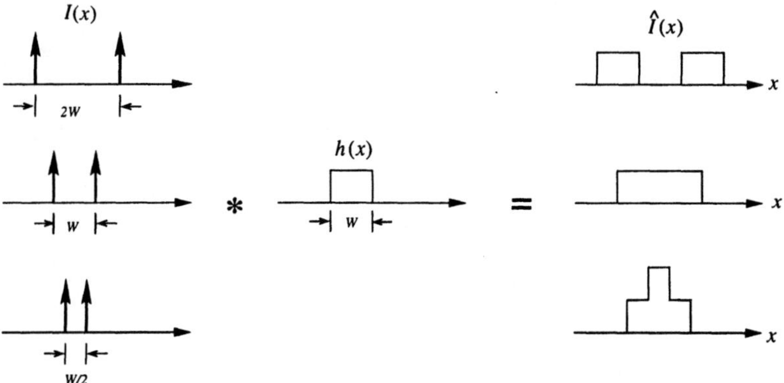

Figure 8.1 The effect of a boxcar point spread function. Note that the two point sources become irresolvable in the resultant image when their separation is not bigger than the width of the boxcar function.

8.1.2 PSF of Fourier Reconstructions

For convenience, we consider the one-dimensional case. Recall from Chapter 6 that given N Fourier samples, the image reconstructed based on the truncated Fourier series is given by

$$\hat{I}(x) = \Delta k \sum_{n=-N/2}^{N/2-1} S(n\Delta k)e^{i2\pi n\Delta k x} \tag{8.5}$$

To derive the underlying PSF, we simply set the true image function $I(x)$ to be a δ-function. Consequently, the measured signal is $S(m\Delta k) = 1$. When we substitute the signal into Eq. (8.5), the following PSF immediately results:

$$h(x) = \Delta k \sum_{n=-N/2}^{N/2-1} e^{i2\pi n\Delta k x} \tag{8.6}$$

Further simplification yields

$$h(x) = \Delta k \frac{\sin(\pi N \Delta k x)}{\sin(\pi \Delta k x)} e^{-i\pi \Delta k x} \tag{8.7}$$

The phase term $e^{-i\pi\Delta k x}$ in Eq. (8.7) can be eliminated, if necessary, with a symmetric coverage of k-space from $-N/2$ to $N/2$ instead of from $-N/2$ to $N/2-1$. In any event, it is often ignored because its effect is insignificant compared with that of the amplitude term.

Note that $h(x)$ is a periodic function with a period $1/\Delta k$. A plot of the amplitude part of $h(x)$ over one period is shown in Fig. 8.2. It is easy to determine from Eq. (8.7) that the width of the main lobe, as measured by the interval between its two zero crossings, is $2/(N\Delta k)$. The effective width of $h(x)$, as calculated from Eq. (8.4) with a change in the integration limits to cover a single period of $h(x)$, is given by

$$W_h = \frac{1}{h(0)} \int_{-\frac{1}{2\Delta k}}^{\frac{1}{2\Delta k}} h(x)dx = \frac{1}{N\Delta k} \qquad (8.8)$$

Therefore, the effective width of $h(x)$ is exactly half the width of its main lobe.

The right-hand side of Eq. (8.8) is known as the Fourier pixel size Δx_{F} in contrast to the usual image digital pixel size Δx. Note that Δx can be made arbitrarily small using zero-padding or other interpolation schemes as discussed in Chapter 6, but the image resolution is fundamentally limited to the Fourier pixel size. Therefore, in order for two point sources to be distinguishable, their separation has to be larger than Δx_{F}. Another implication of Eq. (8.8) is that W_h and N cannot be reduced simultaneously. In other words, we cannot improve image resolution and reduce the number of measured data points at the same time. This assertion is often referred to as the *uncertainty relation* of Fourier imaging, and in practice, one chooses N as large as signal-to-noise ratio and imaging time permit.

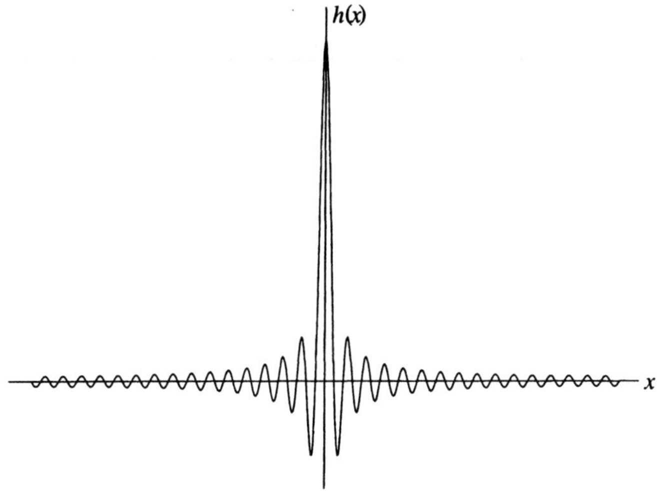

Figure 8.2　Plot of the amplitude part of $h(x)$ given in Eq. (8.7) for $N = 64$.

8.1.3 PSF of Backprojection Reconstructions

The PSF of backprojection reconstruction is given in the following theorems.

Theorem 8.1 *Let $P(p, \phi)$ be the projections of a two-dimensional function $I(x, y)$ and $\hat{I}(x, y)$ be given by*

$$\hat{I}(x, y) = \int_0^\pi P(x \cos \phi + y \sin \phi, \phi) d\phi \tag{8.9}$$

Then,

$$\hat{I}(x, y) = I(x, y) ** \frac{1}{\sqrt{x^2 + y^2}} \tag{8.10}$$

*where ** means two-dimensional convolution.*

Theorem 8.2 *Let $P(p, \theta, \phi)$ be the projections of a three-dimensional function $I(x, y, z)$ and $\hat{I}(x, y, z)$ be given by*

$$\hat{I}(x, y, z) = \frac{1}{2\pi} \int_0^{2\pi} \int_0^\pi P(x \sin \theta \cos \phi + y \sin \theta \sin \phi + z \cos \theta, \theta, \phi) \sin \theta d\theta d\phi \tag{8.11}$$

Then,

$$\hat{I}(x, y, z) = I(x, y, z) *** \frac{1}{\sqrt{x^2 + y^2 + z^2}} \tag{8.12}$$

*where *** represents three-dimensional convolution.*

Equation (8.10) indicates that the PSF of two-dimensional backprojection reconstructions is

$$h(x, y) = \frac{1}{\sqrt{x^2 + y^2}} \tag{8.13}$$

while the PSF of three-dimensional backprojection reconstruction, according to Eq. (8.12), is

$$h(x, y, z) = \frac{1}{\sqrt{x^2 + y^2 + z^2}} \tag{8.14}$$

Equation (8.13) can be derived by considering how projections from a point source get backprojected for image formation. Namely, one can show that

$$\int_0^\pi \delta(x \cos \phi + y \sin \phi) d\phi = \frac{1}{\sqrt{x^2 + y^2}} \tag{8.15}$$

The reader is encouraged to consult reference [32] for an intuitive argument for the relation in Eq (8.15). A more formal proof of Eq. (8.10) is as follows.

$$\hat{I}(x,y) = \int_0^\pi P(x\cos\phi + y\sin\phi, \phi)\,d\phi$$

$$= \int_0^\pi \int_{-\infty}^\infty \mathcal{F}\rho(k,\phi)e^{i2\pi k(x\cos\phi + y\sin\phi)}\,dk\,d\phi$$

$$= \int_0^{2\pi} \int_0^\infty \mathcal{F}\rho(k,\phi)e^{i2\pi k(x\cos\phi + y\sin\phi)}\,dk\,d\phi$$

$$= \int_0^{2\pi} \int_0^\infty k^{-1}\mathcal{F}\rho(k,\phi)e^{i2\pi k(x\cos\phi + y\sin\phi)}\,k\,dk\,d\phi$$

$$= \int_{-\infty}^\infty \int_{-\infty}^\infty \frac{1}{\sqrt{k_x^2 + k_y^2}}\mathcal{F}\rho(k_x,k_y)e^{i2\pi(xk_x + yk_y)}\,dk_x\,dk_y$$

$$= \mathcal{F}^{-1}\left\{ \frac{1}{\sqrt{k_x^2 + k_y^2}} \right\} ** I(x,y)$$

$$= I(x,y) ** \frac{1}{\sqrt{x^2 + y^2}} \tag{8.16}$$

where use of the following identity is made [6]:

$$\mathcal{F}^{-1}\left\{ \frac{1}{\sqrt{k_x^2 + k_y^2}} \right\} = \frac{1}{\sqrt{x^2 + y^2}} \tag{8.17}$$

Equation (8.12) can be proved as follows. Let $I(x,y,z) = \delta(x,y,z)$. Then, $P(p,\theta,\phi) = \delta(p)$. Substituting it into Eq. (8.11) yields

$$h(x,y,z) = \frac{1}{2\pi} \int_0^{2\pi} \int_0^\pi \delta(x\sin\theta\cos\phi + y\sin\theta\sin\phi + z\cos\theta)\sin\theta\,d\theta\,d\phi$$

$$= \frac{1}{2\pi} \int_0^{2\pi} \int_0^\pi \delta(\boldsymbol{r}\cdot\boldsymbol{\mu})\sin\theta\,d\theta\,d\phi$$

$$= \frac{1}{2\pi|\boldsymbol{r}|} \int_0^{2\pi} \int_0^\pi \delta(\boldsymbol{\mu}_r\cdot\boldsymbol{\mu})\sin\theta\,d\theta\,d\phi \tag{8.18}$$

where $\boldsymbol{r} = (x,y,z)$ and $\boldsymbol{\mu} = (\sin\theta\cos\phi, \sin\theta\sin\phi, \cos\theta)$. Due to the symmetry of the problem [16], the integration is independent of the direction of $\boldsymbol{\mu}_r$. For simplicity, suppose μ_r is along the z-axis. Then,

$$\int_0^{2\pi}\int_0^{\pi} \delta(\mu_x \cdot \mu)\sin\theta d\theta d\phi = \int_0^{2\pi}\int_0^{\pi} \delta(\cos\theta)\sin\theta d\theta d\phi$$

$$= 2\pi \int_{-1}^{1} \delta(x)dx$$

$$= 2\pi$$

Substituting this result into Eq. (8.18) immediately gives

$$h(x,y,z) = \frac{1}{|r|} = \frac{1}{\sqrt{x^2 + y^2 + z^2}} \tag{8.19}$$

8.2   Image Noise

Imaging involves measurement and processing of activated signals from an object. Any practical measurement always contains an undesirable component that is uncorrelated with the desired signal. This component is referred to as *noise* or *a random signal*. Noise often arises in an imaging system because of spontaneous fluctuations such as the thermal motion (Brownian motion) of free electrons inside real or equivalent electrical components. Of great concern to imaging scientists is the question of how noise is picked up or generated in an imaging system and how the imaging process handles it—that is, whether it is suppressed or amplified. The first aspect of the topic is related mostly to the imaging system hardware and will not be discussed here. Interested readers are referred to Chen and Hoult's book [13] for an excellent discussion. The second aspect is related to the mathematical and processing principles used for image formation and is discussed in this section. We begin with a review of some fundamental concepts and terminologies of noise signals.

8.2.1   Basic Concepts of Random Signals

8.2.1.1   Random Variables

A characteristic of noise is that it does not have fixed values in repeated measurements. Such a quantity is described mathematically by a random variable and is represented by Greek letters such as ξ. A formal and rigorous definition of a random variable is rather involved and is well beyond the scope of this book. The reader interested in an in-depth discussion is strongly encouraged to consult the excellent book by Papoulis [52].

A simple definition of a random variable is to view it as a function defined over the sample space. As shown in Fig. 8.3, the value of a deterministic variable is a constant, whereas the value of a random variable from a particular measurement is "arbitrary." But if many such measurements are taken, their values follow a certain statistical relationship, known as the *probability density function* (PDF). The PDF of a random variable ξ is often denoted as $p_\xi(x)$, which represents the probability of obtaining a specific value x for ξ in a particular measurement. Since a value will always be obtained from an experiment, the area under any PDF must be one, that is,

$$\int_{-\infty}^{\infty} p_\xi(x)\,dx = 1 \tag{8.20}$$

In practice, $p_\xi(x)$ can take various forms. For example, $p_\xi(x)$ can be a constant or a Gaussian function corresponding to uniform or Gaussian noise. Although a random variable is fully characterized by its PDF, its PDF is not always known in practical situations. We often use parameters such as mean and variance to describe it. In fact, based on the central limit theorem, most measurement noise can be treated as Gaussian noise, in which case the PDF is uniquely defined by its mean and variance.

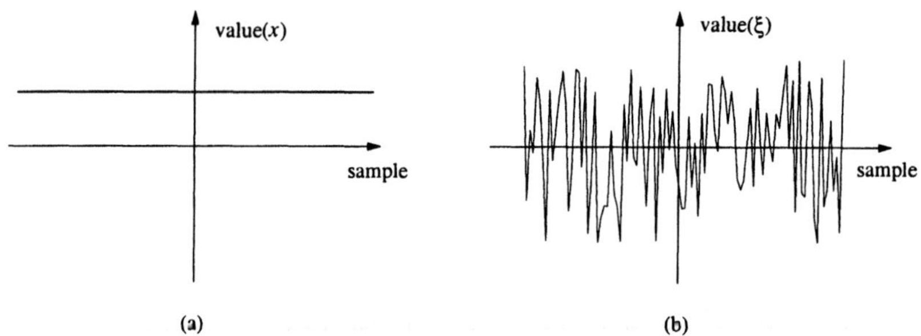

Figure 8.3 Deterministic and random variables as a function of the sample space.

Mean: The mean of a random variable, ξ, is by definition the PDF-weighted average of all possible values of the random variable. It is also called the ensemble average or the mathematical expected value. For a continuous variable, the mean is defined as

$$\bar{\xi} = E\{\xi\} = \int_{-\infty}^{\infty} x p_\xi(x)\,dx \tag{8.21}$$

and for a discrete random variable,

$$\bar{\xi} = E\{\xi\} = \sum_{m} x_m p_\xi(x_m) \tag{8.22}$$

where E is called the mathematical expectation operator. Mean is a first-order statistical moment since it involves only the first power of the random variable.

Variance: The variance of a random variable is defined as

$$\sigma_\xi^2 = \text{var}\{\xi\} = E\{(\xi - \bar{\xi})(\xi - \bar{\xi})^*\} \tag{8.23}$$

which is a second-order statistical moment. The positive number σ_ξ is called the standard deviation, which is a measure of the average deviation from the mean.

■ **Example 8.1**

Assume that ξ is a uniform random variable defined over the interval (x_1, x_2). Then $p_\xi(x) = 1/(x_2 - x_1)$. The mean value of ξ is

$$\bar{\xi} = \int_{-\infty}^{\infty} x p_\xi(x) dx = \frac{1}{x_2 - x_1} \int_{x_1}^{x_2} x dx = \frac{x_1 + x_2}{2}$$

Its standard deviation is

$$\sigma_\xi = \sqrt{\int_{-\infty}^{\infty} (x - \bar{\xi})^2 p_\xi(x) dx}$$

$$= \sqrt{\frac{1}{x_2 - x_1} \int_{x_1}^{x_2} \left(x - \frac{x_1 + x_2}{2} \right)^2 dx}$$

$$= \frac{1}{\sqrt{3}} \frac{x_2 - x_1}{2}$$

■ **Example 8.2**

The PDF of a Gaussian random variable is

$$p_\xi(x) = \frac{1}{\sqrt{2\pi}\sigma} e^{-(x-\mu)^2/2\sigma^2} \tag{8.24}$$

It can be shown, based on the definitions, that $\bar{\xi} = \mu$ and $\sigma_\xi = \sigma$.

Statistical Relationships of Random Variables: Noisy data points or image pixels are often characterized by a large number of random variables. A commonly asked question is: What are the mean and variance of the reconstructed image after mathematical operations such as the Fourier transformation? Or even more simply, what is the resulting noise variance after averaging two neighboring noisy pixels? To answer these questions, we need to know how the random variables involved are related to each other statistically. Two important concepts used for describing the statistical relationship between a pair of random variables are *statistical independence* and *uncorrelatedness*.

For two random variables ξ_1 and ξ_2 if the probability of simultaneously obtaining values x for ξ_1 and y for ξ_2 equals the product of the probabilities of obtaining each separately, that is,

$$p_{\xi_1\xi_2}(x,y) = p_{\xi_1}(x)p_{\xi_2}(y) \tag{8.25}$$

they are said to be statistically independent. Statistical independence is a very strong condition that random variables of practical interest hardly meet. If we are concerned only about their second-order distribution, as is often the case in practice, the interdependence of two random variables can be assessed by a parameter called *correlation coefficient*, which is defined as

$$c_{\xi_1\xi_2} = \frac{E\{(\xi_1 - \bar{\xi}_1)(\xi_2 - \bar{\xi}_2)^*\}}{\sigma_{\xi_1}\sigma_{\xi_2}} \tag{8.26}$$

It is easy to see from the definition that $c_{\xi_1\xi_2}$ takes value in the range $-1 \leq c_{\xi_1\xi_2} \leq 1$. When $c_{\xi_1\xi_2} = 0$, ξ_1 and ξ_2 are said to be *uncorrelated*. In the other extreme that $c_{\xi_1\xi_2} = \pm 1$, ξ_1 and ξ_2 have a linear dependence, namely, $\xi_1 = a\xi_2$ for a certain scaling constant a.

Because uncorrelatedness is only a measure of second-order statistics, one can justify that uncorrelated random variables are not necessarily independent. Conversely, statistically independent random variables are always uncorrelated. For example, if ξ_1 and ξ_2 are independent, their joint PDF can be written as $p_{\xi_1\xi_2}(x,y) = p_{\xi_1}(x)p_{\xi_2}(y)$. Thus,

$$c_{\xi_1\xi_2} = \frac{1}{\sigma_{\xi_1}\sigma_{\xi_2}} \int_{-\infty}^{\infty} \int_{-\infty}^{\infty} (x - \bar{\xi}_1)(y - \bar{\xi}_2)^* p_{\xi_1}(x)p_{\xi_2}(y)\,dx\,dy$$

$$= \frac{1}{\sigma_{\xi_1}\sigma_{\xi_2}} \int_{-\infty}^{\infty} (x - \bar{\xi}_1)p_{\xi_1}(x)\,dx \int_{-\infty}^{\infty} (y - \bar{\xi}_2)^* p_{\xi_2}(y)\,dy$$

$$= \frac{1}{\sigma_{\xi_1}\sigma_{\xi_2}} (\bar{\xi}_1 - \bar{\xi}_1)(\bar{\xi}_2 - \bar{\xi}_2)^*$$

$$= 0$$

■ **Example 8.3**

As an example, we take a look at the resulting mean and variance of a linear combination of many random variables.

Assume that

$$\xi = \sum_{n=1}^{N} c_n \xi_n \tag{8.27}$$

where ξ_n are random variables and c_n are arbitrary deterministic constants. One can prove from the definition that the mean of ξ is equal to

$$E\{\xi\} = \sum_{n=1}^{N} c_n E\{\xi_n\} \tag{8.28}$$

regardless of whether or not the variables ξ_n are correlated.

For the variance, however, the relationship

$$\sigma_\xi^2 = \sum_{n=1}^{N} c_n^2 \sigma_{\xi_n}^2 \tag{8.29}$$

holds only when ξ_n are mutually uncorrelated or independent. For example, consider the case of two real random variables:

$$\begin{aligned}
\operatorname{var}\left\{\sum_{n=1}^{2} c_n \xi_n\right\} &= E\{[(c_1\xi_1 + c_2\xi_2) - (c_1\bar{\xi}_1 + c_2\bar{\xi}_2)]^2\} \\
&= E\{[c_1(\xi_1 - \bar{\xi}_1) + c_2(\xi_2 - \bar{\xi}_2)]^2\} \\
&= c_1^2 E\{(\xi_1 - \bar{\xi}_1)^2\} + 2c_1 c_2 E\{(\xi_1 - \bar{\xi}_1)(\xi_2 - \bar{\xi}_2)\} \\
&\quad + c_2^2 E\{(\xi_2 - \bar{\xi}_2)^2\}
\end{aligned} \tag{8.30}$$

The first and the last terms in Eq. (8.30) are $c_1^2 \sigma_{\xi_1}^2$ and $c_2^2 \sigma_{\xi_2}^2$, respectively. The middle term is zero if ξ_1 and ξ_2 are uncorrelated (or independent).

■ Example 8.4

Making use of the relation in (8.29), one can derive the popular result for signal averaging (an operation frequently encountered in image processing)— N signal averagings yield an improvement by a factor of $\sqrt{N}$ in the signal-to-noise ratio.

Let $\hat{x} = x + \xi$ be a measured quantity containing the true signal x and the noise component ξ with zero mean and standard deviation σ_ξ. The signal-to-noise ratio for $\hat{x}$ from a single measurement is $(\text{S/N})_{\hat{x}} = |x|/\sigma_\xi$. If N measurements are taken such that $\hat{x}_n = x + \xi_n$ are obtained to produce $\hat{y} = \frac{1}{N} \sum_{n=1}^{N} \hat{x}_n = x + \frac{1}{N} \sum_{n=1}^{N} \xi_n$, then the signal-to-noise ratio for $\hat{y}$ is

$$(\text{S/N})_{\hat{y}} = \frac{|x|}{\sqrt{\text{var}\left\{\frac{1}{N} \sum_{n=1}^{N} \hat{x}_n\right\}}} = \sqrt{N}\frac{|x|}{\sigma_\xi} = \sqrt{N}(\text{S/N})_{\hat{x}} \qquad (8.31)$$

assuming that the noise for different measurements is uncorrelated.

8.2.1.2   Random Signals

Random signals picked up in an imaging experiment are described by functions with random values, which are known as *random* (or *stochastic*) *processes*. Denoting $\xi(t)$ as a random process, $\xi(t_0)$ for any time instant t_0 is a random variable, but each sample of $\xi(t)$ is a deterministic function of time $\xi_m(t)$. Hence, $\xi(t)$ can also be considered as a family of time functions such that $\xi(t) = \{\xi_m(t)\}$. For example, the noise signal from a single measurement in practice corresponds to one of these sample functions of an underlying random process, or noise source. If many measurements could be made simultaneously under the "same" conditions, the set of sample functions obtained would define the random process.

As in the case of random variables, we may not always require a complete statistical description of a random process, or we may not be able to obtain it even if desired. In such cases, we work with various statistical moments, either by choice or by necessity. The most important ones are

Mean:
$$\bar{\xi}(t) = E\{\xi(t)\} \qquad (8.32)$$

Variance:
$$\sigma_\xi^2(t) = E\{[\xi(t) - \bar{\xi}(t)][\xi(t) - \bar{\xi}(t)]^*\} \qquad (8.33)$$

and the *correlation function:*

$$R(t, t + \tau) = E\{\xi(t)\xi^*(t + \tau)\} \qquad (8.34)$$

For some random processes, the mean and variance are independent of time, namely, $\bar{\xi}(t) = \bar{\xi}(t_0)$ and $\sigma_\xi(t) = \sigma_\xi(t_0)$; and the correlation function depends only on the time difference τ, namely, $R(t, t + \tau) = R(\tau)$. These processes are termed *wide-sense stationary*. Another important property of random processes is *ergodicity*, which means that time and ensemble averages are interchangeable. For example, if $\xi(t)$ is an ergodic process, then

$$\bar{\xi} = E\{\xi(t)\} =< \xi(t) > \tag{8.35}$$

$$\sigma_\xi^2 = E\{[\xi(t) - \bar{\xi}][\xi(t) - \bar{\xi}]^*\} =< [\xi(t) - \bar{\xi}][\xi(t) - \bar{\xi}]^* > \tag{8.36}$$

$$R(\tau) = E\{\xi(t)\xi^*(t+\tau)\} =< \xi(t)\xi^*(t+\tau) > \tag{8.37}$$

where $< \cdot >$ is the time average operator, defined as

$$< x(t) >= \lim_{T\to\infty} \frac{1}{2T} \int_{-T}^{T} x(t)dt \tag{8.38}$$

Therefore, for ergodic processes, the statistical moments are measurable from any sample function. Noise signals that we deal with in this book will be assumed to fall into this category. Furthermore, for an ergodic process, $R(\tau)$ is a deterministic function of time, and its Fourier transform gives the power spectral density function—a relationship established by the well-known Wiener theorem. If the spectral density function is a constant over the measurement frequency range, the noise is referred to as *white noise* in practice.

8.2.2   Noise Characteristics in the Data Domain

Random noise is an important limiting factor in MR imaging. It gets introduced early on in the signal generation and detection stage and is then processed in the image reconstruction stage. For convenience, we use ξ_d to represent the noise component in the data domain and ξ_I to represent the image noise. In practice, ξ_d depends on a number of factors, particularly the physical configuration of the RF detection system. An in-depth discussion of this topic is beyond the scope of this book; interested readers are referred to [13, 161, 195]. For the present discussion, we simply assume that ξ_d is an additive noise coming from an ergodic, stationary, uncorrelated, white noise process with zero mean and standard deviation σ_d. With this assumption, we have

$$\begin{cases} < \xi_d(k) >= 0 \\ < \xi_d(k)\xi_d^*(k) >= \sigma_d^2 \\ < \xi_d(k)\xi_d^*(k + k_0) > 0 \quad k_0 \neq 0 \end{cases} \tag{8.39}$$

and the noise-corrupted k-space signal can be expressed as

$$\hat{S}(k) = S(k) + \xi_d(k) \tag{8.40}$$

After the image reconstruction step, we have

$$\hat{I}(x) = I(x) + \xi_I(x) \tag{8.41}$$

Clearly, $\xi_I(x)$ depends on the image reconstruction schemes used. This section describes the characteristics of $\xi_I(x)$ in connection with some standard image reconstruction procedures.

8.2.3   Noise in Direct FFT Reconstruction

Assume that N noisy k-space data points are collected and processed using the standard FFT reconstruction algorithm. The image noise is given by

$$\xi_I[m] = \frac{1}{N} \sum_{n=-N/2}^{N/2-1} \xi_d[n] e^{i2\pi mn/N} \qquad -N/2 \le m < N/2 \qquad (8.42)$$

Several properties of $\xi_I[m]$ can be directly derived from Eq. (8.42)

(a)   The image noise $\xi_I[m]$ is of zero mean, namely,

$$E\{\xi_I[m]\} = 0 \qquad\qquad (8.43)$$

(b)   The variance of $\xi_I[m]$ is given by

$$\sigma_I^2 = \frac{1}{N}\sigma_d^2 \qquad\qquad (8.44)$$

(c)   The image noise $\xi_I[m]$ is uncorrelated from pixel to pixel. That is to say

$$E\{\xi_I[m]\xi_I^*[n]\} = 0 \qquad \text{for} \quad m \ne n \qquad (8.45)$$

The result stated in Eq. (8.43) is obvious. Equations (8.44) and (8.45) can be derived directly from the definition. Specifically,

$$E\{\xi_I[m]\xi_I^*[n]\} = \frac{1}{N^2} \sum_{p=-N/2}^{N/2-1} \sum_{q=-N/2}^{N/2-1} E\{\xi_d[p]\xi_d^*[q]\} e^{i2\pi(mp-nq)/N}$$

Noting that $E\{\xi_d[p]\xi_d^*[q]\} = 0$ for $p \ne q$, we have

$$E\{\xi_I[m]\xi_I^*[n]\} = \frac{1}{N^2} \sum_{p=-N/2}^{N/2-1} E\{\xi_d[p]\xi_d^*[p]\} e^{i2\pi(m-n)p/N}$$

$$= \frac{1}{N^2}\sigma_d^2 \sum_{p=-N/2}^{N/2-1} e^{i2\pi(m-n)p/N}$$

$$= \begin{cases} \frac{1}{N}\sigma_d^2 & m = n \\ 0 & \text{otherwise} \end{cases}$$

Remark 8.1 *Eq. (8.44) indicates that, as far as the noise variance is concerned, the FFT processing is equivalent to doing N-point signal averaging.*

Remark 8.2 *The signal-to-noise ratio per pixel of an FFT image is inversely proportional to* $\sqrt{N}$. *That is,*

$$\mathrm{SNR}|_{\mathrm{pixel}} \propto \frac{1}{\sqrt{N}} \tag{8.46}$$

Equation (8.46) can be understood by noting that σ_I decreases as $1/\sqrt{N}$ while the signal strength per pixel decreases as $1/N$ because the pixel size equals $1/(N\Delta k)$.

This point can be made more rigorously by directly calculating the average signal strength per pixel I_{avg} from the Fourier reconstruction. Specifically,

$$I_{\mathrm{avg}}^2 = \frac{1}{N} \sum_{m=-N/2}^{N/2-1} I[m]I^*[m]$$

$$= \frac{1}{N^3} \sum_{m=-N/2}^{N/2-1} \sum_{p=-N/2}^{N/2-1} \sum_{q=-N/2}^{N/2-1} S[p]S^*[q]e^{i2\pi(p-q)m/N}$$

$$= \frac{1}{N^2} \sum_{n=-N/2}^{N/2-1} |S[n]|^2 \tag{8.47}$$

Hence, the average image SNR per pixel is

$$\mathrm{SNR}|_{\mathrm{pixel}} = \frac{I_{\mathrm{avg}}}{\sigma_I} = \frac{\sqrt{\displaystyle\sum_{n=-N/2}^{N/2-1} |S[n]|^2}}{\sqrt{N}\sigma_d} \tag{8.48}$$

Equation (8.46) can be obtained directly from Eq. (8.48) since $\sum_{n=-N/2}^{N/2-1} |S[n]|^2$ stays roughly constant after N reaches a certain value (say, 64), noting that $S[n]$ decays as fast as $1/n$.

Remark 8.3 *Let* $\hat{I}_1[m]$ *be a noise-corrupted FFT image and* $\hat{I}_2[m]$ *be given by*

$$\hat{I}_2[m] = \frac{1}{P} \sum_{p=0}^{P-1} \hat{I}_1(m+p) \tag{8.49}$$

Then, the SNR of $\hat{I}_2[m]$ *is a factor of* $\sqrt{P}$ *better than that of* $\hat{I}_1[m]$.

This statement is a direct consequence of the fact that the noise in $\hat{I}_1[m]$ is uncorrelated from pixel to pixel, as well as the well-known result about such noise discussed in Example 8.3.

8.2.4   Noise in Zero-Padded FFT Reconstruction

With the zero-padded FFT reconstruction algorithm, N noisy data points will produce an arbitrary M (with $M > N$) noisy image points according to the following formula:

$$\xi_I[m] = \frac{1}{N} \sum_{n=-N/2}^{N/2-1} \xi_d[n] e^{i2\pi mn/M} \qquad -M/2 \leq m < M/2 \qquad (8.50)$$

The statistical properties of $\xi_I[m]$ are summarized below.

(a) $\xi_I[m]$ is of zero mean, namely,

$$E\{\xi_I[m]\} = 0 \qquad (8.51)$$

(b)   The variance of $\xi_I[m]$ is given by

$$\sigma_I^2 = \frac{1}{N}\sigma_d^2 \qquad (8.52)$$

(c) $\xi_I[m]$ shows a certain degree of pixel-to-pixel correlation:

$$E\{\xi_I[m]\xi_I^*[n]\} = \frac{1}{N^2}\sigma_d^2 \frac{\sin[\pi(m-n)N/M]}{\sin[\pi(m-n)/M]} e^{-i\pi(m-n)/N} \qquad (8.53)$$

Comparing Eqs. (8.51) and (8.52) to Eqs. (8.43) and (8.44), one can easily see that zero-padding does not affect the mean and variance of the image noise. Hence, the image SNR stays the same even though the digital pixel size is smaller. However, zero-padding does alter the statistical independence of the image noise as evidenced in Eq. 8.53. Because of this property, the result stated in Remark 8.3 does not apply to the situation here. In other words, one may not obtain a factor of $\sqrt{P}$ improvement in SNR by averaging P adjacent pixels in images obtained using the zero-padded FFT reconstruction algorithm.

Before concluding this section, we prove the result given in Eq. (8.53). Specifically, based on the definition, we have

$$E\{\xi_I[m]\xi_I^*[n]\} = \frac{1}{N^2} \sum_{p=-N/2}^{N/2-1} \sum_{q=-N/2}^{N/2-1} E\{\xi_d[p]\xi_d^*()\} e^{i2\pi(mp-nq)/M}$$

$$= \frac{1}{N^2} \sum_{p=-N/2}^{N/2-1} E\{\xi_d[p]\xi_d^*[p]\} e^{i2\pi(m-n)p/M}$$

$$= \frac{1}{N^2}\sigma_d^2 \sum_{p=-N/2}^{N/2-1} e^{i2\pi(m-n)p/M}$$

$$= \frac{1}{N^2}\sigma_d^2 \frac{\sin[\pi(m-n)N/M]}{\sin[\pi(m-n)/M]} e^{-i\pi(m-n)/N}$$

Finally, to gain an intuitive understanding of the noise characteristics of both direct and zero-padded FFT reconstructions, we consider a hypothetical experiment, shown in Fig. 8.4, in which we have a one-dimensional object and four Fourier samples. Direct FFT reconstruction gives an image of four pixels with SNR_0. If the data are zero-filled to eight points, the resultant eight pixels will have the same signal-to-noise ratio SNR_0. Note that in both cases the Fourier pixel size is the same, and so is the signal strength per pixel. If we recollapse the eight pixels to four pixels, no SNR improvement will be gained, since the noise is correlated. On the other hand, if eight phase-encoded measurements were actually collected (for improved resolution), the new image signal-to-noise ratio SNR_1 would be about $SNR_0/\sqrt{2}$. [Actually, it would be slightly higher because of the added signal energy from the new sample points; the exact value can be calculated from Eq. (8.48).] Recollapsing the eight pixels to four will regain the original signal-to-noise ratio, but the imaging time is doubled. Consequently, the SNR efficiency[1] is reduced by a factor of $\sqrt{2}$. Therefore, with the Fourier reconstruction methods, improving spatial resolution with extended k-space sampling will lead to an irreversible loss of SNR efficiency. One is also referred to [134] for a similar argument.

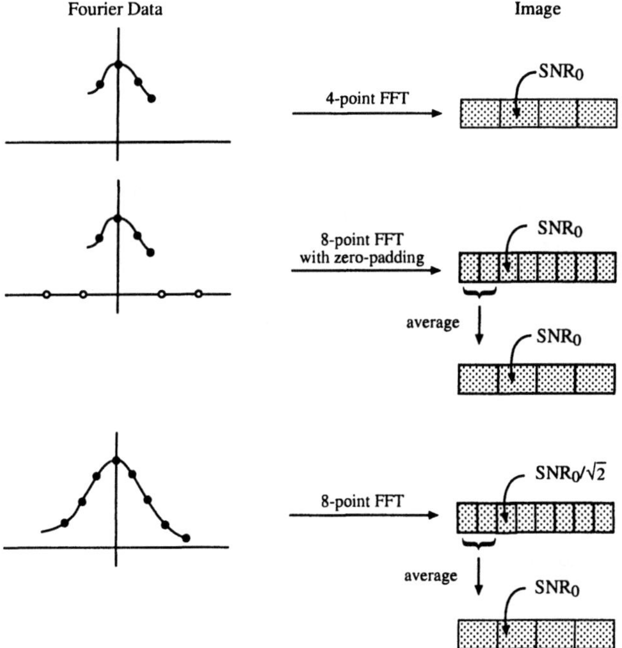

Figure 8.4   Signal-to-noise ratio efficiency of the Fourier imaging method.

---

[1] SNR efficiency is defined as $SNR|_{\text{pixel}}/\sqrt{\text{total imaging time}}$.

8.2.5   Noise in Filtered Backprojection Reconstruction

For simplicity, we consider only two-dimensional filtered backprojection reconstruction using the "M" filter. Let $\xi_d[m,n] = \xi_d[m\Delta k, n\Delta\phi]$ be the additive noise in a measured polar k-space data set consisting of N_ϕ radial lines, each with N_p points. Then, the image noise from filtered backprojection is given by

$$\xi_I(x,y) = \frac{\pi}{N_\phi}\frac{1}{N_p}\sum_{n=-N_\phi/2}^{N_\phi/2-1}\sum_{m=0}^{N_p-1}\frac{|m|}{N_p}\xi_d[m,n]e^{i2\pi mp} \tag{8.54}$$

where $p = x\cos(m\pi/N_\phi) + y\sin(m\pi/N_\phi)$ and Δk is taken to be $1/N_p$. Based on Eq. (8.54), it is easy to show that

$$E\{\xi_I(x,y)\} = 0 \quad \text{if} \quad E\{\xi_d[m,n]\} = 0 \tag{8.55}$$

In other words, the image noise has a zero mean if the mean of the data noise is zero, as is the often the case in practice.

To derive the image noise variance, we further assume that $\xi_d[m,n]$ is uncorrelated from one measurement to another. Under this assumption, we have

$$\text{var}\{\xi_I(x,y)\} = \left(\frac{\pi}{N_\phi N_p}\right)^2\sum_{n=-N_\phi/2}^{N_\phi/2-1}\sum_{m=0}^{N_p-1}\left(\frac{m}{N_p}\right)^2\text{var}\{\xi_d[m,n]\} \tag{8.56}$$

Using the previously established notations: $\text{var}\{\xi_I(x,y)\} = \sigma_I^2$ and $\text{var}\{\xi_d[m,n]\} = \sigma_d^2$, we have

$$\sigma_I^2 = \left(\frac{\pi}{N_\phi N_p}\right)^2\sum_{m=0}^{N_p-1}\sum_{n=-N_\phi/2}^{N_\phi/2-1}\left(\frac{m}{N_p}\right)^2\sigma_d^2$$

$$\approx \frac{\pi^2}{12}\frac{1}{N_p N_\phi}\sigma_d^2 \tag{8.57}$$

where $\sum_{m=0}^{N} m^2 = \frac{1}{6}N(N+1)(2N+1) \approx \frac{1}{3}N^3$ is used.

Note that for two-dimensional Fourier imaging with $N_x \times N_y$ Cartesian points, we have

$$\sigma_I^2 = = \frac{1}{N_x^2 N_y^2}\sum_{n=-N_x/2-1}^{N_x/2}\sum_{m=-N_y/2}^{N_y/2-1}\text{var}\{\xi_d[m,n]\}$$

$$= \frac{1}{N_x N_y}\sigma_d^2 \tag{8.58}$$

where $\xi_d[m,n]$ now represents $\xi_d(m\Delta k_x, n\Delta k_y)$. Therefore,

$$\frac{\sigma_I(\text{FBP})}{\sigma_I(\text{FT})} \approx \frac{\pi}{\sqrt{12}} \tag{8.59}$$

when $N_x N_y = N_p N_\phi$

8.3   Image Artifacts

Image distortions or artifacts often arise in the MR imaging process owing either
to insufficient data or to inaccurate data, or both. An insufficiency of measured
data occurs because of practical physical and temporal constraints in data acquisition. Data distortions are often due to imperfections in the data acquisition
system. Some of these artifacts are obvious and easy to deal with, but many others
are more complex and require careful analysis. Instead of providing a complete
description of all possible image artifacts encountered in practice, we focus on a
few typical ones in this section, analyzing their origin, characteristics, and possible remedies. For a more comprehensive discussion of this topic, the reader is
referred to the review paper by Henkelman and Bronskill [76].

8.3.1   Gibbs Ringing Artifact

The Gibbs ringing artifact is a common image distortion that exists in Fourier
images, which manifests itself as spurious ringing around sharp edges, as illustrated in Fig. 8.5. The maximum undershoot or overshoot of the spurious ringing
is about 9% of the intensity discontinuity and is independent of the number of
data points used in the reconstruction. The frequency of oscillation, however, increases as more data points are used. For this reason, when a large number of
data points is used in practice, the spurious ringing does not cover an appreciable
distance in the reconstructed image and thus becomes "invisible."

The Gibbs ringing artifact is a result of truncating the Fourier series model
owing to finite sampling or missing of high-frequency data. In practice, Gibbs
ringing can occur in both phase- and frequency-encoding directions, but more
often along the phase-encoding direction because temporal constraints often limit
the amount of high-frequency data collected along that direction.

Mathematically, Gibbs ringing is fundamentally related to the convergence
behavior of the Fourier series. Specifically, when $I(x)$ is a smooth function, $\hat{I}(x)$
given in Eq. (8.5) uniformly converges to $I(x)$ as $N \to \infty$ for $x \in$ FOV. More
precisely, if $I(x)$ has continuous derivatives up to and including the pth-order,
then $\hat{I}(x)$ approaches $I(x)$ on the order of $1/N^{p+1}$; namely, as N goes to infinity
$\|\hat{I}(x) - I(x)\|_2$ approaches zero as fast as $1/N^{p+1}$ does. On the other hand, if
$I(x)$ contains step discontinuities, the convergence behavior in the neighborhood
of a point of discontinuity will be "anomalous." Assuming that $I(x)$ has a step
discontinuity at $x = x_0$ such that $I(x_0^+) > I(x_0^-)$, the maximum overshoot location $\tilde{x}_N^+$ in $\hat{I}(x)$ approaches x_0^+ as $N \to \infty$, and

$$\lim_{N \to \infty} \left[\hat{I}(\tilde{x}_N^+) - I(x_0^+) \right] \approx 9\% \left[I(x_0^+) - I(x_0^-) \right] \qquad (8.60)$$

Similarly, for the maximum undershoot, we have

$$\lim_{N \to \infty} \left[\hat{I}(\tilde{x}_N^-) - I(x_0^-) \right] \approx -9\% \left[I(x_0^+) - I(x_0^-) \right] \tag{8.61}$$

Therefore, as $N \to \infty$ the value of the maximum overshoot (undershoot) does not tend to zero but instead tends to a finite limit. The existence of this finite, nonzero, limiting value of the overshoot (undershoot) is due to the nonuniform convergence of $\hat{I}(x)$ to $I(x)$ in the vicinity of discontinuous points of $I(x)$. This nonuniform behavior of the limit $\hat{I}(x) \to I(x)$ as $N \to \infty$ for $x \in$ FOV is formally called the *Gibbs phenomenon*.

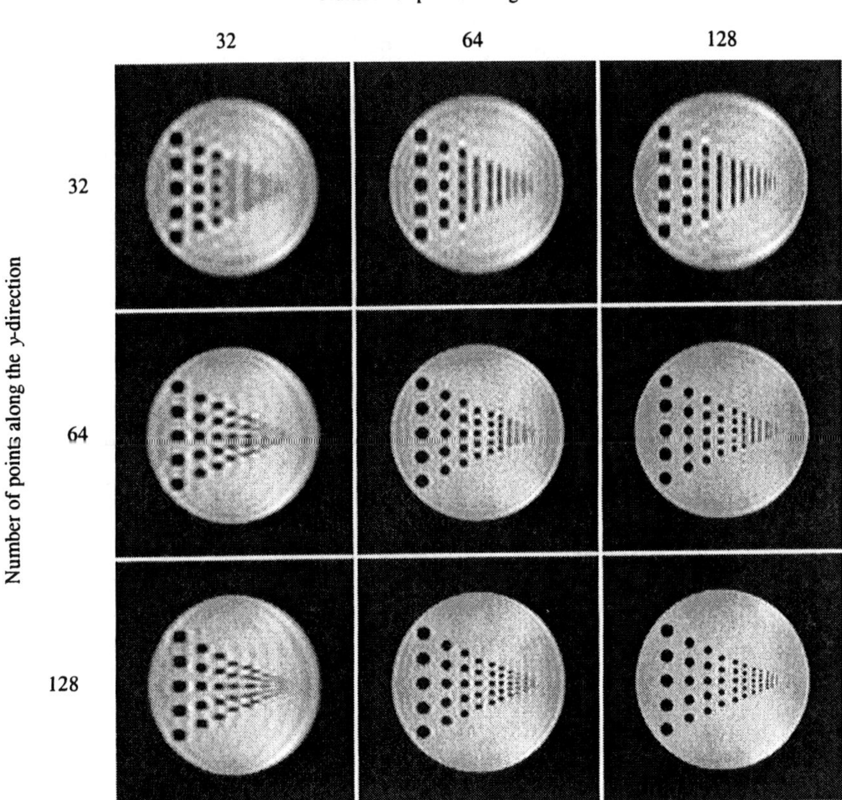

Figure 8.5 Gibbs ringing artifact in Fourier reconstructions. Notice the ringing pattern as a function of number of data points used in the reconstruction.

An obvious way to reduce the Gibbs ringing artifact is to collect more high-frequency data. This may not be possible in practice because of practical physical or temporal constraints on MR data acquisition. Another approach is to filter the

measured data before they are Fourier transformed. This operation is described
by

$$\hat{I}(x) = \Delta k \sum_{n=-N/2}^{N/2-1} S(n\Delta k)w_n e^{i2\pi n\Delta kx} \tag{8.62}$$

where w_n is a preselected filter (often called window) function.

This method is motivated by the understanding that the Gibbs ringing artifact
is directly related to the oscillatory nature of the PSF associated with the rectangular window function implicitly used in the Fourier reconstruction method. With
the reconstruction formula in Eq. (8.62), one can derive that the PSF is

$$h(x) = \Delta k \sum_{n=-N/2}^{N/2-1} w_n e^{i2\pi n\Delta kx} \tag{8.63}$$

Therefore, by properly choosing the window function w_m, one can significantly
suppress the oscillations in $h(x)$, and thus the Gibbs ringing in $\hat{I}(x)$. A variety
of window functions have been proposed for this purpose (see [75] for a comprehensive review). The most popular one is perhaps the Hamming window function
defined in Section 2.3. The PSF associated with the Hamming window function
and its effect on Gibbs ringing reduction are illustrated in Fig. 8.6.

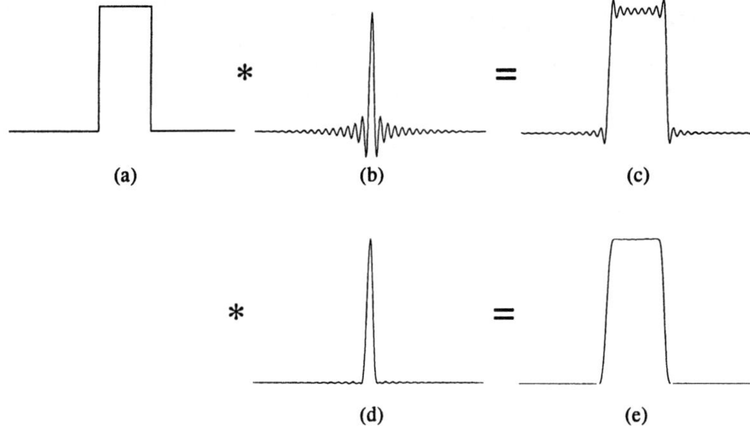

Figure 8.6 (a) True object function, (b-c) the PSF of the rectangular window function
and the corresponding Fourier reconstruction (64 points), (d-e) the PSF of the Hamming
window function and the resulting windowed Fourier reconstruction (64 point).

Although the windowing approach is effective in suppressing the Gibbs ringing, it is at the price of spatial resolution. This point can be understood by examining the effective width of the resulting PSF. Specifically,

$$
W_h = \frac{1}{\Delta k \displaystyle\sum_{m=-N/2}^{N/2-1} w_m} \int_{-\frac{1}{2\Delta k}}^{\frac{1}{2\Delta k}} \Delta k \sum_{m=-N/2}^{N/2-1} w_m e^{i2\pi m \Delta k x} dx
$$

$$
= \frac{1}{\displaystyle\sum_{m=-N/2}^{N/2-1} \left(w_m / w_0 \right) \Delta k}
$$

Since $w_0 \geq w_m$ for any practical window function used for this purpose, we have

$$
W_h \geq \frac{1}{N\Delta k} \tag{8.64}
$$

This equation asserts that the filtering operation is a lossy process in terms of image resolution, as illustrated in Fig 8.7. To overcome this problem, various sophisticated reconstruction methods have been proposed. More discussions of this topic can be found in Chapter 10.

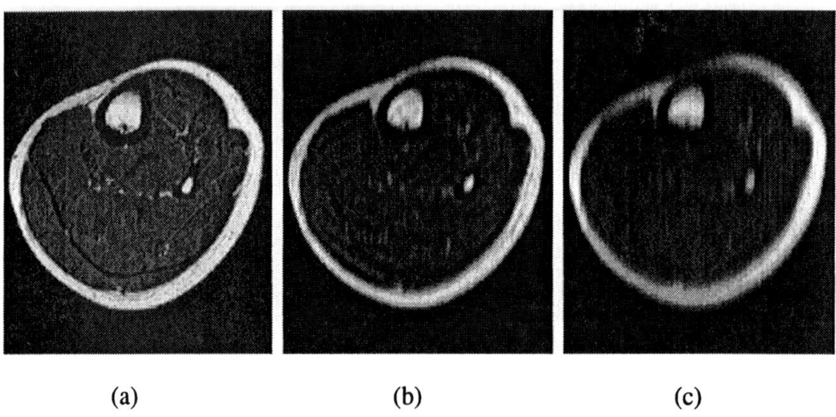

(a)   (b)   (c)

Figure 8.7 Cross-sectional leg images. All the images were reconstructed using the Fourier method with 256 points along the horizontal direction. The vertical direction was reconstructed using the Fourier method with 256 points in (a) and 64 points in (b) but using the Hamming-windowed Fourier method with 64 point in (c). Note the effect of the Hamming filter on Gibbs ringing reduction and the resolution loss.

8.3.2   Aliasing Artifacts

It is well-known that under certain conditions, continuous signals can be completely represented by and recovered from its samples. These conditions are stated in the sampling theorems discussed in Section 5.4. When the sampling conditions are violated, perfect reconstruction is not possible and the resulting image error is known as the *aliasing artifact*. The appearance of aliasing artifacts is dependent on how the samples are taken from a continuous signal. This section focuses on uniform sampling because it is used most often in practice.

Assume that a continuous-time signal $S(t)$ is sampled uniformly at frequency f_s. The Nyquist sampling criterion requires that $S(t)$ is bandlimited to the frequency range $|f| < f_s/2$, which is called the baseband. If this condition is not met, the frequency components outside the baseband will be folded over, thus the term *aliasing*, and become indistinguishable from the frequency components in the baseband. Specifically, the apparent frequency f_a of a component at f is given by

$$f_a = \begin{cases} f - nf_s & \text{if } f > 0 \\ f + nf_s & \text{if } f < 0 \end{cases} \tag{8.65}$$

for an appropriate n such that $|f_a| < f_s/2$.

To better appreciate this relationship, consider $S(t) = \cos(2\pi t)$. Assume that this signal is sampled at $t = n\Delta t$ with $\Delta t = 1.5$. Then, $f_s = \frac{1}{\Delta t} = \frac{2}{3}$, which is below the Nyquist sampling frequency $f_N = 2$. The apparent frequency of $S(t)$ is $f_a = f - f_s = 1 - \frac{2}{3} = \frac{1}{3}$. Therefore, $\cos(2\pi t)$ appears to be the same as $\cos(\frac{2}{3}\pi t)$ when observed at $t = n\frac{3}{2}$, as illustrated in Fig. 8.8.

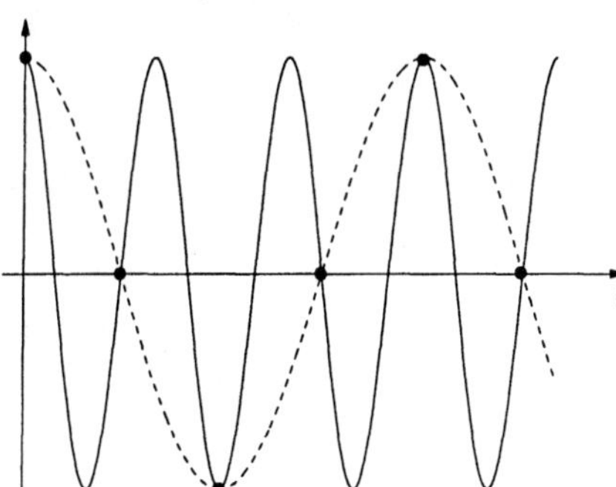

Figure 8.8   Illustration of the undersampling effect on a sinusoidal signal. Notice that the sample values of $\cos(2\pi t)$ and $\cos(\frac{2}{3}\pi t)$ taken at $t = n(\frac{3}{2})$ are the same.

The sampling requirements of k-space signals have been discussed in detail in Section 5.4. The aliasing artifact resulting from undersampling of k-space manifests itself as wrapping-around of the object, as illustrated in Fig. 8.9. This phenomenon can be understood from Eq. (8.65) with the substitution of the frequency variable by the space variable. It is also evident from the following relationship between the Fourier series reconstruction $\hat{I}(x)$ and the true image function $I(x)$ given in Section 6.2:

$$\hat{I}(x) = \sum_{n=-\infty}^{\infty} I\left(x - \frac{n}{\Delta k}\right) \tag{8.66}$$

This relationship is illustrated pictorially in Fig. 8.10.

Note that the appearance of the aliasing artifact is strongly dependent on how sampling is done. As a case in point, angular undersampling in filtered back-projection reconstruction appears as a streaking artifact, as shown in Fig. 8.11. Aliasing artifact becomes less structured (and thus less obvious) for nonuniform sampling. This property is sometimes utilized to reduce the aliasing artifact when signal undersampling cannot be avoided.

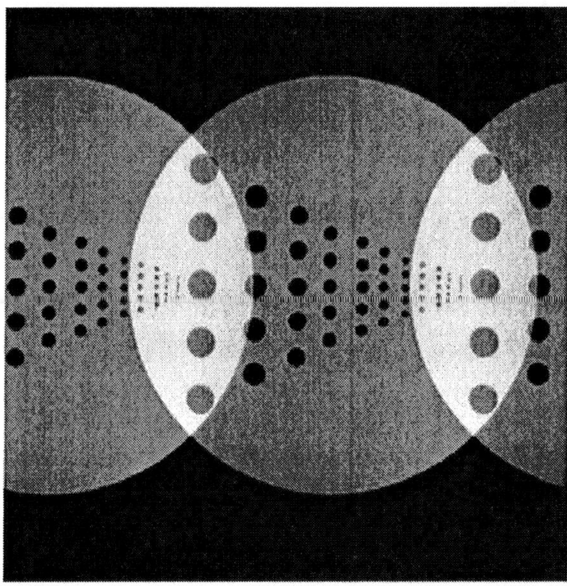

Figure 8.9 Aliasing artifacts due to undersampling along the horizontal direction by a factor of two.

Aliasing artifact is in general difficult to fix after the fact. A common approach to this problem is to prevent it from happening in the data acquisition stage by properly choosing the sampling rate or limiting the measured signal bandwidth (through the use of antialiasing filtering). Some practical anti-aliasing methods along phase-encoding, frequency-encoding, slice-selection directions are discussed at [76].

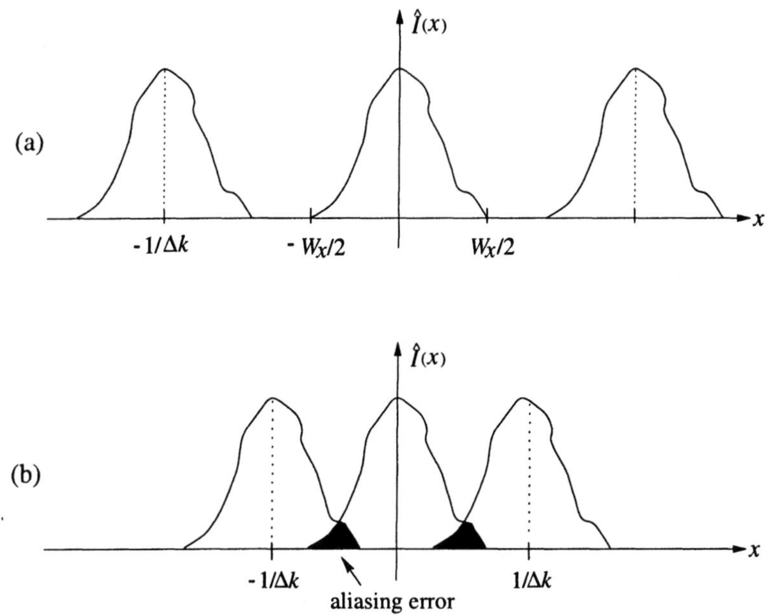

Figure 8.10 The sampling effect on Fourier reconstructions when the Nyquist sampling criterion is met in (a) or violated in (b).

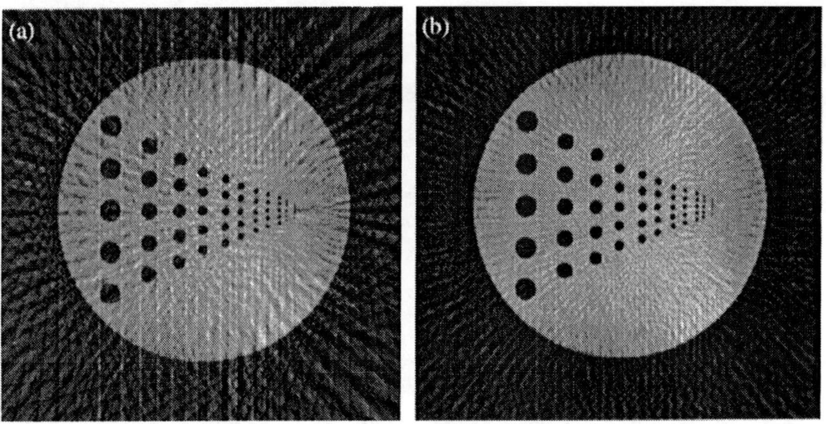

Figure 8.11 Filtered backprojection reconstruction of a phantom image using (a) 32 projections, and (b) 64 projections, taken uniformly from 0 to π. Note that the angular aliasing artifact manifest itself as streaking artifact.

8.3.3 Chemical Shift Artifact

As discussed in Section 3.1.3, the term *chemical shift* refers to the shift in resonance frequency of nuclear spins in different chemical environments. An important example in MRI is that the Larmor frequency of fat protons is shifted to a lower frequency with respect to that of water protons by approximately 3.5 ppm (parts per million). Since spatial position is frequency-encoded in the readout direction in the imaging process, signals from water protons and fat protons in the same spatial location will be assigned to different spatial locations, thus creating a misregistration artifact, as illustrated in Fig. 8.12.

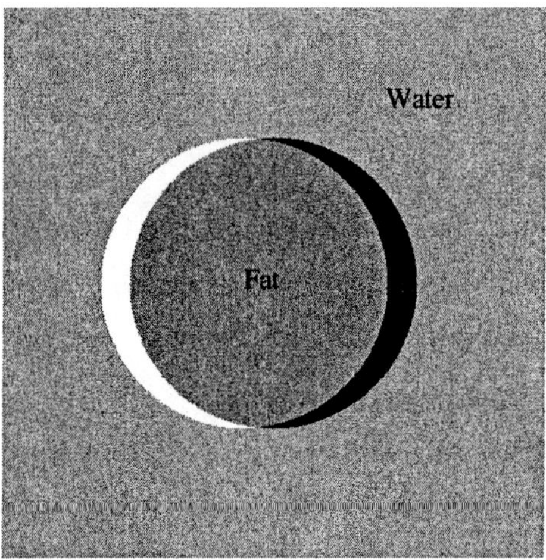

Figure 8.12 Chemical-shift misregistration artifact. Notice that the fat signal is shifted to a lower frequency in the frequency-encoding direction, creating an enhanced rim on the left but a black rim on the right.

The degree of spatial displacement caused by chemical shifts can be readily calculated based on the known experimental parameters. Assume that the main field strength is B_0, the frequency-encoding gradient is G, and the pixel size is Δx. The frequency shift according to Eq. (3.43) is

$$\Delta\omega_c = \gamma\delta B_0 \tag{8.67}$$

where δ is the shielding constant. Since the frequency bandwidth of a pixel is

$$\Delta\omega_x = \gamma G\Delta x \tag{8.68}$$

the amount of spatial displacement, in the unit of a pixel, caused by the chemical shift is

$$\delta_x = \frac{\Delta\omega_c}{\Delta\omega_x} = \frac{\delta B_0}{G\Delta x} \tag{8.69}$$

The exact spatial shift is

$$\Delta x_c = \delta_x \Delta x = \frac{\delta B_0}{G} \tag{8.70}$$

An effective way to reduce the chemical shift artifact is to use a strong readout gradient. According to Eq. (8.69), Δx_c can be made smaller than a pixel with a proper G. This will reduce the chemical shift effect to a negligible level. In practice, however, increasing G will enhance the signal bandwidth and thus sacrifice the signal SNR. Therefore, a compromise between these two parameters has to be reached in practical experimental setups by the user.

Another approach is to use solvent (e.g., fat) suppression techniques. These techniques can significantly reduce the signal from undesirable chemical shift components and thereby minimize the spatial misregistration artifact.

■ Example 8.5

This example calculates the spatial shift between water and fat signals. At $B_0 = 1.5T$, the frequency shift between water and fat protons is

$$\Delta \omega_c = \gamma \delta B_0 = 2.675 \times 10^8 \ \text{rad/s/T} \times 3.5 \times 10^{-6} \times 1.5 \ \text{T}$$
$$= 1.4 \times 10^3 \ \text{rad/s}$$

or

$$\Delta f_c = \frac{\delta \omega_c}{2\pi} = 222 \ \text{Hz}$$

For a gradient of 10 mT/m (1 G/cm), the amount of spatial shift, according to Eq. (8.70), is given by

$$\Delta x_c = \frac{\delta B_0}{G} = \frac{3.5 \times 10^{-6} \times 1.5 \ \text{T}}{10 \times 10^{-3} \ \text{T/m}} = 5.5 \times 10^{-4} \ \text{m} = 0.55 \ \text{mm}$$

For a 80 mm field of 256 pixels,

$$\Delta x = \frac{80 \ \text{mm}}{256} = 0.3125 \ \text{mm}$$

Therefore,

$$\delta_x = \frac{\Delta x_c}{\Delta x} = \frac{0.55}{0.3125} = 1.76 \ \text{pixels}$$

which implies that there will be a 1.76-pixel shift between the water and fat signals from the same spatial location.

8.3.4   Motion Artifacts

In the discussion so far, we have assumed that the object being imaged is stationary during the data acquisition period. In many practical situations, this assumption is not valid, and consequently, image artifacts result. Motion artifacts manifest themselves in a variety of forms, depending on the nature of the object motion and the data acquisition scheme used. The most problematic physiologic motions include blood flow, respiratory motion, cardiac motion, and gross movements of the body. Common motion artifacts are image blurring and ghost (or misregistration), two examples of which are shown in Figs. 8.13 and 8.14. This section discusses some concepts fundamental to understanding motion effects and motion compensation techniques.

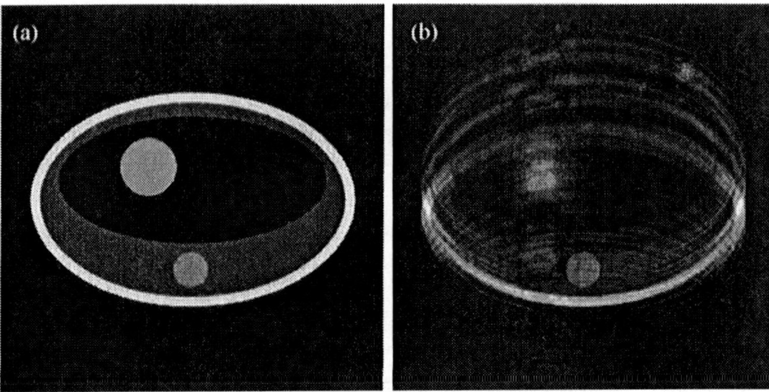

Figure 8.13 Simulated ghost and blurring artifacts due to periodic motion: (a) Ideal snapshot image and (b) artifacted image.

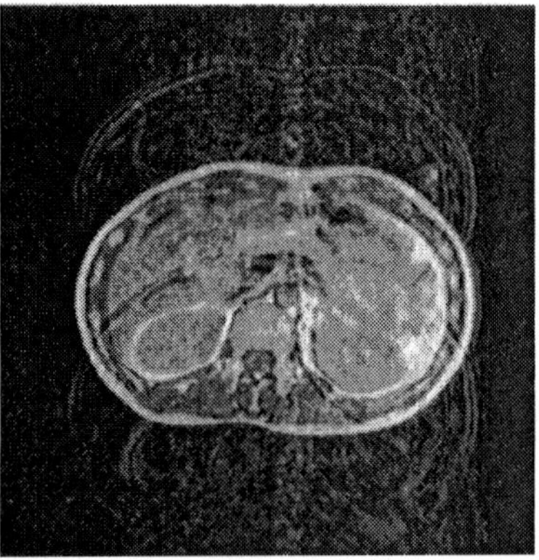

Figure 8.14 Cross-sectional image of the lower abdomen with motion artifacts.

8.3.4.1   Motion Effects along the Readout Direction

Object motion during the readout period can create undesirable phase shifts. To understand this effect, consider the simple case of an object moving with a constant velocity $v = v_x \vec{i} + v_y \vec{j}$. In this case, the object function, $I(x, y, t)$, can be expressed as

$$I(x, y, t) = I[x(t), y(t), t_0] \tag{8.71}$$

where

$$x(t) = x + v_x(t - t_0) \tag{8.72a}$$
$$y(t) = y + v_y(t - t_0) \tag{8.72b}$$

with t_0 being an arbitrary time reference point. In practice, it is convenient to set $t_0 = 0$ and let it be the time instant at which the excitation pulse is applied. We may also rewrite $I[x(t), y(t), 0]$ simply as $I[x(t), y(t)]$ when there is no confusion.

Recall that the phase dispersal of a transverse magnetization introduced by a readout gradient in the rotating frame is given by

$$\phi = \gamma \int_0^t \mathbf{G}(\hat{t}) \cdot \mathbf{r}(\hat{t}) d\hat{t} \tag{8.73}$$

where $r = (x, y)$. The inner product in this expression signifies that ϕ is insensitive to the motion component orthogonal to $\mathbf{G}(t)$. Without loss of generality, we may assume that $\mathbf{G}(t) = G_x(t)\vec{i}$. Then,

$$\phi = \gamma \int_0^t G_x(\hat{t})(x + v_x \hat{t}) d\hat{t}$$
$$= \gamma x \int_0^t G_x(\hat{t}) d\hat{t} + \gamma v_x \int_0^t \hat{t} G_x(\hat{t}) d\hat{t} \tag{8.74}$$

where the first term is a position-dependent phase shift desired for spatial encoding, whereas the second term is an undesirable velocity-dependent phase shift. For notational convenience, we use $\Delta\phi$ to represent the motion-introduced phase shift. With the current motion model, we have

$$\Delta\phi = \gamma v_x \int_0^t \hat{t} G_x(\hat{t}) d\hat{t} \tag{8.75}$$

Clearly, $\Delta\phi$ is dependent on the gradient structure. As an example, consider the gradient function illustrated in Fig. 8.15. It is easy to derive that during the dephasing period $0 \le t \le \tau$,

$$\Delta\phi = -\gamma \int_0^t G_x v_x \hat{t} d\hat{t} = -\frac{1}{2}\gamma G_x v_x t^2 \tag{8.76}$$

and during the data acquisition period $\tau \le t \le 3\tau$,

$$\Delta\phi = -\frac{1}{2}\gamma G_x v_x \tau^2 + \gamma \int_{\tau}^{t} G_x v_x \hat{t} d\hat{t}$$

$$= \frac{1}{2}\gamma G_x v_x \left(t^2 - 2\tau^2\right) \tag{8.77}$$

Inspection of Eq. (8.77) reveals that at the peak of the echo ($t = T_E = 2\tau$),

$$\Delta\phi = \gamma G_x v_x \tau^2 \tag{8.78}$$

Therefore, moving spins are not completely rephased at $t = T_E$ for the given gradient waveform.

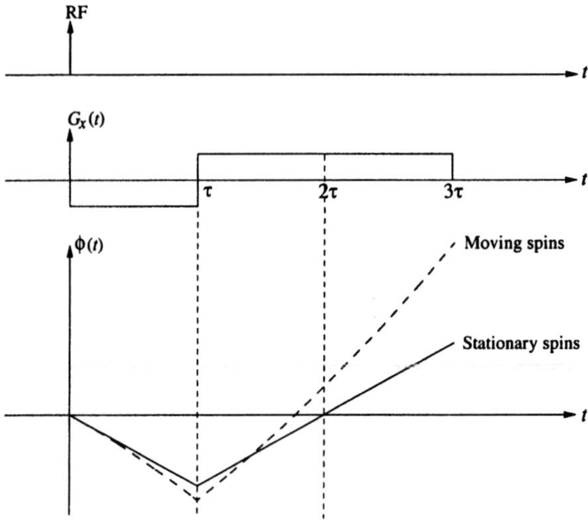

Figure 8.15 (a) A typical readout gradient waveform and (b) the accumulated phase as a function of time by stationary spins and moving spins of a constant velocity along the readout direction.

The imaging effect along the readout direction due to the motion-introduced phase shift can be described by the following point spread function:

$$h(x) = \int_{\tau}^{3\tau} e^{-i\frac{1}{2}\gamma G_x v_x (t^2 - T_E)} e^{i\gamma G_x x(t-2\tau)} dt$$

$$= \int_{\tau}^{3\tau} e^{-i\frac{1}{2}\gamma G_x v_x (t-T_E)^2} e^{i\gamma G_x (x-v_x T_E)(t-T_E)} dt$$

$$= e^{-i\gamma G_x v_x \tau^2} \int_{-\tau}^{\tau} e^{-i\frac{1}{2}\gamma G_x v_x t^2} e^{i\gamma G_x (x-x_s)t} dt \tag{8.79}$$

where $x_s = v_x T_E$ is the distance that the object has moved by the echo time. To gain further insight, we rewrite $h(x)$ as

$$h(x) = e^{-i\gamma G_x v_x \tau^2} e^{i\gamma G_x (x-x_s)^2/v_x} \int_{-\tau}^{\tau} e^{-i\frac{1}{2}\gamma G_x v_x \left(t - \frac{x-x_s}{v_x}\right)^2} dt \qquad (8.80)$$

Noting that

$$\int_{-\infty}^{\infty} e^{-\pi t^2} dt = \frac{1-i}{\sqrt{\pi}} \qquad (8.81)$$

we have

$$\int_{-\tau}^{\tau} e^{-i\frac{1}{2}\gamma G_x v_x t^2} e^{i\gamma G_x (x-x_s)t} dt \approx \int_{-\infty}^{\infty} e^{-i\frac{1}{2}\gamma G_x v_x \left(t - \frac{x-x_s}{v_x}\right)^2} dt$$
$$= \frac{(1-i)\sqrt{\pi}}{\sqrt{\gamma G_x v_x}} \qquad (8.82)$$

Therefore,

$$h(x) \approx \frac{(1-i)\sqrt{\pi}}{\sqrt{\gamma G_x v_x}} e^{-i\gamma G_x v_x \tau^2} e^{i\gamma G_x (x-x_s)^2/v_x} \qquad (8.83)$$

Three imaging effects are evident from Eq. (8.83): *phase shift, spatial shift,* and *blurring*. First, the impact of the phase shift term $e^{-i\gamma G_x v_x \tau^2}$ can be ignored if v_x is a constant. If v_x varies within a voxel, intravoxel dephasing occurs, reducing the signal intensity. If v_x varies from one acquisition to another, it will create significant image artifacts along the phase-encoding direction, as discussed in the next subsection. Second, a point source located at $x = 0$ at the time of the excitation pulse will be shifted to $x = v_x T_E$. This means that the resultant image reflects the location of the object at the echo time. Third, image blurring will result from convolution with $e^{i\gamma G_x (x-x_s)^2/v_x}$.

This analysis can be extended to motion models with higher-order terms. More specifically, let

$$x(t) = \sum_n \frac{1}{n!} x^{(n)}(0) t^n \qquad (8.84)$$

where $x^{(0)}(0), x^{(1)}(0)$, and $x^{(2)}(0)$ corresponds to the initial position, velocity, and acceleration of a moving isochromat. It is easy to show that the phase shift introduced by the nth moment of motion is given by

$$\Delta\phi_n = \frac{1}{n!} x^{(n)}(0) \int_0^t \hat{t}^n G_x(\hat{t}) d\hat{t} \qquad (8.85)$$

The effect of object rotation can be calculated in a similar fashion. For example, assume that an object is undergoing a clockwise rotation with a constant angular velocity ω_0 during the data acquisition period. The object location as a function of time is described by

$$\begin{cases} x(t) = x(0) \cos \omega_0 t + y(0) \sin \omega_0 t \\ y(t) = -x(0) \sin \omega_0 t + y(0) \cos \omega_0 t \end{cases} \tag{8.86}$$

Correspondingly, the phase accumulated by a spin isochromat during the data acquisition period is given by

$$\phi = \int_0^t \left[x(0) \cos \omega_0 \hat{t} + y(0) \sin \omega_0 \hat{t} \right] G_x(\hat{t}) d\hat{t} \tag{8.87}$$

8.3.4.2 Motion Effects along the Phase-Encoding Direction

Before we analyze motion effects along the phase-encoding direction, it is useful to notice a couple of differences between phase encoding and frequency encoding regarding object motion. First, the sampling rate along the phase-encoding direction is at least two orders of magnitude slower than that along the frequency-encoding (readout) direction. Second, there is no phase accumulation from one phase-encoding step to the next.[2] Although the first point indicates that object motion is more troublesome along the phase-encoding direction than along the readout direction, the second property makes motion effects along the phase-encoding direction easier to analyze.

To further illustrate the second point, consider constant-velocity object motion along the phase-encoding direction. Assume that a constant phase-encoding gradient along the x-direction is turned on at t_n for a duration of τ. Then, according to Eq. (8.73), we have

$$\phi_n = \gamma \int_{t_n}^{t_n + \tau} G_n(x + v_x t) dt$$

$$= \gamma G_n x \tau + \gamma G_n v_x \tau (t_n + \tau/2)$$

$$= 2\pi k_n x + 2\pi k_n v_x (t_n + \tau/2) \tag{8.88}$$

where $k_n = \gamma/(2\pi) G_n \tau$. In contrast to Eq. (8.77), the motion-introduced phase shift along the phase-encoding direction is

$$\Delta \phi = 2\pi k_n v_x (t_n + \tau/2) = 2\pi k_n v_x t_n + 2\pi k_n v_x v_x \tau/2 \tag{8.89}$$

The second linear phase shift term can be ignored because the resulting spatial displacement $v_x \tau/2$ is usually insignificant. As a result, we can rewrite $\Delta\phi$ simply as

$$\Delta \phi = 2\pi k_n v_x t_n \tag{8.90}$$

---

[2]This statement does not apply to fast imaging methods discussed in Chapter 9.

Equation (8.90) can be obtained directly from the Fourier shift theorem. Specifically, ignoring the readout direction and treating phase encoding as being instantaneous (i.e., $\tau \approx 0$), we can express the imaging equation as

$$S(k_n) = \int_{-\infty}^{\infty} I(x, t_n) e^{-i2\pi k_n x} dx \tag{8.91}$$

Expressing $I(x, t_n)$ as $I_0(x - v_x t_n)$ with $I_0(x)$ being the snapshot of $I(x, t)$ at $t = 0$, we immediately get

$$S(k_n) = e^{-i2\pi k_n v_x t_n} \int_{-\infty}^{\infty} I_0(x) e^{-i2\pi k_n x} dx$$

$$= e^{-i2\pi k_n v_x t_n} S_0(k_n) \tag{8.92}$$

from which the motion-introduced phase-shift term is evident.

It is useful to generalize Eq. (8.91) by explicitly writing the signal as a function of k and t such that

$$S(k, t) = \int_{-\infty}^{\infty} I(x, t) e^{-i2\pi k x} dx \tag{8.93}$$

This so-called (k, t)-space treatment provides significant insight into the behavior of motion effects along the phase-encoding direction.[3] To illustrate this concept, consider periodic object motion for which the object function can be expressed as

$$I(x, t) = \sum_{m} \hat{I}_m(x) e^{i2\pi m f_0 t} \tag{8.94}$$

where f_0 is the fundamental frequency of the object motion. The corresponding joint space-frequency distribution is given by

$$\hat{I}(x, f) = \sum_{m} \hat{I}_m(x) \delta(f - m f_0) \tag{8.95}$$

Inspection of Eq. (8.93) indicates that to generate motion-artifact-free snapshot images from $I(x, t)$, it is necessary to traverse the entirety of k-space instantaneously. In practice, it takes a finite time (say, $\Delta t = N_{\text{acq}} T_R$, where N_{acq} is the number of acquisitions per encoding) from collecting one phase-encoding measurement to another. As a consequence, (k, t)-space is effectively sampled as in Fig. 8.16a when the phase-encoding measurements are taken in a linear order.

---

[3] Equation (8.93) is not applicable to the readout direction because of the phase accumulation effect.

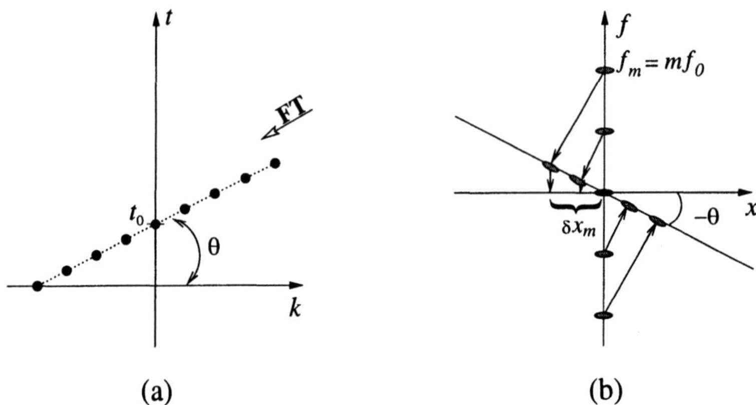

(a)   (b)

Figure 8.16 (a) Tilted sampling trajectory in (k, t)-space, and (b) the resulting projection image. Note that the projection angle is $-\theta$ instead of θ predicted by the projection-slice theorem because here t is related to f by the inverse Fourier transform, while k is related to x by the forward transform.

To understand how motion artifacts arise from the tilted sampling trajectory, we first consider Fourier reconstruction from the hypothetical continuous data along this trajectory. Based on the result derived in Example 8.6, direct Fourier reconstruction from the data along the tilted trajectory is given by

$$\tilde{I}[p] = \iint \hat{I}(x, f)e^{i2\pi f t_0}\delta(x\cos\theta - f\sin\theta - p)dxdf \qquad (8.96)$$

Substituting Eq. (8.95) into Eq. (8.96) yields

$$\tilde{I}[p] = \iint \sum_m \hat{I}_m(x)\delta(f - mf_0)e^{i2\pi f t_0}\delta(x\cos\theta - f\sin\theta - p)dxdf$$

$$= \sum_m e^{i2\pi m f_0 t_0}\int \hat{I}_m(x)\delta(x\cos\theta - mf_0\sin\theta - p)dx$$

$$= \frac{1}{|\cos\theta|}\sum_m e^{i2\pi m f_0 t_0}\hat{I}_m\left(\frac{p}{\cos\theta} + mf_0\tan\theta\right) \qquad (8.97)$$

For convenience, we further project $\tilde{I}[p]$ onto the x-axis by setting $x = p\cos\theta$, which gives

$$\tilde{I}(x) = \tilde{I}(p\cos\theta) = \frac{1}{|\cos\theta|}\sum_m e^{i2\pi m f_0 t_0}\hat{I}_m(x + mf_0\tan\theta) \qquad (8.98)$$

It is clear from Eq. (8.98) that the mth frequency component in the projection image is shifted by

$$\delta x_m = mf_0\tan\theta \qquad (8.99)$$

In the ideal case that $\theta = 0$, $\delta x_m = 0$. Then, according to Eq. (8.94), we have

$$\tilde{I}(x) = I(x, t_0) \tag{8.100}$$

which is an ideal snapshot of $I(x, t)$. In practice, however, $\theta \neq 0$, different motion frequency components will be misregistered in the reconstruction, resulting in the well-known "ghosting" artifact. Next, we further characterize the ghosting artifact with respect to the discrete data.

We first recall the definition of a few quantities. Assume that N phase-encoding measurements at $k = (n - N/2)\Delta k$ are collected at $t = n\Delta t$, for $n = 0, 1, \ldots, N - 1$. We have

$$\text{Fourier pixel size:} \qquad \Delta x_{\text{F}} = \frac{1}{N\Delta k}$$

$$\text{Field of view:} \qquad W_x = N\Delta x_{\text{F}}$$

$$\text{Imaging time:} \qquad T_{\text{acq}} = N\Delta t$$

Then,

$$\tan\theta = \frac{\Delta t}{\Delta k} = \frac{N\Delta t}{N\Delta k} = T_{\text{acq}}\Delta x_{\text{F}} \tag{8.101}$$

Substituting it into Eq. (8.99) yields

$$\delta x_m = m f_0 T_{\text{acq}} \Delta x_{\text{F}} \tag{8.102}$$

or

$$\frac{\delta x_m}{\Delta x_{\text{F}}} = m f_0 T_{\text{acq}} \tag{8.103}$$

Because Δx_{F} is the effective width of the underlying point spread function, it is apparent that the spatial displacement for the mth harmonic will not create noticeable ghosting artifacts if

$$\delta x_m \leq \Delta x_{\text{F}}/2 \tag{8.104}$$

By making use of the result in Eq. (8.102), the condition in Eq. (8.104) can be equivalently expressed as

$$T_{\text{acq}} \leq \frac{1}{2m f_0} \tag{8.105}$$

An interesting interpretation of Eq. (8.105) is that if T_{acq} satisfies the Nyquist criterion with respect to $m f_0$, the mth harmonic will not create significant ghosting artifacts. Ghosting artifacts from all lower-order harmonics are also negligible, as they satisfy Eq. (8.105) automatically.

When the condition in Eq. (8.105) is violated, distinct ghosts may appear. The center location of the ghost image resulting from the mth harmonic is specified by Eq. (8.99). Some alternative expressions are also useful. For example,

$$\delta x_m = m \left(\frac{T_{\text{acq}}}{T} \right) \Delta x_{\text{F}} \tag{8.106}$$

where $T = 1/f_0$ is the period of the object motion, and

$$\delta x_m = m \left(\frac{\Delta t}{T} \right) W_x \tag{8.107}$$

Notice that when a ghost image moves outside the field of view, it will be folded over. Its new position inside the field of view can be calculated from the following equation:

$$\hat{x} = \begin{cases} x + \delta x_m - nW_x, & \text{if } x + \delta x_m > W_x/2 \\ x + \delta x_m + nW_x, & \text{if } x + \delta x_m < -W_x/2 \end{cases} \tag{8.108}$$

for an appropriate n such that $|\hat{x}| < W_x/2$.

This analysis can be easily extended to a general motion model. Specifically, starting again with Eq. (8.96) but treating $\hat{I}(x, f)$ as a general function, we have, similarly to Eq. (8.98), that

$$\tilde{I}(x) = \frac{1}{|\cos\theta|} \int e^{i2\pi f t_0} \hat{I}(x + f\tan\theta, f) df \tag{8.109}$$

Therefore, as with periodic motion, motion artifact in general is a result of spatial misregistration of various frequency components. Clearly, $\tilde{I}(x) = I(x, t_0)$ only when $\theta = 0$.

Although Eq. (8.109) is valid for Fourier imaging of a general moving object, it cannot be directly applied to other imaging schemes with different (k, t)-space trajectories. As an example, consider projection-reconstruction imaging in which sequential radial scanning of k-space is used. It has been shown [141] that with this imaging scheme, motion-introduced data inconsistencies from one projection to another result in streaking (instead of ghosting) artifacts, as illustrated in Fig. 8.17. For a detailed comparison of motion effects between standard Fourier imaging and projection-reconstruction imaging, the reader is referred to [141].

■ **Example 8.6**

This example derives the result in Eq. (8.96). We first express $S(k, t)$ as

$$S(k, t) = \iint I(x, f) e^{-i2\pi(kx - ft)} dx df$$

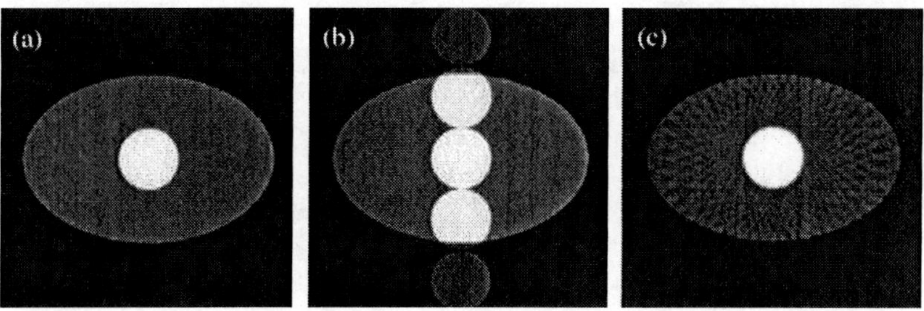

Figure 8.17 A comparison of motion effects in standard Fourier imaging and projection-reconstruction imaging: (a) ideal snapshot from a simulated phantom in which the intensity of the central region varies sinusoidally, (b) Fourier reconstruction (phase encoding along the vertical direction), and (c) filtered backprojection reconstruction.

We next evaluate $S(k, t)$ along the tilted line shown Fig. 8.16b to get a one-dimensional signal $\tilde{S}(k_t)$. Noting that the tilted line is defined by

$$\begin{cases} k = k_t \cos\theta \\ t = k_t \sin\theta + t_0 \end{cases}$$

we have

$$\tilde{S}(k_t) = S(k_t \cos\theta, k_t \sin\theta + t_0)$$

$$= \iint I(x, f) e^{-i2\pi(xk_t \cos\theta - fk_t \sin\theta - ft_0)} \, dx df$$

$$= \iint I(x, f) e^{i2\pi f t_0} e^{-i2\pi k_t(x \cos\theta - f \sin\theta)} \, dx df$$

Finally, inverse-Fourier transforming $\tilde{S}(k_t)$ yields

$$\tilde{I}[p] = \int \tilde{S}(k_t) e^{i2\pi k_t p} \, dk_t$$

$$= \iint \left[I(x, f) e^{i2\pi f t_0} \int e^{-i2\pi k_t(x \cos\theta - f \sin\theta - p)} \, dk_t \right] dx df$$

$$= \iint I(x, f) e^{i2\pi f t_0} \delta(x \cos\theta - f \sin\theta - p) \, dx df$$

■ **Example 8.7**

This example examines the misregistration artifact with oblique flow. Consider the case in Fig. 8.18, where a blood vessel runs obliquely through the image plane. A flowing isochromat initially located at $(0,0)$ when an RF pulse is applied $(t = t_0)$ will be at different positions when it is subsequently phase- and frequency-encoded. Assume that phase encoding along the x-axis is applied instantaneously at $t = t_1$ and frequency-encoding along the y-axis is applied at $t = t_2$ (taken to be the middle point of the frequency-encoding period). The flowing isochromat will be then located at $(x_1, y_1) = (v_x t_1, v_y t_1)$ and $(x_2, y_2) = (v_x t_2, v_y t_2)$, respectively. Consequently, the encoded position will be (x_1, y_2), and the isochromat appears to be at this *wrong* position in the reconstructed image. The amount of misregistration depends on the angle of the vessel relative to the phase-encoding and frequency-encoding axes and the time separation between encoding along the two axes. The artifact does not occur if the vessel runs along the imaging axes and can be suppressed by reducing the time delay between phase and frequency encoding.

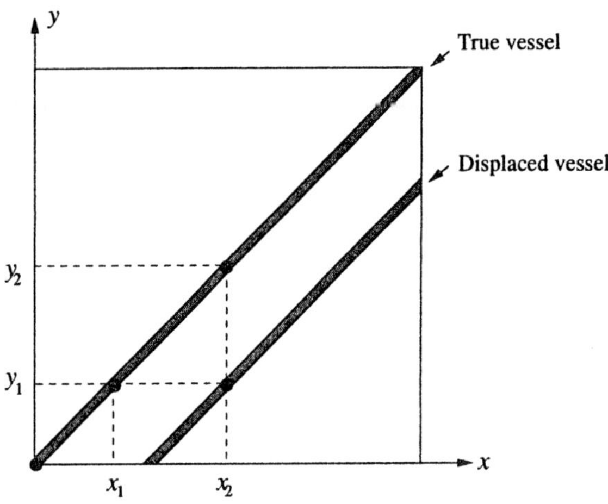

Figure 8.18   Illustration of oblique flow artifact.

8.3.4.3 Some Motion-Compensation Methods

This subsection describes some basic methodologies for motion compensation. Practical imaging schemes often involve the use of a combination of them. Since implementation of motion-compensation strategies is application-dependent, this subsection will not dwell on these issues.

Gradient Moment Nulling: According to Eq. (8.85), the phase accumulated by the nth moment of motion in the time interval between an RF pulse and the peak of the subsequent echo is

$$\Delta\phi_n = \frac{1}{n!}x^{(n)}(0)\int_0^{T_E} t^n G_x(t)dt \tag{8.110}$$

where the integral is the nth moment of the gradient function $G_x(t)$. Therefore, if a special gradient waveform is chosen such that

$$\int_0^{T_E} t^n G_x(t)dt = 0 \tag{8.111}$$

then

$$\Delta\phi_n = 0 \tag{8.112}$$

Such a technique is called *gradient moment nulling*. A special case is first moment nulling, in which

$$\Delta\phi_1 = v_x \int_0^{T_E} t G_x(t)dt = 0 \tag{8.113}$$

It is easy to show that this condition is met by the gradient waveform shown in Fig. 8.19.

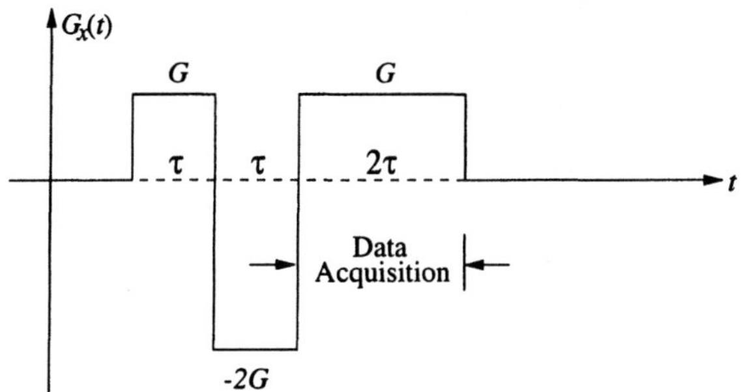

Figure 8.19   A typical velocity-compensated gradient waveform

For some practical applications, it is desirable to null a particular moment or all the moments of order N or less. That is,

$$\Delta\phi_n = \int_0^{T_E} t^n G_x(t)dt = 0 \qquad \text{for } n = n_0 \tag{8.114}$$

or

$$\Delta\phi_n = \int_0^{T_E} t^n G_x(t)\,dt = 0 \qquad \text{for } n = 0, 1, \ldots, N \tag{8.115}$$

A variety of numerical algorithms have been proposed for designing gradient waveforms with the above property. For a comprehensive review, the reader is referred to [72].

With gradient moment nulling, the motion-introduced phase shifts for the central k-space data are made to be zero or negligible. This property is particularly important when motion characteristics are changing from one acquisition to another.

Navigator Echoes: Navigator echoes are companion echo signals collected immediately before or after a regular imaging echo. Different from imaging echoes, navigators are collected from the same k-space location so that variations among them reflect the object motion. Based on how they are mapped to k-space, navigators are classified into two types: *linear navigators* and *circular navigators*. Other forms of navigators are also possible but have not been widely used.

Linear navigators, as the name implies, are collected along a straight line in k-space, usually along one of the imaging axes, such as the k_x- or k_y-axis [135]. To see how motion parameters can be determined from such signals, let $S_n(k_x, 0)$, $n = 0, 1, \ldots$, represent a set of navigators collected from a moving object $I(x, y, t)$ at times $t = t_n$. For bulk object translation,

$$I(x, y, t_n) = I(x + \Delta x_n, y + \Delta y_n, t_0) \tag{8.116}$$

Based on the projection-slice theorem, we have

$$\begin{aligned}
\mathcal{F}^{-1}\{S_n(k_x, 0)\}(x) &= \int_{-\infty}^{\infty} I(x + \Delta x_n, y + \Delta y_n, t_0)\,dy \\
&= \int_{-\infty}^{\infty} I(x + \Delta x_n, y, t_0)\,dy
\end{aligned} \tag{8.117}$$

Therefore,

$$\mathcal{F}^{-1}\{S_n(k_x, 0)\}(x) = \mathcal{F}^{-1}\{S_0(k_x, 0)\}(x + \Delta x_n) \tag{8.118}$$

from which Δx_n can be determined.

One may notice from Eq. (8.118) that $S_n(k_x, 0)$ are insensitive to object displacements along the y-direction, provided that the object does not move outside the field of view. To determine Δy_n, we need to collect another set of linear navigators along the k_y-axis denoted as $S_n(0, k_y)$. Similarly to Eq. (8.118), one can show that

$$\mathcal{F}^{-1}\{S_n(0, k_y)\}(y) = \mathcal{F}^{-1}\{S_0(0, k_y)\}(y + \Delta y_n) \tag{8.119}$$

In practice, one may assume that the object motion is steady enough so that motion characteristics are similarly reflected in both the imaging echo and the companion navigator echoes for each acquisition. Then, the motion parameters estimated from the navigators can be used to correct for the acquisition-to-acquisition motion for the imaging data before image reconstruction is performed. A notable problem with linear navigators is that they are not efficient in tracking translations, for two sets of navigators are needed to track planar object displacements. In addition, linear navigators cannot handle object rotations of any kind.

To overcome the problem with linear navigators, navigator signals collected along a circular k-space trajectory, as shown in Fig. 8.20, have been proposed [139]. A desirable property of circular navigators is that global in-plan motion of an object, both rotational and rotational, can be determined from a single set of circular navigator signals.

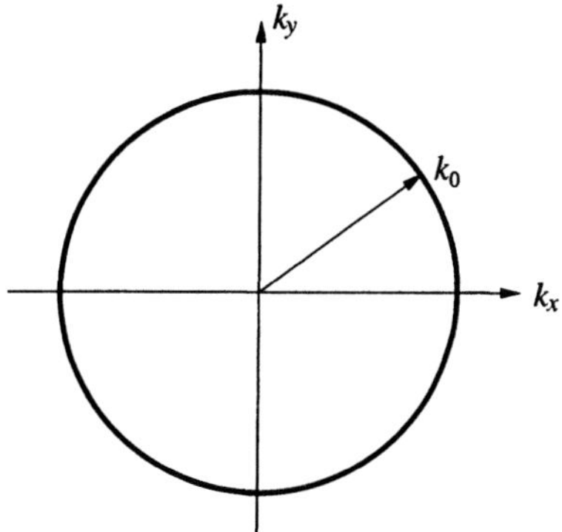

Figure 8.20 K-space trajectory of circular navigator signals.

To see how motion parameters can be extracted from circular navigators, consider two circular navigator signals $S_1(k_0, \theta)$ and $S_2(k_0, \theta)$ collected from $I_1(x, y)$ and $I_2(x, y)$ with

$$I_2(x, y) = I_1(x \cos \theta_0 + y \sin \theta_0 - x_0, -x \sin \theta_0 + y \cos \theta_0 - y_0) \qquad (8.120)$$

It is easy to show that

$$S_2(k_0, \theta) = S_1(k_0, \theta - \theta_0)e^{-i2\pi k_0[x_0 \cos(\theta-\theta_0)+y_0 \sin(\theta-\theta_0)]} \qquad (8.121)$$

This equation indicates that rotation of the object can be measured as a relative shift of the magnitude profile of the circular navigator signals, while translations are encoded in their phase difference. Therefore, one can decouple the determination of translation parameters from that of the rotation parameter. More specifically, one can first determine θ_0 from the correlation function of $|S_1(k_0, \theta)$ and

$|S_2(k_0, \theta)|$. Then, from Eq. (8.121) we have

$$
\begin{aligned}
\Phi(\theta) &= \angle S_1(k_0, \theta) - \angle S_2(k_0, \theta - \theta_0) \\
&= 2\pi k_0 [x_0 \cos(\theta - \theta_0) + y_0 \sin(\theta - \theta_0)]
\end{aligned}
\tag{8.122}
$$

With $\Phi(\theta)$, x_0 and y_0 can be determined easily. Specifically, if $\Phi(\theta)$ is known for $0 \le \theta \le 2\pi$, as is the case when the navigators cover a complete circle, x_0 and y_0 can be determined using the following formulas:

$$
x_0 = \frac{1}{2\pi^2 k_0} \int_0^{2\pi} \Phi(\theta) \cos(\theta - \theta_0) d\theta
\tag{8.123a}
$$

$$
y_0 = \frac{1}{2\pi^2 k_0} \int_0^{2\pi} \Phi(\theta)(\sin\theta - \theta_0) d\theta
\tag{8.123b}
$$

In practice, $\Phi(\theta)$ cannot be extracted from $S_1(k_0, \theta)$ and $S_2(k_0, \theta - \theta_0)$ directly using trigonometric functions because of the well-known phase-wrapping problem. To eliminate the need to solve the associated phase-unwrapping problem, one can extract $\partial\Phi(\theta)/\partial\theta$ instead. Specifically, let

$$
p(\theta) = e^{i\Phi(\theta)} = \frac{S_1(k_0, \theta)S_2^*(k_0, \theta - \theta_0)}{|S_1(k_0, \theta)S_2(k_0, \theta - \theta_0)|}
\tag{8.124}
$$

Then,

$$
\frac{dp(\theta)}{d\theta} = ie^{i\Phi(\theta)}\frac{d\Phi(\theta)}{d\theta}
\tag{8.125}
$$

and

$$
\frac{d\Phi(\theta)}{d\theta} = -ip^*(\theta)\frac{dp(\theta)}{d\theta}
\tag{8.126}
$$

where $dp(\theta)/d\theta$ can be evaluated using an FFT-based algorithm [191]. Noting that

$$
\frac{d\Phi(\theta)}{d\theta} = -2\pi k_0 x_0 \sin(\theta - \theta_0) + 2\pi k_0 y_0 \cos(\theta - \theta_0)
\tag{8.127}
$$

the translation parameters can now be determined using the following formulas:

$$
x_0 = \frac{-1}{2\pi^2 k_0} \int_0^{2\pi} \frac{d\Phi(\theta)}{d\theta} \sin(\theta - \theta_0) d\theta
\tag{8.128a}
$$

$$
y_0 = \frac{1}{2\pi^2 k_0} \int_0^{2\pi} \frac{d\Phi(\theta)}{d\theta} \cos(\theta - \theta_0) d\theta
\tag{8.128b}
$$

There are several practical issues in using circular navigators for motion estimation. First, determination of the optimal radius k_0 of the circular trajectory is nontrivial. Second, $p(\theta)$ is not properly defined in Eq. (8.124) when

$|S_1(k_0,\theta)S_2(k_0,\theta)| \approx 0$. Further discussion of these and other issues can be found at [159].

Ghost Phase Cancellation (GPC): The GPC method proposed by Xiang and Henkelman is an elegant way to utilize the phase property of the ghost component for suppression of ghost artifacts [271, 273]. The basic idea of GPC is the pixel-by-pixel decomposition of a measure ghosted complex image I into two components: the desired time-averaged image $\hat{I}_0$ and the undesirable ghost image g. Assuming that J images are acquired, we can express each of them as

$$I_j = \hat{I}_0 + g_j \qquad j = 1, 2, \ldots, J \tag{8.129}$$

which give rise to J equations containing $(J+1)$ unknowns for each pixel. To solve for $\hat{I}_0$ from Eq. (GPC-decomposition), additional information is required. In practice, the J data sets are acquired in a manner so that the g_j are related to each other by a simple phase shift, thus the name *ghost phase cancellation*. To understand how this is done, consider the three-point GPC method [271]. In this method, three data frames ($J = 3$) are acquired in a time-interleaved fashion. Many time-interleaving schemes are available, an example of which is shown in Fig. 8.21. According to Eq. (8.98) (with omission of the scaling constant), the three images obtained from these data by direct Fourier reconstruction are given by

$$I_1(x) = \hat{I}_0(x) + \sum_{m \neq 0} e^{i2\pi m f_0 t_0} \hat{I}_m(x + \delta x_m) \tag{8.130a}$$

$$I_2(x) = \hat{I}_0(x) + \sum_{m \neq 0} e^{i2\pi m f_0 (t_0 + \Delta t)} \hat{I}_m(x + \delta x_m) \tag{8.130b}$$

$$I_3(x) = \hat{I}_0(x) + \sum_{m \neq 0} e^{i2\pi m f_0 (t_0 + 2\Delta t)} \hat{I}_m(x + \delta x_m) \tag{8.130c}$$

where $\hat{I}_m$ represents the mth harmonic and δx_m is defined in Eq. (8.99).

If we further assume that no more than one ghost harmonic is present at any location (i.e., no overlap of ghosts), Eq. (8.130) can then be simplified to

$$I_1(x) = \hat{I}_0(x) + e^{i2\pi m f_0 t_0} \hat{I}_m(x + \delta x_m) \tag{8.131a}$$

$$I_2(x) = \hat{I}_0(x) + e^{i2\pi m f_0 (t_0 + \Delta t)} \hat{I}_m(x + \delta x_m) \tag{8.131b}$$

$$I_3(x) = \hat{I}_0(x) + e^{i2\pi m f_0 (t_0 + 2\Delta t)} \hat{I}_m(x + \delta x_m) \tag{8.131c}$$

where it is understood that m is an arbitrary integer whose value is x-dependent. Comparing Eq. (8.131) to Eq. (8.129) yields

$$g_1(x) = e^{i2\pi m f_0 t_0} \hat{I}_m(x + \delta x_m) \tag{8.132a}$$

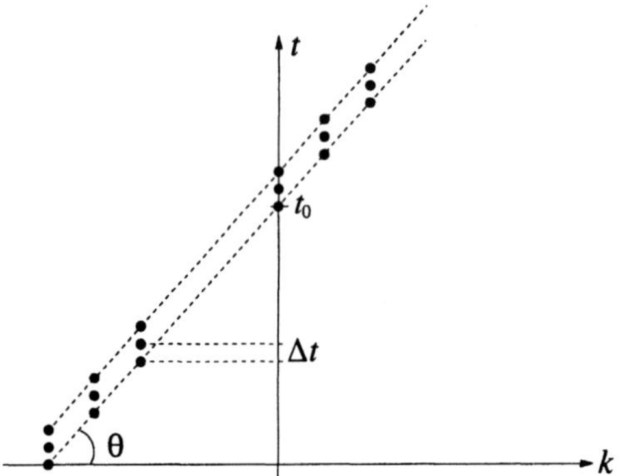

Figure 8.21 Three data frames acquired in a time-interleaved fashion for use in the three-point GPC method.

$$g_2(x) \;=\; e^{i2\pi m f_0(t_0 + \Delta t)}\,\hat{I}_m(x + \delta x_m) \tag{8.132b}$$

$$g_3(x) \;=\; e^{i2\pi m f_0(t_0 + 2\Delta t)}\,\hat{I}_m(x + \delta x_m) \tag{8.132c}$$

Inspection of Eq. (8.132) indicates that

$$|g_1| = |g_2| = |g_3| \tag{8.133}$$

and

$$g_1 \cdot g_3 = g_2^2 \tag{8.134}$$

Equation (8.134) is a key formula for the three-point GPC method, with which the following closed-form solution to Eq. (8.129) results:

$$\hat{I}_0 = \frac{(I_1 \cdot I_3) - I_2^2}{I_1 + I_3 - 2I_2} \tag{8.135}$$

and

$$g_1 \;=\; \frac{(I_1 - I_2)^2}{I_1 + I_3 - 2I_2} \tag{8.136a}$$

$$g_2 \;=\; \frac{(I_2 - I_1)(I_3 - I_2)}{I_1 + I_3 - 2I_2} \tag{8.136b}$$

$$g_3 \;=\; \frac{(I_3 - I_2)^2}{I_1 + I_3 - 2I_2} \tag{8.136c}$$

The desired time-averaged image $\hat{I}_0$ can be calculated from Eq. (8.135) pixel by pixel. However, when the denominator is zero or very close to zero, the formula should be evaluated with caution. It is suggested [271] that at each point $\hat{I}_0$

is calculated according to the formula only when the value of the denominator is above the noise level; otherwise, $\hat{I}_0$ is computed simply as the complex average of the three measured images.

Based on the concept of ghost-phase cancellation, a simpler and more effective 2-point ($J = 2$) method has also been proposed. The reader is referred to [274] for a detailed discussion of the original 2-point GPC method and to [117, 118, 119] for its improvements. To illustrate the performance of the GPC method, two axial images of the lower abdomen are shown in Fig. 8.22. As can be seen from Fig. 8.22b, the GPC method significantly reduces the ghost artifact present in the original image shown in Fig. 8.22a. In general, this level of ghost suppression may not be obtainable because $\hat{I}_0$ produced by GPC is ghost-free only when I_j are corrupted with isolated ghost artifacts. The GPC method is less effective for removing overlapped and/or aliased ghosts because the phase of those ghost components does not satisfy the assumptions of the GPC model.

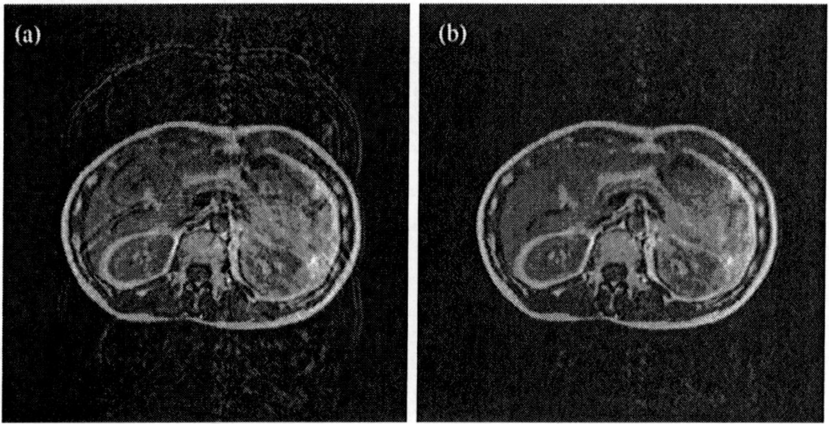

Figure 8.22   Axial images of the lower abdomen: (a) Magnitude image from one of the two time-interleaved scans, and (b) de-ghosted image by the two-point GPC method. (Images courtesy of Dr. Q.-S. Xiang.)

Dynamic Imaging by Model Estimation (DIME): Given a dynamic object, DIME aims to capture the entire spatiotemporal distribution within the imaging time window instead of obtaining a motion-artifact-free snapshot or a time-averaged image. In doing so, DIME collects a sequence of data frames. An example of (k, t)-space coverage with these data frames is shown in Fig. 8.23, where the frame rate is

$$\Delta T = N \Delta t \tag{8.137}$$

Based on the discussion in the previous sections, ΔT is expected to be larger than the Nyquist sampling interval with respect to the dynamic signal changes. Therefore, traditional signal interpolation methods cannot be used to generate data on the desired rectilinear trajectories. To overcome the temporal undersampling problem, DIME represents temporal signal changes at each point by a generalized harmonic model,

$$I(r, t) = \sum_{m=1}^{M(r)} c_m(r) e^{i2\pi f_m(r)t} \tag{8.138}$$

where M is the model order and f_m are the motion frequencies. This model can theoretically handle both periodic and nonperiodic motions with rigid-body or non-rigid-body changes. Specifically, any periodic motion can be described by this model with $f_m = m f_0$; for nonperiodic motions with line frequency spectra, f_m takes on arbitrary real numbers. More complex motions such as those with continuous spectra can also be handled in this model by allowing f_m to take on complex values.

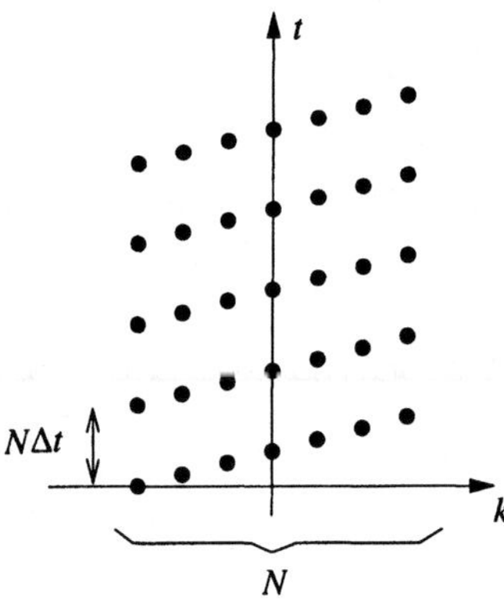

Figure 8.23   Coverage of (k, t)-space with multiple data frames in DIME.

The general model given in Eq. (8.138) assumes no spatial correlation of the time variations at different locations. This is certainly not the case for any practical application. Specifically, $\{f_m(r_1)\}$ and $\{f_m(r_2)\}$ will have many identical frequency components. For notational simplicity, we can remove the r-dependence from M and f_m by rewriting Eq. (8.138) as

$$I(r, t) = \sum_{m=1}^{M} c_m(r) e^{i2\pi f_m t} \tag{8.139}$$

where now M is the total number of motion frequency components for the entire object and $\{f_m\}$ accounts for all the possible motion frequencies present. With this model, the measured data are given by

$$S(\boldsymbol{k}, t) = \int_{-\infty}^{\infty} I(\boldsymbol{r}, t) e^{-i2\pi \boldsymbol{k} \cdot \boldsymbol{r}} d\boldsymbol{r}$$

$$= \sum_{m=1}^{M} \left[\int_{-\infty}^{\infty} c_m(\boldsymbol{r}) \, e^{-i2\pi \boldsymbol{k} \cdot \boldsymbol{r}} d\boldsymbol{r} \right] e^{i2\pi f_m t}$$

$$= \sum_{m=1}^{M} \hat{c}_m(\boldsymbol{k}) e^{i2\pi f_m t} \tag{8.140}$$

where

$$\hat{c}_m(\boldsymbol{k}) = \int_{-\infty}^{\infty} c_m(\boldsymbol{r}) e^{-i2\pi \boldsymbol{k} \cdot \boldsymbol{r}} d\boldsymbol{r} \tag{8.141}$$

Equation (8.140) indicates that the measured data for each $\boldsymbol{k}$ value can also be described by a generalized harmonic model. By introducing this data model, we effectively convert the dynamic imaging problem to a parameter identification problem. In order to uniquely determine the model parameters, sufficient data have to be collected in $(\boldsymbol{k}, t)$-space. Because of the inherent time-sequential constraint and the underlying undersampling problem, data need to be acquired optimally to avoid image artifacts. An important property of this model is that if the motion frequencies are known a priori, the coefficients can be determined exactly in most cases even when $(\boldsymbol{k}, t)$-space is undersampled along the time axis. Specifically, it is easy to show that for a given $\boldsymbol{k}$ value, if L data points are taken at $t_1, t_2, \ldots, t_L$, then $\hat{c}_m(\boldsymbol{k})$ can be uniquely recovered from the measured data as long as

$$\boldsymbol{E}_m \neq \boldsymbol{E}_n, \qquad \text{for } m \neq n \tag{8.142}$$

where

$$\boldsymbol{E}_m \doteq \left(\, e^{i2\pi f_m t_1} \quad e^{i2\pi f_m t_2} \quad \cdots \quad e^{i2\pi f_m t_L} \, \right) \tag{8.143}$$

If the temporal sampling is uniform such that $t_l = l\Delta t$, this condition can be restated as:

$$2\pi f_m \Delta t \neq 2\pi f_n \Delta t + p2\pi \qquad \text{for } m \neq n \text{ and any integer } p \tag{8.144}$$

This property significantly relaxes the burden on data acquisition.

The data acquisition step of DIME is characterized by the collection of two data sets: one for determining the motion frequencies and the other for determining the amplitude parameters. Because of the above reconstruction condition, the amplitude parameters can be determined from the regularly collected imaging data shown in Fig. 8.23, although they may be temporally undersampled. To accurately determine the motion frequencies f_m, however, $(\boldsymbol{k}, t)$-space data whose temporal sampling rate satisfies the Nyquist criterion are needed. Since the frame sampling interval in Fig. 8.23 often violates the Nyquist criterion, DIME acquires an auxiliary data set with high temporal resolution. In practice, these data can be collected in a variety of ways. For example, in cardiac imaging the ECG signal can be used to estimate the motion frequencies associated with cardiac motion. However, for MRI the most convenient approach is to collect these data while acquiring the dynamic imaging data using the well-known navigator excitation protocol [135]. Assuming that one imaging signal and one navigator signal are collected for each excitation, the navigator signals can be acquired along a particular vertical line in (k, t)-space as shown in Fig. 8.24a. It is clear that the effective temporal sampling interval for this signal is Δt, which normally satisfies the Nyquist criterion. There are also many other ways to distribute the navigator signals. Two examples are shown in Fig. 8.24b-c, in which the navigator signals are phase-encoded to cover several k-space lines either sequentially or in a parallel fashion. The advantage of these data collection schemes is their improved motion sensitivity since some motion components may not be observable at certain k-space locations because $\hat{c}_m(k) = 0$ for these values of k.

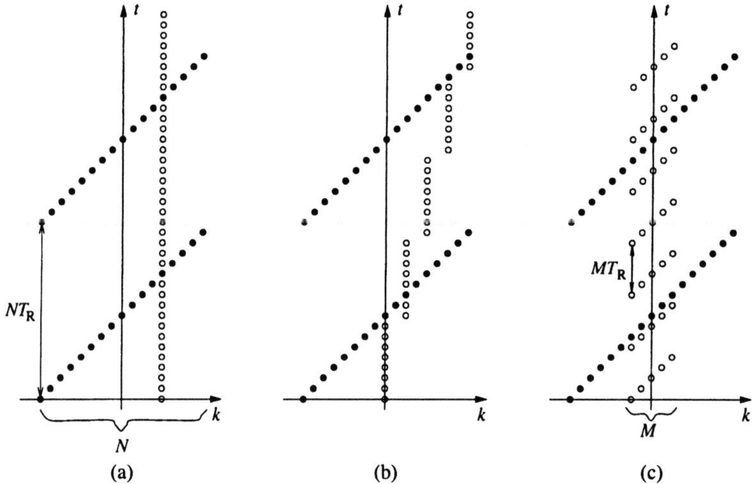

Figure 8.24   Different schemes for covering (k, t)-space with dynamic imaging ($\bullet$) and navigator signals ($\circ$).

Image reconstruction with DIME consists of three major steps. First, the motion frequencies f_m are determined from the navigator signals. By taking advantage of the special structure of the model, one can use a linear prediction based method to gain computational efficiency [179]. Second, once the frequencies f_m are known, the amplitude parameters $\hat{c}_m(k)$ can be determined easily by fitting the model in Eq. (8.140) to the measured imaging data using any of the standard linear least-squares solvers [31]. Third, after the model parameters are available, the signal in the entire (k, t)-space is defined and we can, in principle, generate a continuous movie of dynamic signal changes. In practice, a sequence of "snapshot" data frames with temporal resolution Δt is generated using the signal model in Eq. (8.140). With these data, the snapshot dynamic images can be reconstructed using the conventional Fourier method.

A set of DIME results are shown in Figs. 8.25 to illustrate its performance. The experimental data were collected by connecting a lemon to a platform that was translated within the coil along the main axis of the scanner. The platform was displaced periodically along the readout direction by a computer-controlled stepping motor through a distance of 8 mm at a frequency of 0.216 Hz. A spin-echo sequence with $T_R = 450$ ms was used to collect data as in Fig. 8.24a, with imaging and navigator echoes at $T_E = 30$ ms and $T_E = 60$ ms, respectively. Thirty-two 128×128 frames of imaging data were collected. As can be seen in Fig. 8.25b, the direct Fourier reconstruction from the motion-corrupted data contains serious motion artifacts. Averaging 32 frames of such motion-corrupted imaging data yielded the result in Fig. 8.25c. As expected, averaging removes the ghosting artifacts quite well because of the phase cancellation effect [271], but considerable blurring remains because the result is a time-averaged image. "Snapshot" images generated by DIME exhibited no obvious blurring or ghosting artifacts, as shown in the example snapshot in Fig. 8.25d.

8.3.5   Artifacts Due to Corrupted Data

Various types of data distortions can occur in practice. This section discusses two examples to illustrate that simple distortions in the raw k-space data can result in serious image artifacts.

8.3.5.1   Data Clipping Artifact

Data clipping is graphically shown in Fig. 8.26. It occurs when the received signal is larger than the receiver system (specifically, the analog-to-digital converter) can handle. Because k-space data peak at the origin, data clipping represents a loss of low-frequency data. The resulting image artifact can then be understood by modeling the data distortion as the subtraction of a sharp spike at the central k-space. Because the Fourier transform of a sharp spike is a broad spike, the resulting image, as the difference between the correct image and a broad spatial component, will suffer an intensity distortion. An example of this image artifact is shown in Fig. 8.27. In practice, data clipping is fixed through hardware adjustments to lower the receiver gain. Some post-processing methods have also been proposed to reduce the image artifact from clipped data. The interested reader is referred to [167] for a discussion of this topic.

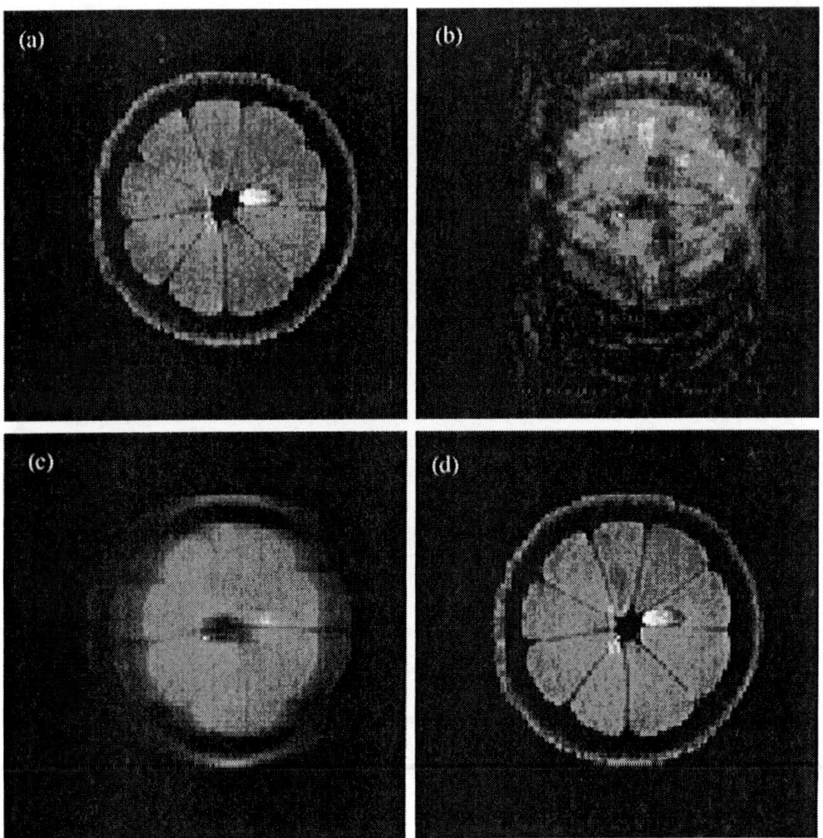

Figure 8.25 Results of a rigid-body motion experiment, showing (a) the stationary lemon, (b) the Fourier reconstruction, (c) the average of 32 images (d) a snapshot image generated by DIME.

8.3.5.2 Noisy Spike Artifacts

Raw k-space data are sometimes corrupted with noisy spikes of various origins. The resulting image artifact is in the form of striations running across the image. The pattern of the striation artifact depends on the shape and location of the spikes. Consider the simple case of a noisy spike located at (k_{x_0}, k_{y_0}). Representing it as a δ-function

$$e(k_x, k_y) = A\delta(k_x - k_{x_0}, k_y - k_{y_0}) \tag{8.145}$$

The resulting image error is

$$\epsilon(x, y) = Ae^{i2\pi(k_{x_0}x + k_{y_0}y)} \tag{8.146}$$

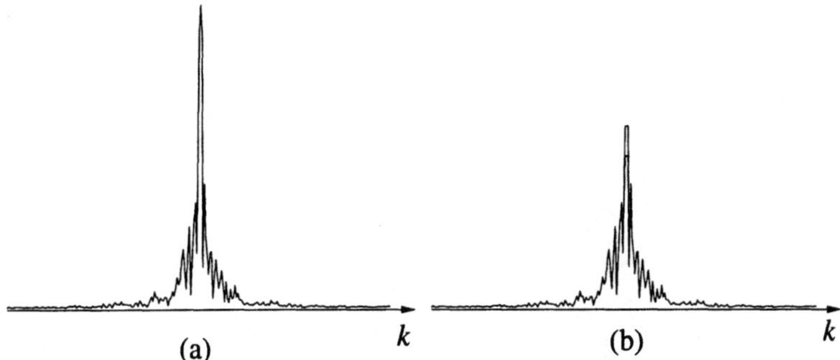

Figure 8.26 An illustration of data clipping.

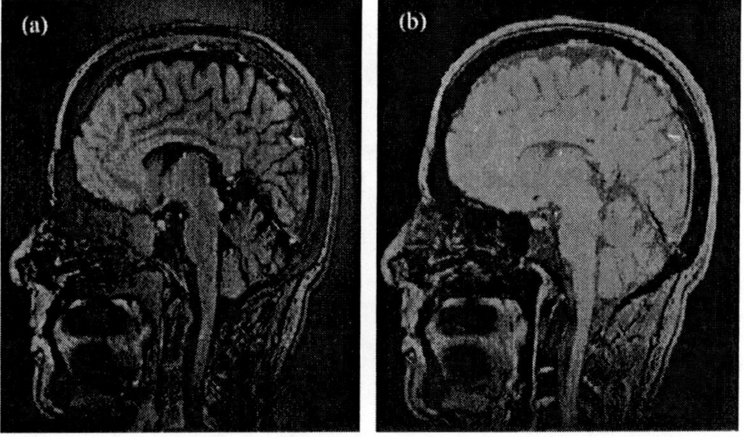

Figure 8.27 Head images: (a) with the data clipping artifact and (b) without the artifact.

The width (or frequency) and orientation of the resulting striations are directly related to the location of the spike as determined by Eq. (8.146). More specifically,

$$k_0 = \sqrt{k_{x_0}^2 + k_{y_0}^2} \tag{8.147}$$

specifies the striation frequency, and

$$\varphi_0 = \arctan\left(\frac{k_{y_0}}{k_{x_0}}\right) \tag{8.148}$$

determines the orientation of the striations.

Examples of the striation artifact resulting from a noisy spike located at two different k-space locations are shown in Fig. 8.28. This type of artifact can often be handled using a post-processing method. Specifically, noisy spikes can sometimes be identified by examining the k-space data and then be removed before image reconstruction is performed.

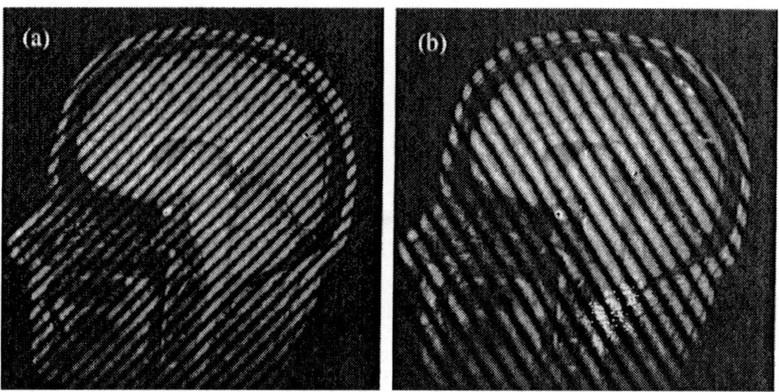

Figure 8.28 Head images showing the striation artifact due to a single noisy spike located at different positions of k-space. The noisy spike is located at $(-0.09, -0.09)$ for (a) and and at $(-0.05, 0.05)$ for (b).

Exercises

8.1   What is the underlying assumption made regarding the imaging process so that the output of an imaging system is equal to the convolution of its point spread function and the true object function?

8.2   Prove Eq. (8.3) using the superposition rule and the convolution property of the δ-function.

8.3   Assume that the point spread function of an unknown imaging system is (a) $h(x) = \Pi(x)$, and (b) $h(x) = \Lambda(2x)$. For each case,

   (a)   Determine the resolution limit of the system.

   (b)   Sketch the resulting image if the true object function is $\rho(x) = \delta(x) + \delta(x - 1)$.

8.4   For an unknown imaging system, briefly discuss how one experimentally determines its point spread function.

8.5   MR signals are subject to T_2 or T_2^* decay during the readout period. Calculate the PSF of the T_2-decay function assuming that the signal can be expressed as

$$S(t) = \int_{-\infty}^{\infty} I(x)e^{-t/T_2}e^{-i\gamma G_x x t}\,dx \qquad t \geq 0$$

8.6   The backprojection reconstruction technique requires projection data taken at projection angles in the range $0 \leq \theta_n \leq \pi$. If projections were taken for $0 \leq \theta_n \leq 2\pi$ and were all projected by simply extending the upper integration limit in the backprojection integral from π to 2π, determine whether the following statements are true or false.

   (a)   An identical image would be obtained.

   (b)   The $1/r$ blurring would remain the same.

   (c)   The "star" artifact would be reduced.

   (d)   The image SNR would be improved a factor of $\sqrt{2}$.

8.7   Justify that the "cross-power" of two *uncorrelated* random variables ξ_1 and ξ_2 is zero, that is,

$$\sigma_{\xi_1\xi_2}^2 = E\{(\xi_1 - \mu_{\xi_1})(\xi_2 - \mu_{\xi_2})^*\} = 0$$

8.8   Justify that if $\xi_1, \xi_2, \cdots, \xi_N$ are *mutually uncorrelated* ($\sigma^2_{\xi_m \xi_n} = 0$, for $m \neq n$), then the mean and variance of the new random variable $\xi = \sum_{n=1}^{N} \xi_n$ are

$$\mu_\xi = E\{\xi\} = \sum_{n=1}^{N} \mu_{\xi_n}$$

$$\sigma^2_\xi = E\{(\xi - \mu_\xi)(\xi - \mu_\xi)^*\} = \sum_{n=1}^{N} \sigma^2_{\xi_n}$$

8.9   Prove that the correlation function $R(\tau)$ of a stationary process $\xi(t)$ has a complex-conjugate symmetry, that is,

$$R(\tau) = R^*(-\tau).$$

8.10   For two uncorrelated random variables ξ_1 and ξ_2, the mean and variance of $\xi = \xi_1 + \xi_2$ are $\mu = \mu_1 + \mu_2$ and $\sigma^2 = \sigma_1^2 + \sigma_2^2$, respectively. Assume that $\mu_1 = \mu_2 = 0$ and that ξ_1 and ξ_2 are correlated. What is the variance ($\hat{\sigma}^2$) for ξ? Is $\hat{\sigma}$ always larger than σ? Give one example for $\hat{\sigma} > \sigma$ and one for $\hat{\sigma} < \sigma$.

8.11   Gibbs ringing is characteristic of Fourier imaging methods. No matter how many encodings are taken, it is present in the reconstructed image as long as finite sampling is used. True or false? Why?

8.12   Windowing the Fourier data can help reduce Gibbs ringing (at the expense of spatial resolution). What is its effect on image S/N as compared to the rectangular window? (Derive the S/N value for an arbitrary window function.)

8.13   Show the relationship given in Eq. (8.65).

8.14   Calculate the aliased version of the following signals:

(a) $S(t) = \sin(2\pi t + 23°)$ for $f_s = 1$ and 1.5, respectively.

(b) $S(t) = \sin(2\pi t) + 2\cos(\pi t) + 4\sin(4\pi t)$ for $f_s = 1$, 2 and 3, respectively.

8.15   Assume that in a phase-encoding experiment, the desired phase-encoding gradients are $G_n = n\Delta G_0$. What will happen to the reconstructed image if the gradient system malfunctions such that the effective gradients applied are

(a) $G_n = 0$

(b) $G_n = n(\Delta G_0/2)$

(c) $G_n = n(2\Delta G_0)$

(d) $G_n = n(\Delta G_0/2) + \delta G$

8.16 Discuss the chemical shift effect along the phase-encoding direction.

8.17 Explain why the chemical shift artifact is more serious in higher fields than in lower fields.

8.18 Given the following object, sketch the reconstructed image showing the chemical shift artifact, assuming that the object is phase-encoded along the vertical direction but frequency-encoded along the horizontal direction.

(a) Region A contains pure fat ($\rho_f = 1$) and region B contains pure water ($\rho_w = 2$).

(b) Region A contains pure water ($\rho_w = 1$) and region B contains pure fat ($\rho_f = 2$).

(c) Region A contains pure water ($\rho_w = 1$) and region B contains half water and half fat ($\rho_w = 1$ and $\rho_f = 1$).

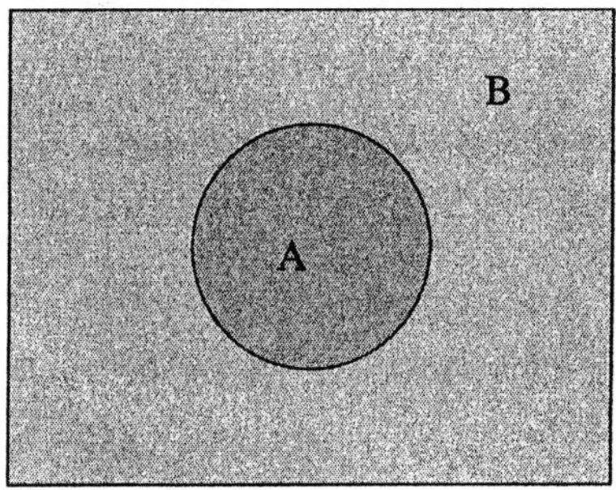

8.19 Inhomogeneities in the main magnetic field can often have deteriorative effects on image quality. Consider a one-dimensional case in which the object is a boxcar function and an unknown field gradient G_u exists across the object in a poorly shimmed main magnetic field. Calculate the reconstructed image function assuming that frequency encoding is used and the continuous signal is measured. Discuss the effect of the inhomogeneity by comparing the result with what would be obtained without the field inhomogeneity.

8.20 The Fourier signal for an image function $\rho(x) = \frac{1}{2}[\delta(x-x_0)+\delta(x+x_0)]$ is $S(k) = \cos 2\pi x_0 k$. Assume that $S(k)$ is uniformly sampled at $k = m\Delta k$, $-\infty < m < \infty$.

(a) What is the Fourier reconstruction from $S(m\Delta k)$ for $\Delta k = \frac{2}{3x_0}$? Note that the Fourier reconstruction is defined as

$$\hat{\rho}(x) = \begin{cases} \Delta k \displaystyle\sum_{m=-\infty}^{\infty} S(m\Delta k)e^{i2\pi m\Delta kx} & x \in [-\frac{1}{2\Delta k}, \frac{1}{2\Delta k}] \\ 0 & \text{otherwise.} \end{cases}$$

(b) What is the corresponding Fourier signal of this reconstructed image function?

8.21 Prove the point spread function for the Fourier reconstruction to be

$$h(x) = \Delta k \sum_{m=-N/2}^{N/2-1} e^{i2\pi m\Delta kx} = \Delta k \frac{\sin(\pi N\Delta kx)}{\sin(\pi \Delta kx)}e^{-i\pi \Delta kx}$$

by verifying that

$$\mathcal{F}^{-1}\left\{\Delta kS(k)\sum_{m=-N/2}^{N/2-1}\delta(k-m\Delta k)\right\} = \int_{-\infty}^{\infty} \rho(\tau)h(x-\tau)d\tau,$$

where $S(k) = \mathcal{F}\{\rho(x)\}$.

8.22 John just got an "A" in his MRI course and wanted to impress his girl friend Sue with his MRI skills. He performed a two-dimensional phase-encoded imaging experiment to get the head image of his classmate Joe, shown in (a). He was very excited since everything he learned from the class worked, and he immediately went off to get Sue. When they returned, Joe was gone, and the image had disappeared from the screen. John reprocessed the k-space data, but this time produced the image in (b). He was quite embarrassed but assured Sue that Joe had played a practical joke on him by corrupting the k-space data. To justify his claim, he went through his k-space data file point by point. Equipped with the theories he learned from class, he soon uncovered Joe's contaminations of the data. After processing the "corrected" k-space data, he reconstructed the image in (c).

(a) What kind of image artifact is present in image (b)?

(b) How did Joe corrupt the k-space data? Be specific and give justifications.

(c) What correction to the contaminated k-space data resulted in the reconstruction shown in image (c)? Justify your answer.

(d)   What do you think John should do to reproduce an image like that in (a)? (Be scientific.) Why?

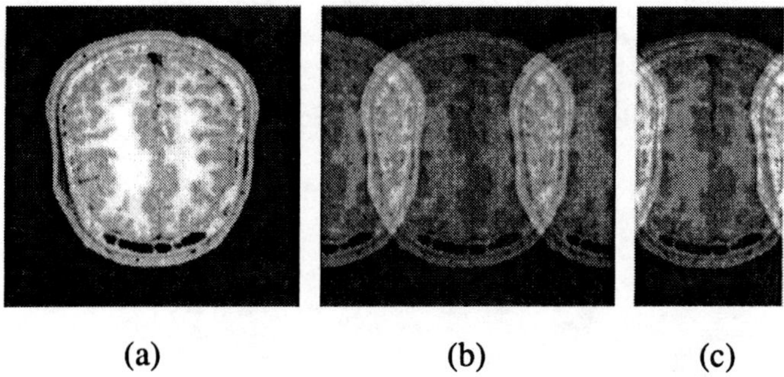

(a)   (b)   (c)

8.23   Assume that you collect N data points (with symmetric and uniform sampling) in the Fourier space from a one-dimensional rectangular object of width W_1 and unit intensity.

(a)   Qualitatively plot the Fourier reconstruction from the data.

(b)   Calculate and plot the reconstructed image if the point spread function is approximated by a rectangular window function of width $W_2 = 1/(N\Delta k)$ and amplitude $1/W_2$ (assuming $W_1 = 5W_2$).

(c)   If one is interested only in the intensity measurement, what is the average image intensity over the reconstructed object? What is the systematic measurement error?

(d)   Assume that the data noise standard deviation is σ, what is the measurement error introduced to the average intensity by the noise? What would this error be if $N/2$ encodings were collected with two signal averagings?

8.24   Assume that $(2N + 1)$ noisy data points, say $d_n = S_n + \xi_n$ from $-N \le n \le N$, are collected in k-space from a real object function $\rho(x)$. Let

$$\rho_1[m] = \sum_{n=-N}^{N} d_n e^{i2\pi mn/(2N+1)}$$

$$\rho_2[m] = \sum_{n=-N}^{-1} d_n^*) e^{-i2\pi mn/(2N+1)} + \sum_{n=0}^{N} d_n e^{i2\pi mn/(2N+1)}$$

Justify that the SNR of $\rho_1(m)$ is better than that of $\rho_2(m)$ by a factor of $\sqrt{2}$.

8.25 Prove that the point spread function of the direct backprojection method is $1/r = 1/\sqrt{x^2 + y^2}$ by verifying that

$$\mathcal{B}\{\mathcal{R}\{\delta(x,y)\}\} = \frac{1}{\sqrt{x^2 + y^2}}$$

8.26 Derive the relationship given in Eq. (8.121).

8.27 Assume that two circular navigator signals $S_1(k_0, \theta)$ and $S_2(k_0, \theta)$ are collected from $\rho_1(x,y)$ and $\rho_2(x,y)$ with

$$\rho_2(x,y) = \rho_1(\hat{x}, \hat{y})$$

where

$$
\begin{aligned}
\hat{x} &= (x - x_0)\cos\theta_0 + (y - y_0)\sin\theta_0 \\
\hat{y} &= -(x - x_0)\sin\theta_0 + (y - y_0)\cos\theta_0 - y_0
\end{aligned}
$$

Show that

$$S_2(k_0, \theta) = S_1(k_0, \theta - \theta_0)e^{-i2\pi k_0(x_0\cos\theta + y_0\sin\theta)}$$

8.28 Derive the formula given in Eq. (8.135).

8.29 Show that the following expression is equivalent to that given in Eq. (8.135):

$$I_0 = \frac{I_1 + I_2 + I_3}{3} - \frac{3(I_1^2 + I_2^2 + I_3^2) - (I_1 + I_2 + I_3)^2}{6(I_1 + I_3 - 2I_2)}$$

8.30 In special cases, the GPC method can produce a ghost-free, time-averaged image $\hat{I}_0$ from two ghosted complex images I_1 and I_2. Let

$$
\begin{aligned}
I_1 &= \hat{I}_0 + g_1 \\
I_2 &= \hat{I}_0 + g_2
\end{aligned}
$$

and

$$g_2 = g_1 e^{i\theta}$$

Derive an expression for $\hat{I}_0$ in terms of I_1, I_2 and, θ.

Chapter 9

Fast-Scan Imaging

There is nothing that nuclear spins will not do for you, as long as you treat them as human beings.

Erwin Hahn

Fast imaging is one of the most interesting and important areas of MRI. This chapter is devoted to a systematic discussion of this topic. Before proceeding, let us first examine the range of possibilities to improve imaging speed over the conventional imaging method. From the discussion presented in Chapter 5, it is easy to derive that the total data acquisition time for a spin-echo imaging experiment is

$$T_{\mathrm{acq}} = N_{\mathrm{acq}} N_{\mathrm{enc}} T_{\mathrm{R}} \tag{9.1}$$

where N_{acq} is the number of signal acquisitions (or signal averagings) for each encoded signal, N_{enc} is the number of encodings, and T_{R} is the time interval between two consecutive encoded signals. Clearly, T_{acq} can be shortened by reducing N_{acq}, N_{enc}, and T_{R}, individually or simultaneously. The cost of reducing N_{acq} is a loss of signal-to-noise ratio, and the absolute limit is reached when $N_{\mathrm{acq}} = 1$. To achieve high-speed imaging, one has to find a way to significantly reduce $(N_{\mathrm{enc}} T_{\mathrm{R}})$. We discuss how this is accomplished in several popular fast-scan imaging methods, including fast spin-echo imaging, fast gradient-echo imaging, echo-planar imaging, and burst imaging.

9.1 Fast Spin-Echo Imaging

Conceptually, fast spin-echo (FSE) imaging is a simple extension of the basic spin-echo imaging method. It uses the CPMG sequence discussed in Chapter 4 to generate multiple spin echoes, each of which is individually phase- or frequency-encoded to cover k-space. This section describes the basic concept and some practical limitations of FSE imaging.

9.1.1   Basic Concept

To illustrate the basic FSE imaging concept, consider the data acquisition sequence shown in Fig. 9.1, in which M echo signals are generated for each 90° excitation pulse. If these signals are encoded differently, M k-space lines will be generated for each excitation. Assume that a total of N_{enc} encodings are required to cover k-space. Then, the number of excitations necessary is given by

$$N_{\mathrm{ex}} = \frac{N_{\mathrm{enc}}}{M} \tag{9.2}$$

Hence, a factor of M improvement in imaging speed is obtained over the conventional single-echo imaging method. The value of M is limited by the T_2 value of the object being imaged. In practice, $M = 8$ or 16, or even higher is possible [81].

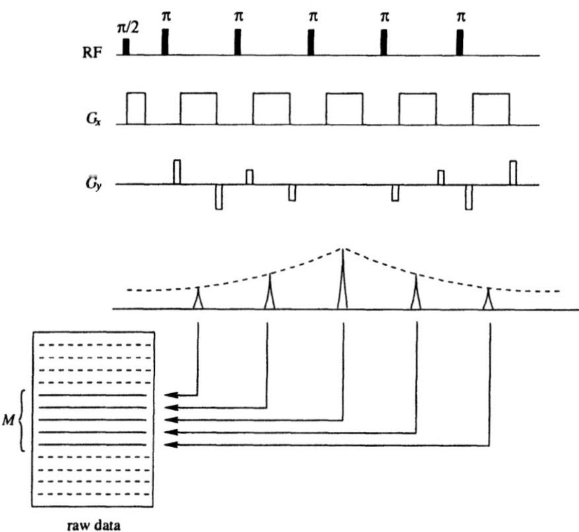

Figure 9.1   A representative FSE imaging sequence that generates M spin echoes after a 90° pulse. These echoes are individually encoded to produce M data lines in k-space.

A first question that arises with FSE imaging is how to encode the echo train. Encoding a train of echoes is a little bit more tricky than encoding a single echo because the encoding effect of one echo is carried over to the subsequent ones in the echo train. To avoid this complication, one often uses phase rewinding.

Specifically, as shown in Fig. 9.1, each echo is first phase-encoded with G_{pe}, and the phase dispersal thus introduced is rewound at the end of the echo by applying a rephasing gradient $-G_{\mathrm{pe}}$. It is possible, of course, to eliminate phase rewinding if the phase accumulation effect is properly accounted for.

Encoding ordering (or distribution of the echo trains in k-space) is also important in FSE imaging because of the inherent T_2 decay during the formation of the echo train. Referring to the timing diagram in Fig. 9.2, the amplitude of the nth echo in the echo train has the following characteristic exponential T_2-weightings:

$$E_n = e^{-nT_{\mathrm{E}}/T_2} \qquad n = 1, 2, \dots, M \tag{9.3}$$

These weightings have different effects on image contrast and resolution, depending on how the echoes are mapped to k-space.

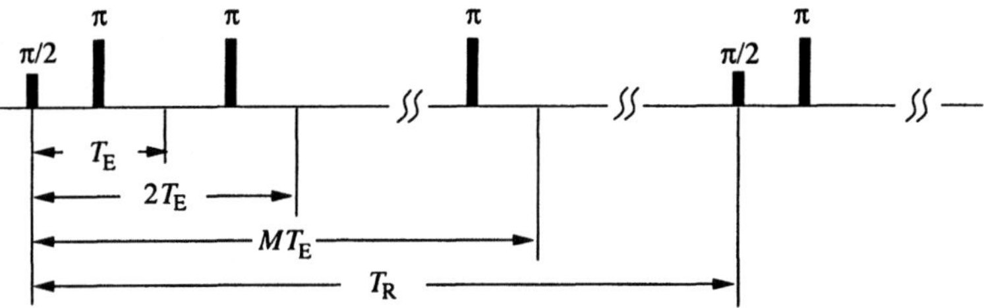

Figure 9.2 Timing of an FSE imaging sequence.

Let $S_{mn}(t)$ represent the nth echo from the mth excitation. These signals can be mapped to k-space according to the following interleaved scheme along the phase-encoding direction:

$$k_{mn} = \left[m - 1 + (n-1)N_{\mathrm{ex}} - \frac{N_{\mathrm{enc}}}{2} \right] \Delta k \qquad m = 1, 2, \dots, N_{\mathrm{ex}}$$
$$n = 1, 2, \dots, M \tag{9.4}$$

The resulting k-space coverage is shown in Fig. 9.3.

Corresponding to the k-space coverage in Fig. 9.3, the data along the phase-encoding direction will carry a T_2-weighting, as illustrated in Fig. 9.4a. Alternatively, the weighting function in Fig. 9.4b results if the following phase-encoding ordering scheme is used:

$$k_{mn} = \begin{cases} -\left[m - 1 + (n-1)\frac{N_{\mathrm{ex}}}{2} \right] \Delta k & m = 1, 2, \dots, \frac{N_{\mathrm{ex}}}{2} \\ & n = 1, 2, \dots, M \\ \left[m - N_{\mathrm{ex}}/2 + (n-1)\frac{N_{\mathrm{ex}}}{2} \right] \Delta k & m = \frac{N_{\mathrm{ex}}}{2} + 1, \dots, N_{\mathrm{ex}} \\ & n = 1, 2, \dots, M \end{cases} \tag{9.5}$$

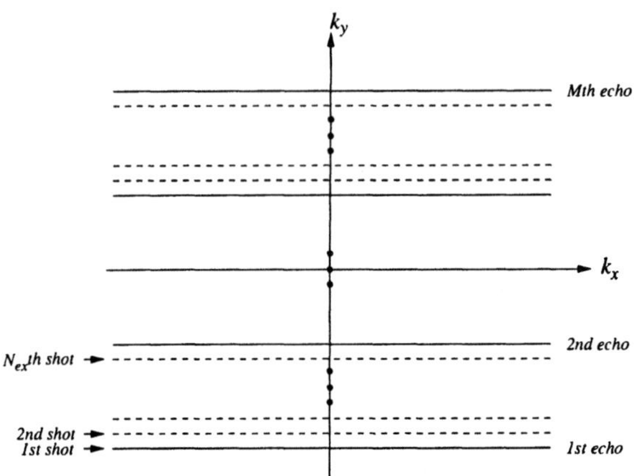

Figure 9.3 K-space coverage of the phase-encoding ordering scheme described by Eq. (9.4).

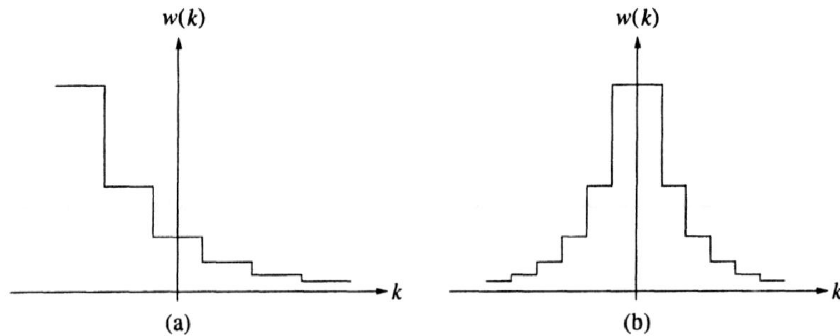

Figure 9.4 Two T_2-weighting functions for k-space data acquired with an FSE imaging sequence.

Although the phase-encoding ordering schemes in Eqs. (9.4) and (9.5) give the same k-space coverage, the resulting image contrast is different. Since image contrast is determined primarily by the central k-space data, it is obvious that the phase-encoding ordering scheme in Eq. (9.4) will produce stronger T_2-weighted contrast than the scheme described by Eq. (9.5). By the same analysis, one can produce variable degrees of T_2-weighting by properly ordering the phase-encoding steps and adjusting the inter-echo spacing.

Although the original FSE imaging sequence, known as RARE (Rapid Acquisition with Relaxation Enhancement), was proposed by Hennig et al. for fast T_2-weighted imaging [156], the FSE imaging sequence is capable of producing the full range of SE contrast. For example, one can adjust T_R in the same way as in spin-echo imaging to generate T_1-weighted images. Similarly, proton density-weighted images can be obtained using a long T_R and a short $\widehat{T}_E$, the effective echo time for the central k-space data.

9.1.2 Practical Issues

FSE imaging has several practical limitations. The first is due to the fact that a number of π pulses are applied in a short time interval in the FSE sequence, which may deposit excessive RF power on the object being imaged. This problem can be alleviated by reducing the length of the echo train. The second limitation is image blurring and ringing artifact along the phase-encoding direction due to the inherent T_2 decay during the formation of the echo train. Although T_2 decay occurs in both the readout and phase-encoding directions, its effect in the latter direction is more pronounced because the time interval between the first and the last echo is several times longer than a typical readout time interval. In addition, the T_2-weighting function along the phase-encoding direction is discontinuous, resulting in an oscillatory PSF, an example of which is shown in Fig. 9.5b.

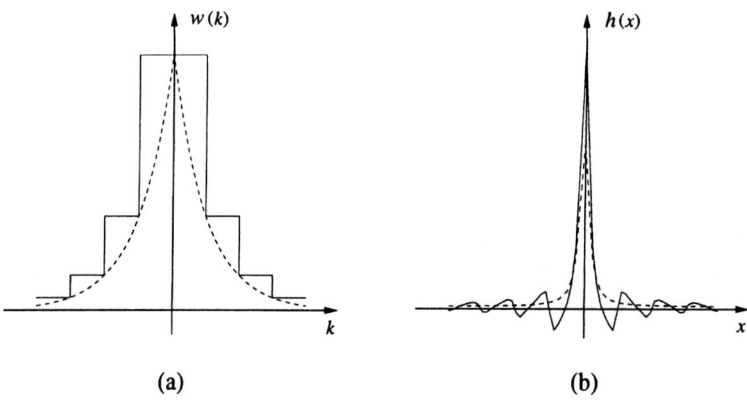

Figure 9.5 T_2-weighting function and the corresponding PSF. Note the oscillations present in the PSF associated with the discontinuous T_2-weighting function.

The ringing artifact can be suppressed by removing the discontinuities in the T_2-weighting function. A post-processing method was proposed in [285] to deal with the problem. Neglecting the T_2 decay along the readout direction, we can express the k-space data obtained from an FSE sequence as

$$S(k_x, k_y) = \int_{-\infty}^{\infty} \int_{-\infty}^{\infty} \rho(x, y) e^{-T_E(k_y)/T_2(x,y)} e^{-i2\pi(k_x x + k_y y)} dx\, dy \qquad (9.6)$$

where x and y denote the readout and phase-encoding directions, respectively, and $T_E(k_y)$ represents the effective echo time for each phase-encoding step. If we further assume that T_2 variations along the phase-encoding direction are small, we can treat T_2 as a function of x only. Therefore, after reconstruction along the readout direction, we have

$$\hat{S}(x, k_y) = e^{-T_{\mathrm{E}}(k_y)/T_2(x)} \int_{-\infty}^{\infty} \rho(x, y) e^{-i2\pi k_y y} dy \qquad (9.7)$$

Equation (9.7) suggests a simple correction scheme. That is, if $T_2(x)$ is known, the T_2-weighting function along the k_y-direction can be eliminated by multiplying $\hat{S}(x, k_y)$ by

$$w(k_y) = e^{T_{\mathrm{E}}(k_y)/T_2(x)} \qquad (9.8)$$

Since $w(k_y)$ is a high-pass filter, this step may result in a loss of signal-to-noise ratio. If the goal is to remove the discontinuities in the T_2-weighting function, the following modulation function should be used:

$$w(k_y) = e^{-\widehat{T}_{\mathrm{E}}(k_y)/T_2(x)} \qquad (9.9)$$

where $\widehat{T}_{\mathrm{E}}(k_y)$ is dependent on the phase-encoding ordering scheme. For the scheme given in Eq. (9.4), it is easy to show that

$$\widehat{T}_{\mathrm{E}}(n\Delta k_y) = (n-1)_{N_{\mathrm{enc}}} \frac{T_{\mathrm{E}}}{N_{\mathrm{enc}} T_2(x)} \qquad n = 1, 2, \ldots, N_{\mathrm{enc}} \qquad (9.10)$$

where $(n-1)_{N_{\mathrm{enc}}}$ denotes $(n-1)$ modulo N_{enc}.

Now the question is how to determine $T_2(x)$. The approach proposed in [285] applies an extra excitation to generate a set of echoes, called *auxiliary echoes*, with the same inter-echo spacing, say T_{E}. These auxiliary echoes are acquired in the absence of the phase-encoding gradient, and they provide M projections of the object along the frequency-encoding direction. Under the ideal condition, these projections differ only by a weighting factor $e^{-nT_{\mathrm{E}}/T_2(x)}$. Therefore, fitting the T_2 exponential function point-by-point through this set of projections will give the desired T_2 values.

In addition to the T_2 decay, phase inconsistency in the echo train can also lead to image artifacts. One source of phase inconsistency is due to the fact that the transverse magnetization may be recalled at different spatial positions by the refocusing pulses. Specifically, assuming that all the refocusing pulses are 180°_φ pulses and ignoring the T_2 decay, we find that the nth echo in the echo train is related to the first one by

$$S_n(t) = S_1(t) e^{-i2(n-1)\varphi} \qquad (9.11)$$

Additional phase errors may also exist if the directionality of the refocusing pulses fluctuates and eddy current exists due to gradient switching. If the phase error is not properly accounted for, it will introduce image artifact. One approach to handle this problem is to estimate the phase errors from the auxiliary echoes and remove them from the imaging data before the image reconstruction algorithm is applied. Further discussion of this topic can be found in [285].

9.2 Fast Gradient-Echo Imaging

Gradient-echo imaging with a long T_R has been discussed in Section 7.5, and a generic pulse sequence is shown in Fig. 7.6. Similar to conventional spin-echo imaging, gradient-echo imaging collects one k-space line per excitation pulse, and, as such, it does not offer any significant speed improvement if a long T_R is used. In this section, we discuss fast gradient-echo imaging methods that operate in the regime of very short T_Rs.

When a spin system is excited by a train of periodic RF pulses with repetition time $T_R \ll T_2$, the spin system will reach a dynamic equilibrium, known as the steady state. A number of steady-state gradient-echo imaging sequences have been proposed. Based on how the transverse magnetization is handled after each excitation, these methods are conveniently grouped into two classes: spoiled steady-state imaging methods and true steady-state imaging methods. As the nomenclature suggests, methods in the first class establish a steady-state longitudinal magnetization but destroy or "spoil" any residual transverse magnetization before a new RF pulse is applied. Methods in the second allow both the longitudinal and transverse components to reach a dynamic equilibrium state. In the following sections, we describe the basic concepts of both types of steady-state imaging methods.

9.2.1 Spoiled Steady-State Imaging

To understand the concept of spoiled steady-state imaging, we consider the FLASH (Fast Low Angle SHot) sequence [154] shown in Fig. 9.6. This sequence is also known as the spoiled GRASS (Gradient Refocused Acquisition in the Steady State). Note that in this sequence, the residual transverse magnetization after data collection is destroyed by a spoiler gradient pulse applied along the slice-selection direction. Specifically, the amplitude of the spoiler gradient is varied from one excitation to another in order to avoid coherent buildup of the transverse magnetization. Spoiling is a key element of this imaging scheme since other components are similar to the counterparts in the long-T_R imaging sequence. In addition to the gradient spoiling method used in this sequence, effective RF spoiling methods have also been developed, which incrementally step the phase of the RF pulses. More detailed discussion of the topic is beyond the scope of this text. The interested reader is referred to [66, 127].

We next derive signal expressions for a spoiled steady-state experiment. Steady-state signals from a sequence of repetitive pulses have been derived in Section 7.5, where it is assumed that $T_R \gg T_2$ such that $M_{x'y'}^{(n)}(0_-) = 0$. In the present discussion, $T_R \ll T_2$ and, hence, $M_{x'y'}^{(n)}(0_-) \neq 0$. This means that the transverse magnetization generated by a pulse has not been completely dephased when the next pulse is applied. With spoiled steady-state imaging methods, this residual transverse magnetization is destroyed using various spoiling methods be-

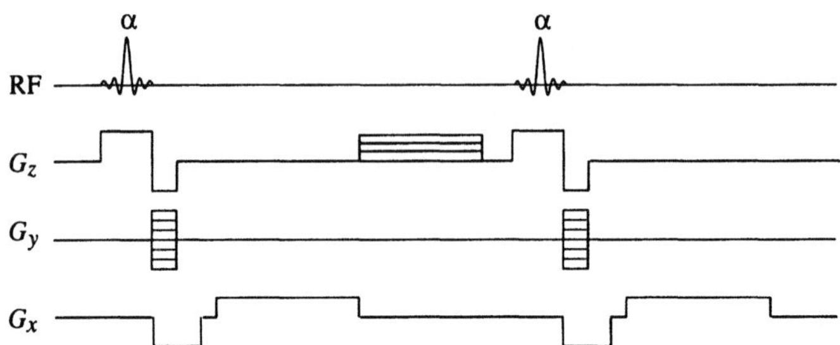

Figure 9.6 Two-dimensional FLASH sequence. Note that the residual transverse magnetization after data collection is destroyed by a spoiler gradient pulse in the slice-selection direction. The amplitude of the spoiler gradient is varied from one excitation to another to avoid build-up of transverse coherence.

fore a new pulse is applied. Consequently, we have, as in the long-T_R case,

$$M_{x'y'}^{(n)}(0_-) = 0 \tag{9.12}$$

Equation (9.12) is called the *perfect spoiling condition.*

When perfect spoiling is achieved, the signal expressions for long T_Rs given in Section 7.5 apply to the situation here. That is,

$$M_{z'}^{ss}(0_-) = \frac{M_z^0(1 - e^{-T_R/T_1})}{1 - \cos \alpha e^{-T_R/T_1}} \tag{9.13}$$

and

$$M_{x'y'}^{ss}(0_+) = \frac{M_z^0(1 - e^{-T_R/T_1})}{1 - \cos \alpha e^{-T_R/T_1}} \sin \alpha \tag{9.14}$$

Equations (9.13) and (9.14) indicate that the amplitude of spoiled steady-state signals is dependent on the flip angle α and the repetition time T_R. For a fixed T_R, one can maximize $M_{x'y'}^{ss}(0_-)$ by properly choosing α. This optimal angle, now known as the *Ernst angle*, is customarily denoted by α_E. It is easy to derive from Eq. (9.14) that

$$\cos \alpha_E = e^{-T_R/T_1} \tag{9.15}$$

or

$$\alpha_E = \cos^{-1}\left(e^{-T_R/T_1}\right) \tag{9.16}$$

In steady-state imaging experiments, it is desirable that data acquisition start after the steady state has been reached. Otherwise, image artifacts can result because signals carry different T_1-weightings while a spin system is approaching the steady state. We next evaluate how many pulses are necessary for a spin system to reach a spoiled steady state.

Recall that the longitudinal magnetization before the nth pulse is given by

$$M_{z'}^{(n)}(0_-) = M_z^0(1 - e^{-T_R/T_1}) + M_{z'}^{(n-1)}(0_-)\cos\alpha e^{-T_R/T_1} \qquad (9.17)$$

For simplicity, we introduce two new variables E_1 and E_2 such that

$$\begin{cases} E_1 = e^{-T_R/T_1} \\ E_2 = e^{-T_R/T_2} \end{cases} \qquad (9.18)$$

Then, Eq. (9.17) can be written as

$$M_{z'}^{(n)}(0_-) = M_z^0(1 - E_1) + M_{z'}^{(n-1)}(0_-)\cos\alpha E_1 \qquad (9.19)$$

Solving this difference equation yields

$$M_{z'}^{(n)}(0_-) = M_z^0(1 - E_1)\frac{1 - (\cos\alpha E_1)^n}{1 - \cos\alpha E_1} + M_z^0(\cos\alpha E_1)^n \qquad n \geq 1 \quad (9.20)$$

The convergence error, defined as the difference between $M_{z'}^{(n)}(0_-)$ and the desired steady-state value $M_{z'}^{ss}(0_-)$, can be calculated as

$$\Delta M_{z'}^{(n)}(0_-) = M_{z'}^{(n)}(0_-) - M_{z'}^{ss}(0_-)$$

$$= M_z^0\frac{(E_1 - 1)(\cos\alpha E_1)^n}{1 - \cos\alpha E_1} + M_z^0(\cos\alpha E_1)^n$$

$$= M_z^0\frac{(\cos\alpha E_1)^n E_1(1 - \cos\alpha)}{1 - \cos\alpha E_1} \qquad (9.21)$$

It is often useful to normalize this error against the steady-state value. The resulting relative convergence error is given by

$$\frac{\Delta M_{z'}^{(n)}(0_-)}{M_{z'}^{ss}(0_-)} = \frac{(\cos\alpha E_1)^n E_1(1 - \cos\alpha)}{1 - E_1} \qquad (9.22)$$

From this formula, one can determine the number of pulses needed to drive a spin system to the steady state within an acceptable error. The calculation can be further simplified in the case that $\alpha = \alpha_E$, for which

$$\frac{\Delta M_{z'}^{(n)}(0_-)}{M_{z'}^{ss}(0_-)} = E_1^{2n+1} \qquad (9.23)$$

Image contrast behavior of spoiled steady-state imaging can be understood from Eq. (9.14). Specifically, the gradient echo amplitude can be expressed as

$$A_E = \frac{M_z^0(1 - e^{-T_R/T_1})}{1 - \cos\alpha e^{-T_R/T_1}}\sin\alpha e^{-T_E/T_2^*} \qquad (9.24)$$

indicating that T_1-weighted, T_2^*-weighted, and spin density-weighted contrast can be generated with an appropriate choice of the sequence parameters: T_R, T_E, and α. For example, to enhance T_1-weighting, one uses a short T_E (minimizing T_2^* effect), short T_R (maximizing T_1 effect), and large α (maximizing T_1 effect). Similarly, for T_2^*-weighted contrast, one uses a long T_R, a long T_E, and a small α; for spin density-weighted contrast, one uses a long T_R, short T_E, and a small α.

■ Example 9.1

The T_1 value for white matter in the brain is approximately 600 ms at 1.5 T. Assuming $T_R = 40$ ms, calculate α_E and the number of pulses needed to get $M_{z'}^{(n)}(0_-)$ within 99% of the steady-state value.

The desired Ernst angle can be calculated directly from Eq. (9.16)

$$\alpha_E = \cos^{-1}\left(e^{-40/600}\right) = 20.7°$$

According to Eq. (9.23), we have

$$n = -\frac{T_1}{2T_R} \ln\left(\frac{\Delta M_{z'}^{(n)}(0_-)}{M_{z'}^{ss}(0_-)}\right) - \frac{1}{2}$$

$$= -\frac{600}{2 \times 40} \ln(0.01) - \frac{1}{2}$$

$$\approx 34$$

Therefore, about 34 preparatory pulses are necessary to get $M_{z'}^{(n)}(0_-)$ within 99% of its steady-state value.

9.2.2   Steady-State Imaging

When T_R is on the order of T_2 and no attempt is made to spoil the transverse magnetization, both the longitudinal and transverse magnetizations will reach a steady state. This phenomenon, called *steady-state free precession* (SSFP), was first studied by Carr [116] in 1958 and later used for imaging.

We shall first derive expressions for the SSFP signal and then discuss steady-state imaging methods. Recall the previously established abbreviations: $E_1 = e^{-T_R/T_1}$ and $E_2 = e^{-T_R/T_2}$. The magnetization immediately before the $(n+1)$th pulse is related the magnetization immediately after the nth pulse by

$$M_r^{(n+1)}(0_-) = \mathbf{P}M_r^{(n)}(0_+) + (1 - E_1)M^0 \tag{9.25}$$

where

$$M_r = \begin{bmatrix} M_{x'} \\ M_{y'} \\ M_{z'} \end{bmatrix} \qquad M^0 = \begin{bmatrix} 0 \\ 0 \\ M_z^0 \end{bmatrix} \tag{9.26a}$$

$$\mathbf{P} = \begin{bmatrix} E_2 \cos \Phi & E_2 \sin \Phi & 0 \\ -E_2 \sin \Phi & E_2 \cos \Phi & 0 \\ 0 & 0 & E_1 \end{bmatrix} \tag{9.26b}$$

in which Φ is the clockwise precession angle (relative to the x'-axis) that the magnetization vector has accumulated in the interval after the nth pulse and before the $(n + 1)$th pulse.

Assume that the pulses are applied along the x'-axis. Then,

$$M_r^{(n+1)}(0_+) = \mathbf{R}_{x'}(\alpha) M_r^{(n+1)}(0_-) \tag{9.27}$$

Substituting Eq. (9.25) into Eq. (9.27) yields

$$M_r^{(n+1)}(0_+) = \mathbf{R}_{x'}(\alpha) \mathbf{P} M_r^{(n)}(0_+) + (1 - E_1) \mathbf{R}_{x'}(\alpha) M^0 \tag{9.28}$$

Similarly, one can derive

$$M_r^{(n+1)}(0_-) = \mathbf{P} \mathbf{R}_{x'}(\alpha) M_r^{(n)}(0_-) + (1 - E_1) M^0 \tag{9.29}$$

Setting

$$M_r^{(n+1)}(0_-) = M_r^{(n)}(0_+) = M_r^{ss}(0_-) \tag{9.30a}$$

$$M_r^{(n+1)}(0_+) = M_r^{(n)}(0_+) = M_r^{ss}(0_+) \tag{9.30b}$$

we immediately obtain the following governing equations for the steady-state magnetization:

$$M_r^{ss}(0_-) = \mathbf{P} \mathbf{R}_{x'}(\alpha) M_r^{ss}(0_+) + (1 - E_1) M^0 \tag{9.31a}$$

$$M_r^{ss}(0_+) = \mathbf{R}_{x'}(\alpha) \mathbf{P} M_r^{ss}(0_+) + (1 - E_1) \mathbf{R}_{x'}(\alpha) M^0 \tag{9.31b}$$

Solutions to Eq. (9.31) can be found to be

$$M_r^{ss}(0_-) = (1 - E_1) \left[\mathbf{I} - \mathbf{P} \mathbf{R}_{x'}(\alpha) \right]^{-1} M^0 \tag{9.32a}$$

$$M_r^{ss}(0_+) = (1 - E_1) \left[\mathbf{I} - \mathbf{R}_{x'}(\alpha) \mathbf{P} \right]^{-1} \mathbf{R}_{x'}(\alpha) M^0 \tag{9.32b}$$

where $\mathbf{I}$ is a 3×3 identity matrix. These solutions can be written more explicitly as

$$\begin{cases} M_{x'}(0_-) = M_z^0 (1 - E_1) E_2 \sin \alpha \sin \Phi / D \\ M_{y'}(0_-) = M_z^0 (1 - E_1)(E_2 \sin \alpha \cos \Phi - E_2^2 \sin \alpha)/D \\ M_{z'}(0_-) = M_z^0 (1 - E_1)[1 - E_2 \cos \Phi - E_2 \cos \alpha(\cos \Phi - E_2)]/D \end{cases} \tag{9.33}$$

and

$$
\begin{cases}
M_{x'}(0_+) = M_z^0(1 - E_1)E_2 \sin \alpha \sin \Phi/D \\
M_{y'}(0_+) = M_z^0(1 - E_1)(1 - E_2 \cos \Phi) \sin \alpha/D \\
M_{z'}(0_+) = M_z^0(1 - E_1)[E_2(E_2 - \cos \Phi) + (1 - E_2 \cos \Phi) \cos \Phi]/D
\end{cases}
$$

$$(9.34)$$

where

$$
D = (1 - E_1 \cos \alpha)(1 - E_2 \cos \Phi) - (E_1 - \cos \alpha)(E_2 - \cos \Phi)E_2 \quad (9.35)
$$

Equation (9.34) shows that the SSFP signal is a complicated function of α, E_1, E_2, and Φ. Ernst and Anderson [136] found that the optimal flip angle for producing the maximum transverse magnetization is given by

$$
\cos \alpha_{\mathrm{opt}} = \frac{E_1 + E_2(\cos \Phi - E_2)/(1 - E_2 \cos \Phi)}{1 + E_1 E_2(\cos \Phi - E_2)/(1 - E_2 \cos \Phi)} \quad (9.36)
$$

This expression can be obtained by differentiating $M_{y'}^{\mathrm{ss}}(0_+)$ with respect to α and setting the result to zero. In fact, it can be shown that

$$
\left.\frac{dM_{x'}^{\mathrm{ss}}(0_+)}{d\alpha}\right|_{\alpha=\alpha_{\mathrm{opt}}} = \left.\frac{dM_{y'}^{\mathrm{ss}}(0_+)}{d\alpha}\right|_{\alpha=\alpha_{\mathrm{opt}}} = \left.\frac{dM_{x'y'}^{\mathrm{ss}}(0_+)}{d\alpha}\right|_{\alpha=\alpha_{\mathrm{opt}}} = 0 \quad (9.37)
$$

A number of steady-state imaging methods have been proposed and found to have practical use. As an example, a two-dimensional FISP (Fast Imaging with Steady-state Precession) sequence (developed by Siemens Medical Systems, Inc.) is shown in Fig. 9.7. Compared with the FLASH sequence in Fig. 9.6, one can see that the imaging gradients in the FISP sequence are completely balanced so that the net effect of each imaging gradient is constant from one excitation cycle to the next. To understand the contrast behavior of this imaging scheme, we examine the special case of $\Phi = \pi$. This condition is achieved with alternating pulses (for example, pulses applied alternately along x'- and $-x'$-directions) and negligible field inhomogeneities. Under this condition, $M_{x'}(0_+) = 0$, and

$$
M_{x'y'}^{\mathrm{ss}}(0_+) = M_{y'}^{\mathrm{ss}}(0_+) = \frac{M_z^0(1 - E_1) \sin \alpha}{(1 - E_1 \cos \alpha) - E_2(E_1 - \cos \alpha)} \quad (9.38)
$$

For $T_R \ll T_2, T_1$, the following approximations can be invoked:

$$
E_1 \approx 1 - \frac{T_R}{T_1} \quad (9.39a)
$$

$$
E_2 \approx 1 - \frac{T_R}{T_2} \quad (9.39b)
$$

Consequently, Eq. (9.38) can be rewritten as

$$
M_{x'y'}^{\mathrm{ss}}(0_+) = \frac{M_z^0 \sin \alpha}{1 + T_1/T_2 - (T_1/T_2 - 1) \cos \alpha} \quad (9.40)
$$

For $\alpha = 90°$, Eq. (9.40) simplifies to

$$M^{ss}_{x'y'}(0_+) = M^0_z \frac{T_2}{T_1 + T_2} \qquad (9.41)$$

or further to

$$M^{ss}_{x'y'}(0_+) = M^0_z \frac{T_2}{T_1} \qquad (9.42)$$

noting that $T_1 \gg T_2$.

Equations (9.41) and (9.42) indicate that FISP images carry a T_2/T_1 contrast. Hence, FISP produces strong signals from tissues with long T_2 and short T_1. For $T_R \ll T_2$, the FISP signal is essentially independent of the T_R value. This implies that FISP can be run at a very short T_R without sacrificing SNR, a unique feature of steady-state imaging. For $T_1 > T_R \gg T_2$, FISP behavior approaches that of FLASH. This can be understood from the fact that $M^{ss}_{x'y'}(0_+)$ given in Eq. (9.34) will collapse to Eq. (9.14). There are many other implementations of steady-state imaging; the reader is referred to [73] for a comprehensive review.

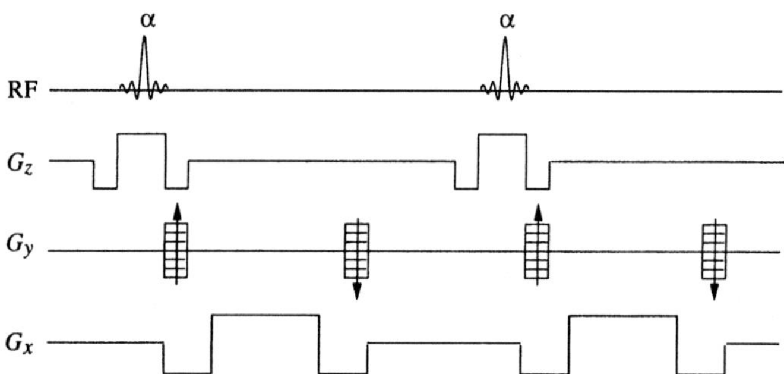

Figure 9.7 Two-dimensional FISP sequence. Note that all the gradients are balanced from cycle to cycle and the pulses are applied alternately along the x'- and $-x'$-directions.

9.3   Echo-Planar Imaging

Echo-planar imaging (EPI) is the first ultra high-speed imaging technique proposed by Mansfield in 1977 [197]. Since then, many of its variants have been proposed. Nowadays, the term is broadly used to refer to the class of high-speed imaging methods that collect a "complete" set of two-dimensional encodings during the free induction decay period following a single excitation pulse. Hence, echo-planar imaging has become a synonym for single-shot imaging, although multishot EPI methods with interlaced k-space coverage are also in common use.

A key concept of echo-planar imaging is the use of time-varying gradients to traverse k-space. In the ensuing discussion, we discuss three popular k-space trajectories: zigzag trajectory, rectilinear trajectory, and spiral trajectory.

9.3.1 Zigzag Trajectory

To understand how k-space is covered with a single excitation, consider first the original EPI method proposed by Mansfield [197], which is shown in Fig. 9.8. This imaging scheme involves the use of a pair of frequency-encoding gradients during the readout period: a small constant gradient and a rapidly alternating gradient. The alternating gradient generates a series of gradient echoes during the free precession period, thus making fast imaging possible.

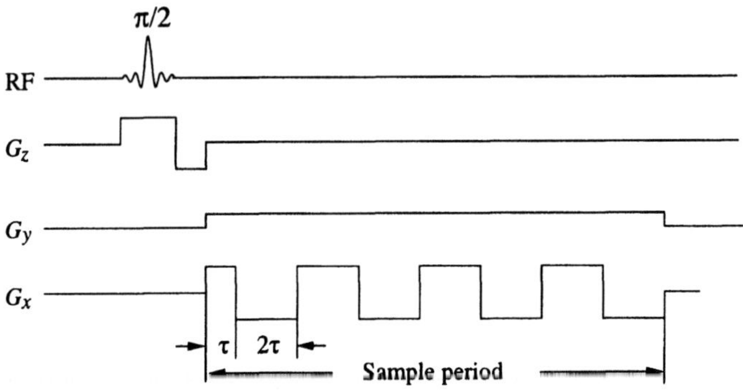

Figure 9.8 An EPI sequence that performs two-dimensional frequency-encoding by a constant gradient and an alternating gradient.

Recall that

$$k(t) = \gamma \int_0^t G(\tau)d\tau \tag{9.43}$$

it is easy to derive that

$$k_y(t) = \gamma G_y t \tag{9.44a}$$

$$k_x(t) = \begin{cases} \gamma G_x t, & 0 < t < \tau \\ \gamma G_x(2\tau - t) & \tau < t < 3\tau \\ \gamma G_x(t - 4\tau) & 3\tau < t < 5\tau \\ \quad \vdots \end{cases} \tag{9.44b}$$

Therefore, each gradient echo generated by this sequence is mapped to a tilted k-space line, resulting in a zigzag trajectory shown in Fig. 9.9. Note that the zigzag trajectory traverses only the top half of k-space. To get full k-space coverage, one needs to form a spin echo or a gradient echo. This can be done easily by applying a 180° pulse after the 90° excitation pulse or turning on a negative G_y gradient before data acquisition starts (see Problem 9.28).

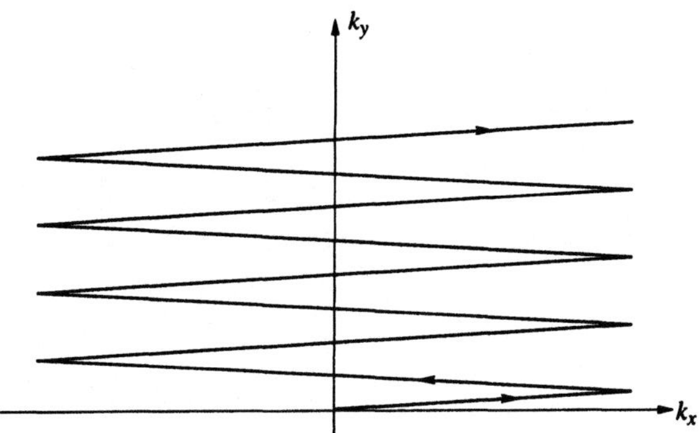

Figure 9.9   The zigzag k-space trajectory for the EPI pulse sequence given in Fig. 9.8.

A practical problem with the zigzag trajectory is that it requires special image reconstruction algorithms because k-space is sampled in a nonuniform fashion along the k_y-direction. One way to solve this image reconstruction problem is to use the interlaced sampling theory discussed in Section 5.4. More specifically, for a fixed k_x value, the signal variation along the k_y-axis can be represented by $S(k_y)$, which is sampled nonuniformly as shown in Fig. 9.10. Breaking the sampled points of $S(k_y)$ into two sequences, one containing the odd-indexed points and the other containing the even-indexed points, we have

$$S_o[n] = S(2n\Delta k_y) \tag{9.45}$$

and

$$S_e[n] = S(2n\Delta k_y + \delta) \tag{9.46}$$

In the ideal case of infinite sampling, the Fourier reconstructions from $S_o[n]$ and $S_e[n]$, according to Eq. (6.10), are given by

$$I_o(y) = \sum_n I\left(y - \frac{n}{2\Delta k_y}\right) \tag{9.47}$$

and

$$I_e(y) = \sum_n e^{in\pi\delta} I\left(y - \frac{n}{2\Delta k_y}\right) \tag{9.48}$$

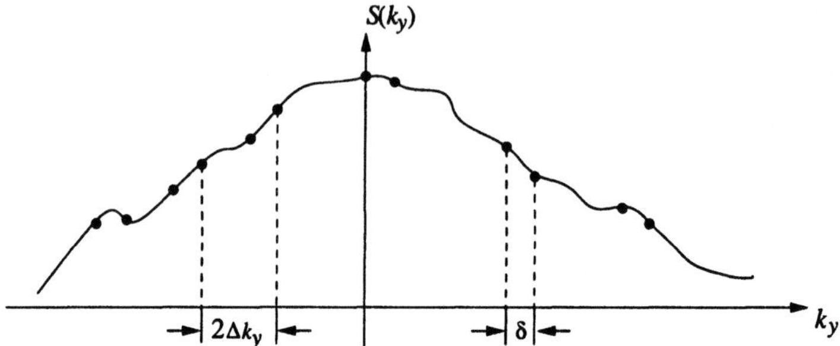

Figure 9.10   Sampling of the k-space signal along the k_y-direction for a fixed k_x value by a zigzag trajectory. Note that δ is a function of k_x.

Assume that Δk_y is chosen to be the critical Nyquist sampling interval, as is the case in practice. Then, $I_o(y)$ and $I_e(y)$ will be aliased versions of $I(y)$, as shown in Fig 9.11. However, this aliasing artifact can be removed by properly recombining $I_o(y)$ and $I_e(y)$.

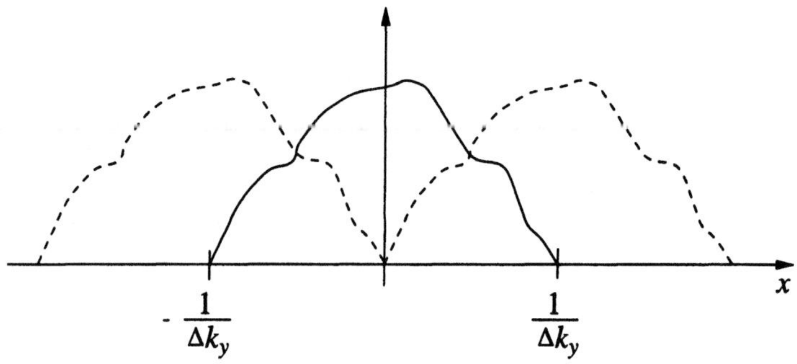

Figure 9.11   Fourier reconstruction from the odd-indexed or even-indexed data points of the sampled signal shown in Fig. 9.10.

Specifically, in the interval of $0 \le y \le 1/(2\Delta k_y)$, we have

$$I_o(y) \;=\; I(y) + I\left(y - \frac{1}{2\Delta k_y}\right) \tag{9.49a}$$

$$I_e(y) \;=\; I(y) + e^{i\pi\delta} I\left(y - \frac{1}{2\Delta k_y}\right) \tag{9.49b}$$

and in the interval of $-1/(2\Delta k_y) \leq y \leq 0$, we have

$$I_o(y) = I(y) + I\left(y + \frac{1}{2\Delta k_y}\right) \tag{9.50a}$$

$$I_e(y) = I(y) + e^{-i\pi\delta}I\left(y + \frac{1}{2\Delta k_y}\right) \tag{9.50b}$$

Simple algebraic manipulations yield

$$I(y) = \begin{cases} \dfrac{e^{i\pi\delta}}{e^{i\pi\delta} - 1}I_o(y) + \dfrac{1}{e^{i\pi\delta} - 1}I_e(y) & 0 \leq y \leq 1/(2\Delta k_y) \\[2ex] \dfrac{e^{-i\pi\delta}}{e^{-i\pi\delta} - 1}I_o(y) + \dfrac{1}{e^{-i\pi\delta} - 1}I_e(y) & -1/(2\Delta k_y) \leq y \leq 0 \end{cases} \tag{9.51}$$

In the practical case of finite sampling, $I_o(y)$ and $I_e(y)$ can be reconstructed using the conventional FFT reconstruction algorithm discussed in Chapter 6, which are then recombined together, according to Eq. (9.51), to give $I(y)$.

9.3.2 Rectilinear Trajectory

It is possible to provide orthogonal sampling of k-space using an EPI sequence. One such sequence, proposed by Pykett and Rzedzian in 1987 [227], is considered here. As shown in Fig. 9.12, this sequence phase-encodes individual gradient echoes using a series of blipped G_y pulses. Note that in contrast to conventional imaging, the phase-encoding gradient here has a constant amplitude and need not be stepped incrementally because the transverse magnetization accumulates phase dispersal imparted by each phase-encoding blip. This phase accumulation effect does not occur in conventional imaging since a fresh transverse magnetization is generated for each phase-encoding step.

An advantage of this data acquisition scheme over the zigzag scheme given in Fig. 9.8 is that it gives the usual rectilinear k-space trajectory; therefore, no special image reconstruction algorithm is required. However, since the entire sampling process needs to be completed on a time scale on the order of T_2^*, the phase-encoding blip needs to be applied very rapidly and with a sufficiently high amplitude to impart the required phase warp. Therefore, special gradient hardware is often needed to implement this pulse sequence.

Figure 9.13 illustrates the k-space trajectory of the EPI sequence with blipped phase-encoding gradients. Note that the gradients applied in the interval between the 90° and 180° pulses correspond to the progression from the k-space origin to the highest spatial frequency point. The ensuing 180° pulse then moves the transverse magnetization to the conjugate k-space position.

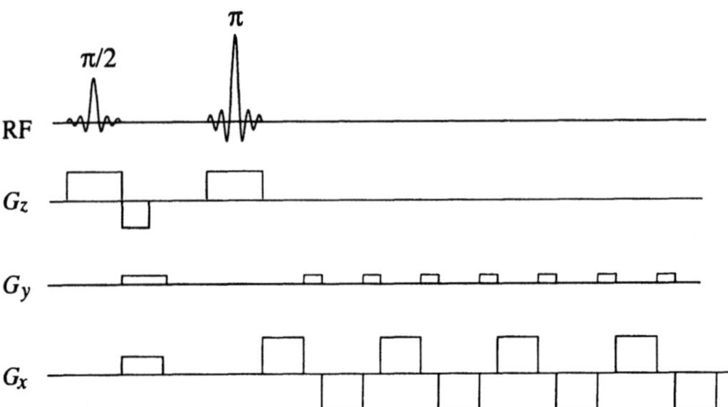

Figure 9.12 An EPI sequence with phase-encoding along the y-direction using blipped gradient pulses.

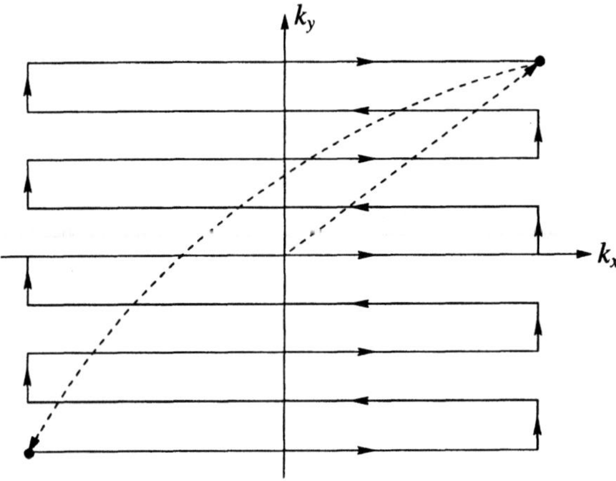

Figure 9.13 K-space trajectory for the EPI sequence given in Fig. 9.12.

9.3.3 Spiral Trajectory

A single-shot imaging method with much less demanding requirements on gradient hardware is shown in Fig. 9.14. This method uses a pair of increasing sinusoidal gradients to traverse k-space in a spiral fashion (Fig. 9.15); hence it is known as spiral imaging [85, 204]. This method completely eliminates rapid gradient switching required in the previous sequences.

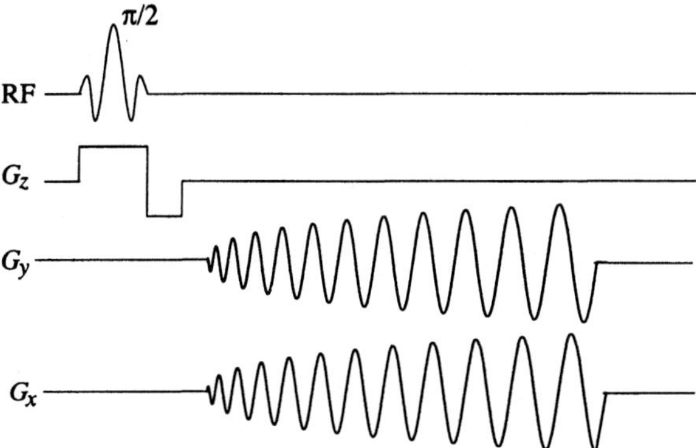

Figure 9.14 A spiral EPI sequence.

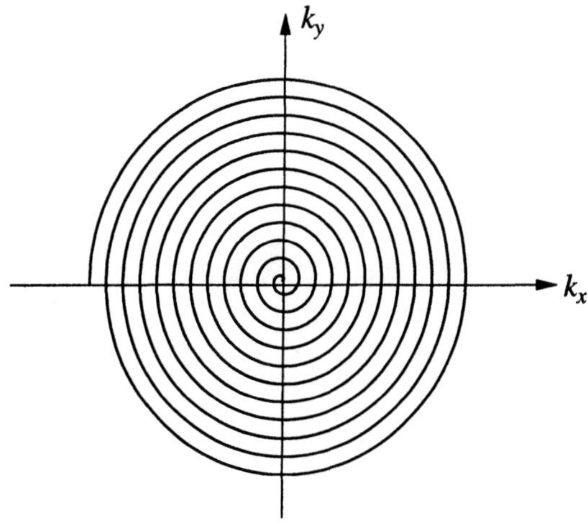

Figure 9.15 K-space trajectory of the spiral EPI sequence shown in Fig. 9.14.

A spiral trajectory in the (k_x, k_y)-plane is described by[1]

$$\mathbf{k}(t) = A\omega(t)e^{i\omega(t)} \tag{9.52}$$

where $\mathbf{k} \triangleq k_x + ik_y$, and $\omega(t)$ is some function of time. Selecting $\omega(t)$ is an

---

[1] For interlaced spiral imaging, the nth spiral is described by $\mathbf{k}(t) = A\omega(t)e^{i[\omega(t)+\varphi_0]}$, where $\varphi_0 = 2\pi(n-1)/N_i$ with N_i being the total number of interlaced spirals.

important step in spiral sequence design. One example of $\omega(t)$ is

$$\omega(t) = \omega_0 t \tag{9.53}$$

The corresponding k-space trajectory is described by

$$\mathbf{k}(t) = A\omega_0 t e^{i\omega_0 t} \tag{9.54}$$

or simply (because A is a parameter to be determined),

$$\mathbf{k}(t) = At e^{i\omega_0 t} \tag{9.55}$$

The required gradient function is given by

$$\mathbf{G}(t) = \frac{1}{\gamma}\frac{d}{dt}\mathbf{k}(t)$$
$$= Ae^{i\omega_0 t} + iAt\omega_0 e^{i\omega_0 t} \tag{9.56}$$

where $\mathbf{G}(t) \triangleq G_x + iG_y$. The corresponding x and y channel gradients are

$$G_x(t) = A\cos\omega_0 t - At\omega_0 \sin\omega_0 t \tag{9.57a}$$
$$G_y(t) = A\sin\omega_0 t + At\omega_0 \cos\omega_0 t \tag{9.57b}$$

The spiral path defined by this pair of gradients has a constant angular velocity, as is evident from Eq. (9.55). This means that more time is spent in the central region of k-space than in the outer region. In fact, the scanning velocity of this data acquisition scheme in the outer region of k-space may become too large to be practical because of limited gradient strength. This problem can be overcome with spiral trajectories of a constant linear velocity. One such trajectory is obtained by setting

$$\omega(t) = \omega_0\sqrt{t} \tag{9.58}$$

Correspondingly,

$$\mathbf{k}(t) = A\sqrt{t}\,e^{i\omega_0\sqrt{t}} \tag{9.59}$$

and

$$\mathbf{G}(t) = \frac{A}{2t}e^{i\omega_0\sqrt{t}} + \frac{A}{2}\omega_0 e^{i\omega_0\sqrt{t}} \tag{9.60}$$

At the outer region of k-space (for large values of T), we have

$$\mathbf{G}(t) \approx \frac{A}{2}\omega_0 e^{i\omega_0\sqrt{t}} \tag{9.61}$$

which means that the magnitude of $\mathbf{G}(t)$ becomes a constant.

One problem with this gradient function is that it has a pole at $t = 0$. Therefore, it is basically impossible to implement it in practice because of limited gradient strength and risetime. A more practical spiral trajectory is defined by

$$\mathbf{k}(t) = At\sqrt{1 + t/T}\,e^{i\omega_0 t\sqrt{1+t/T}} \tag{9.62}$$

where T is a time parameter to be determined such that $\mathbf{k}(t)$ has constant angular velocity for $t \ll T$ and a constant linear velocity for $t \gg T$.

Data acquired along a spiral trajectory entail special algorithms for image reconstruction. In practice, a data interpolation scheme [168, 212] is often applied to map the spiral data to a rectangular grid, after which the data are processed by the conventional Fourier reconstruction algorithm. The interpolation problem can be alleviated using a square spiral trajectory (see Problem 9.29) for which only one-dimensional interpolation is needed.

9.3.4   Discussion

With current gradient technology, EPI methods can acquire a two-dimensional image with scan times on the order of 50 ms. This capability overcomes a significant problem of image degradation due to physiological motion. In addition, the effective T_R in single-shot EPI methods is infinitely long, resulting in images characterized by true T_2 or T_2^* contrast.

Despite these advantages, EPI methods have several characteristic limitations. First, the maximum attainable resolution is limited by the T_2^* value. Specifically, the T_2^*-PSF can be written as

$$h(x) = \frac{\gamma G_x T_2^*}{-1 + i\gamma G_x T_2^* x} \tag{9.63}$$

Although this PSF may be negligible along the readout direction, it can result in significant blurring in the other direction because data acquisition takes place over a time span much bigger than T_2^*. In addition, EPI images can suffer from significant image artifacts due to off-resonance effects and gradient errors. More in-depth discussion of these topics can be found in [66, 70, 137].

9.4   Burst Imaging

Burst imaging is another class of ultra-fast imaging methods, which generate a series of RF echoes sufficient to form a two-dimensional image with a single shot of a string of RF pulses, called "burst" pulse [157] or DANTE (Delays Alternating with Nutations for Tailored Excitation) pulse [69, 193, 282]. Since burst imaging is not yet a mature imaging technique, this section presents only a brief discussion of the fundamental concepts without dwelling on the implementation details.

Consider the basic burst imaging sequence shown in Fig. 9.16. This sequence was coined DUFIS (DANTE Ultrafast Imaging Sequence) by Lowe and Wysong [193]. As can be seen, the burst pulse consists of a train of uniformly spaced, identical, low-flip-angle RF pulses. The burst pulse is applied in the presence of a constant gradient field. Following the burst pulse, a 180° pulse is applied

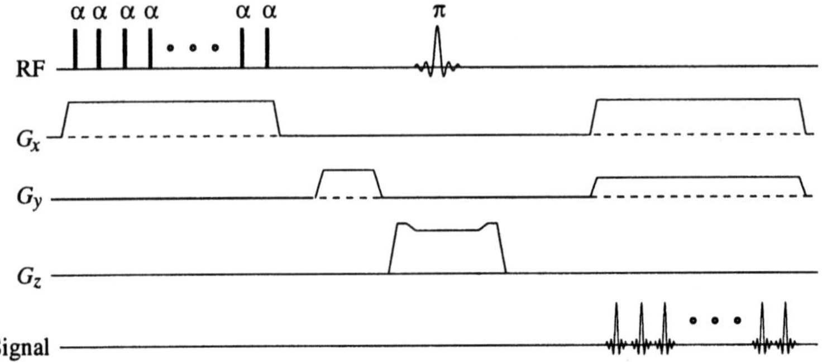

Figure 9.16 A burst imaging sequence. An echo train is formed after the slice-selective 180° pulse. Each echo is spatially encoded using two constant gradients.

to rephase the transverse magnetization. By making the 180° pulse frequency-selective, one can selectively refocus the transverse magnetization in a particular slice, thereby achieving slice selection.

To see how fast imaging is accomplished with this excitation scheme, we examine the signals generated by it. One may recall from Section 4.3.3 that n RF pulses applied to a spin system can generate up to $(3^{n-1} - 1)/2$ echoes after the last pulse. In the present case, the subpulses in a burst pulse are uniformly spaced; therefore, many of the signal pathways coincide, resulting in a much smaller set of echoes. To illustrate this point, a special case is analyzed using the extended phase diagram in Fig. 9.17, where the burst pulse contains six subpulses. As can be seen, five echoes form after the burst pulse and before the refocusing pulse. The same signal pathways generate another five echoes after the refocusing pulse. These echoes are called higher-order echoes because they result from interactions between two or more subpulses. In addition to these higher-order echoes, there are six primary echoes resulting from the interactions between the individual subpulse and the 180° refocusing pulse. By tracking the signal pathways, one can see that the first five primary echoes contain higher-order echoes except for the last one that is a pure primary echo. But, for convenience, we call them all primary echoes. Note in this example that fewer higher-order echoes will be formed if the 180° is moved closer to the burst pulse, but the length of the primary echo train stays the same. Because the higher-order echoes are much smaller in amplitude compared to the primary echoes and show significant variability among them [282], only the primary echoes are captured for imaging in this excitation scheme. Therefore, it is generally assumed that for a burst pulse with N_p subpulses, N_p echo signals are generated.

The signals generated by a burst pulse can be encoded in a number of ways. An example is shown in Fig. 9.16 where the echo signals are acquired in the presence of two constant gradients. The resulting k-space coverage is shown in

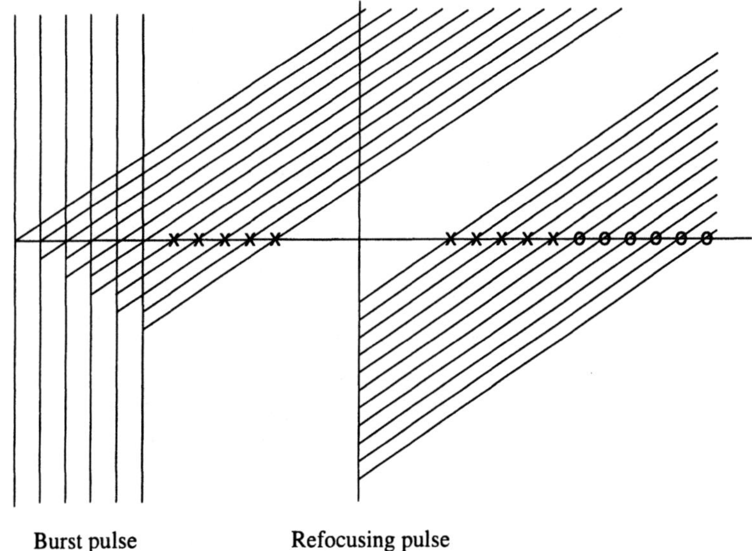

Burst pulse   Refocusing pulse

Figure 9.17 Extended phase graph for a burst imaging sequence with six subpulses and a 180° refocusing pulse. Note that five higher-order echoes (marked by "X") are formed after the burst pulse and before the refocusing pulse. The same signal pathways generate another five higher-order echoes after the refocusing pulse. In addition to these higher-order echoes, there are six primary echoes (marked by "o") resulting from the interactions between the individual subpulse and the 180° refocusing pulse. The longitudinal magnetization is not shown in the phase graph.

Fig. 9.18, which corresponds to the zigzag EPI trajectory in Fig. 9.9. One can justify that isotropic resolution can be achieved if

$$G_y\tau = G_x N_p \tau \tag{9.64}$$

where τ is the subpulse spacing of the burst pulse.

In contrast to the EPI methods, burst imaging does not require gradient switching, thereby eliminating the associated problems. In addition, burst imaging uses RF echoes, so it is less sensitive to field inhomogeneities. A major drawback of the burst imaging scheme shown in Fig. 9.16 is its poor signal-to-noise ratio. This can be understood from the nonuniform excitation profile of the burst pulse. As the burst pulse is essentially a DANTE pulse, its excitation profile can be analyzed approximately using the Fourier approach. As illustrated in Fig. 9.19, a burst pulse is highly frequency-selective. In the presence of a gradient, an object will be excited in spatial strips, leaving much of the magnetization unused. To alleviate this problem, burst pulses with phase or frequency modulation have been proposed. The reader is referred to [69] for a detailed discussion.

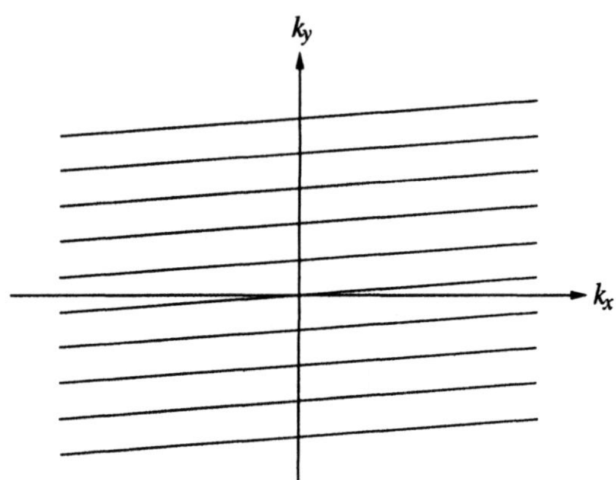

Figure 9.18 K-space coverage of the burst imaging sequence given in Fig. 9.16.

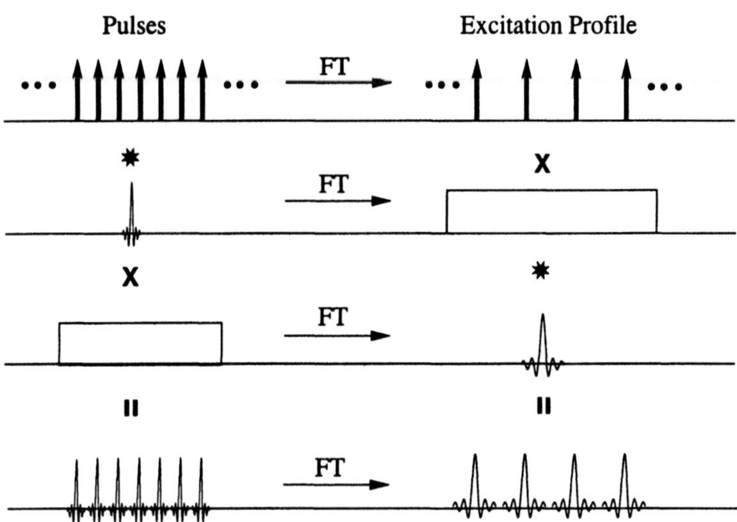

Figure 9.19 Excitation profiles of a train of uniformly spaced low-flip-angle pulses as predicted by the Fourier analysis.

Exercises

9.1   Assume that the echo train length is 16 in an FSE imaging sequence. How many k-space lines are collected per excitation pulse?

9.2   What is a rewinder gradient? Design an FSE imaging sequence without the use of phase rewinding.

9.3   Why is T_2-blurring along the phase-encoding direction much more serious in FSE imaging than in conventional SE imaging?

9.4   Discuss how the first three spin-echo signals generated by the following sequence are mapped to k-space:

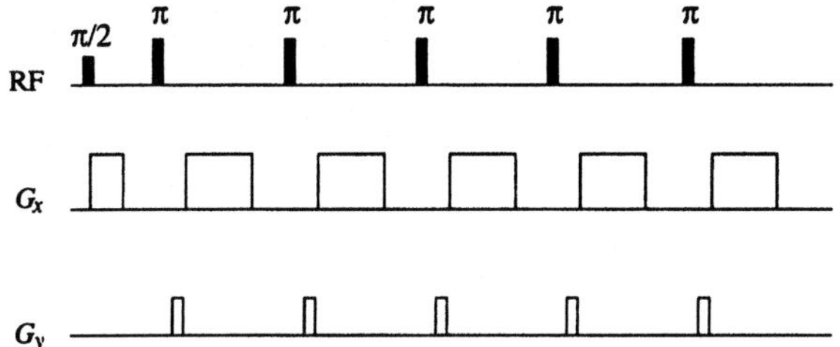

9.5   The following fast imaging sequence developed by GE researchers is known as GRASE (gradient and spin echo). Discuss how imaging speed improvement over the conventional SE imaging method is achieved using this scheme by highlighting its similarities to and differences from the standard FSE imaging method.

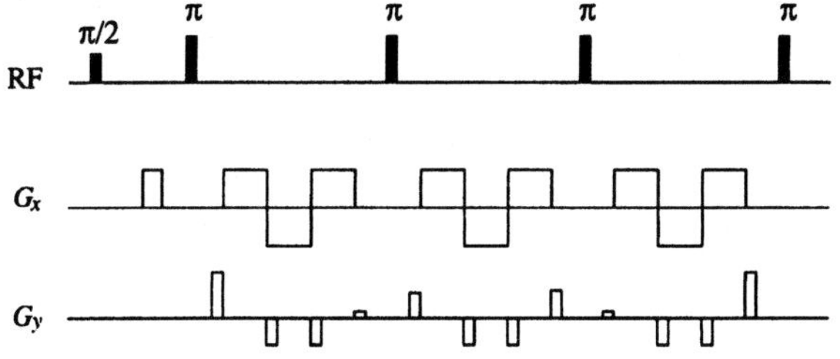

9.6   Sketch the resulting T_2-weighting function for the following phase-encoding ordering scheme for an FSE imaging sequence:

$$k_{mn} = \left[(m-1)N_{\text{ex}} + n - 1 - \frac{N_{\text{enc}}}{2} \right] \Delta k \qquad m = 1, 2 \cdots, N_{\text{ex}}$$

$$n = 1, 2, \cdots, M$$

9.7   Use numerical methods to calculate the PSFs of the T_2-weighting functions shown in Fig. 9.4.

9.8   Determine a phase-encoding ordering scheme for the FSE imaging sequence so that the k-space data carry the following T_2-weighting along the phase-encoding direction:

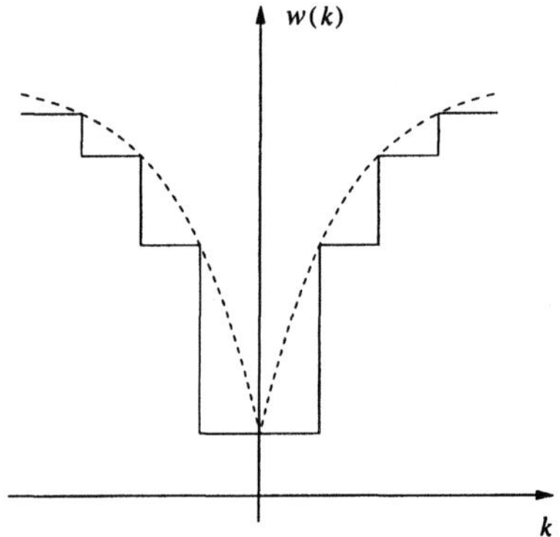

9.9   A spin system at thermal equilibrium is excited by the sequence shown in (a) to generate three spin echoes from a single slice along z. Design the x and y gradients so that the echo signals are mapped to the radial k-space trajectories shown in (b). (Be specific about the gradient functions!)

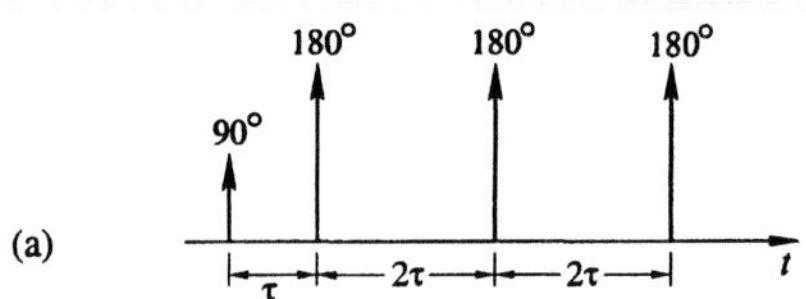

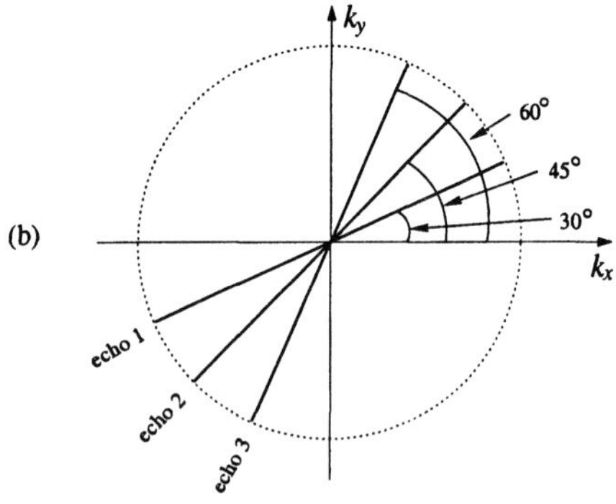

9.10 Derive the Ernst angle formula given in Eq. (9.16). For $T_R \ll T_1$, show that $\alpha_E \approx \sqrt{2T_R/T_1}$ and that $M_{x'y'}^{ss}(0_+) \approx \frac{1}{2} M_z^0 \alpha_E$.

9.11 Solve the difference equation in Eq. (9.19).

9.12 What is spoiling in fast gradient-echo imaging?

9.13 The T_1 values for cerebrospinal fluid, white matter, and gray matter are approximately 4500 ms, 600 ms, and 950 ms at 1.5 T. Assume $T_R = 40$ ms and $\alpha = \alpha_E$ in a spoiled steady-state experiment. How many pulses are needed for each tissue to drive $M_z^{(n)}(0_-)$ to within 10% of the steady-state value?

9.14 In the regime of short-T_R steady-state imaging, 90° pulses do not necessarily give the best SNR. Calculate $M_{x'y'}^{ss}(90°)/M_{x'y'}^{ss}(\alpha_E)$ for a spoiled steady-state imaging experiment with $T_R = 40$ ms and $T_1 = 600$ ms.

9.15 Discuss how to generate T_1-weighted, T_2^*-weighted, and spin-density-weighted contrast in FLASH imaging.

9.16 Explain why elimination of T_1-weighting requires a shorter T_R with FLASH than with conventional spin-echo imaging.

9.17 Explain why it is not suitable to form spin echoes in short-T_R imaging with small flip-angle excitations.

9.18 Discuss the similarities and differences between FLASH imaging and spin-echo imaging in creating T_1-weighted image contrast.

9.19 Prove the following identity:

$$\mathbf{I} - \mathbf{R}_{x'}(\alpha)\mathbf{P} = \begin{bmatrix} 1 - E_2 \cos \Phi & -E_2 \sin \Phi & 0 \\ E_2 \sin \Phi \cos \alpha & 1 - E_2 \cos \Phi \cos \alpha & -E_1 \sin \alpha \\ -E_2 \sin \Phi \sin \alpha & E_2 \cos \Phi \sin \alpha & 1 - E_1 \cos \alpha \end{bmatrix}$$

where $\mathbf{P}$ is defined in Section 9.2.2.

9.20 Prove the relation in Eq. (9.37).

9.21 Show that $M_{y'}(0_+)$ given in Eq. (9.34) becomes independent of the precession angle Φ for $\alpha = \alpha_E = \cos^{-1}(-T_R/T_1)$.

9.22 Show that similar to Eq. (9.38), we have for $\Phi = 0$

$$M_{x'y'}^{ss}(0_+) = M_{y'}^{ss}(0_+) = \frac{M_z^0(1 - E_1)\sin \alpha}{(1 - E_1 \cos \alpha) + E_2(E_1 - \cos \alpha)}$$

9.23 Derive the signal expression in Eq. (9.40) from Eq. (9.38).

9.24 Discuss why FISP becomes equivalent to FLASH when T_R is long compared to T_2.

9.25 Discuss why with FISP at $T_R \ll T_2$, it is better, in terms of SNR, to run two acquisitions at a shorter T_R than one acquisition with a longer T_R.

9.26 Show that for $\Phi = \pi$ and $T_R \ll T_2$, Eqs. (9.36) and (9.40) can be simplified to

$$\cos \alpha_{\text{opt}} \approx \frac{T_1 - T_2}{T_1 + T_2}$$

and

$$M_{x'y'}(0_+)\Big|_{\alpha=\alpha_{\text{opt}}} \approx \frac{1}{2} M_z^0 \sqrt{\frac{T_2}{T_1}}$$

9.27 Discuss the similarities and differences between spoiled steady-state imaging and true steady-state imaging.

9.28 Determine and sketch the k-space trajectory for the following EPI sequences.

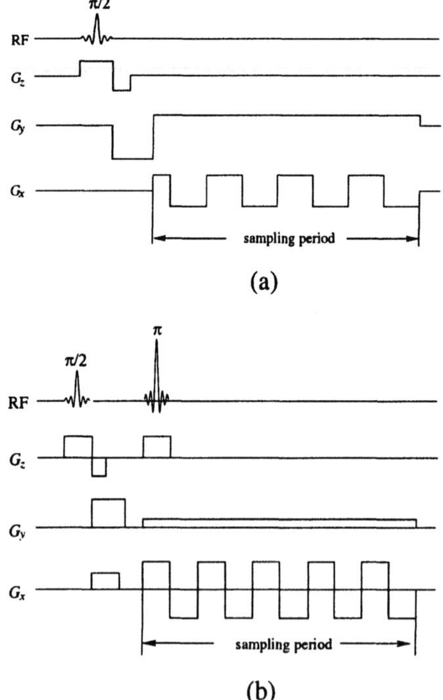

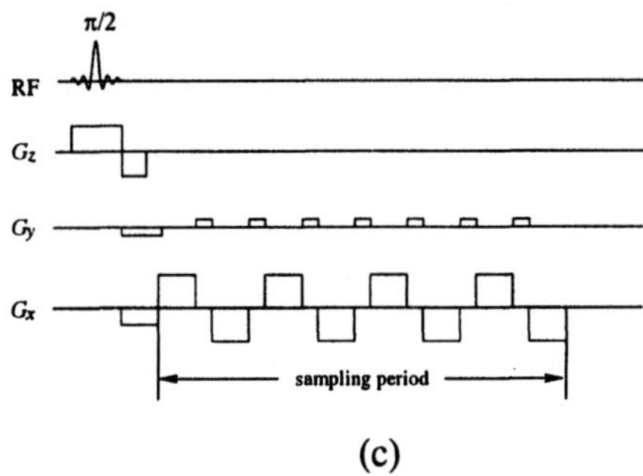

(c)

9.29 Design an EPI pulse sequence that gives the following square spiral k-space trajectory:

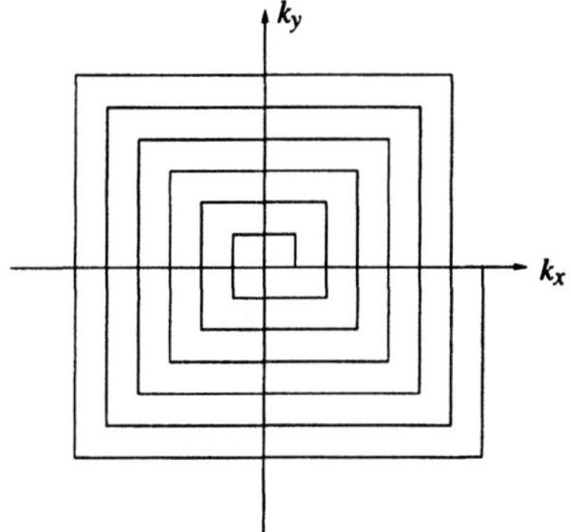

9.30 Interlaced spiral scans are often used to reduce the T_2-decay effect and gradient requirement limitations. Design a pulse sequence to give the following interlaced spiral trajectory:

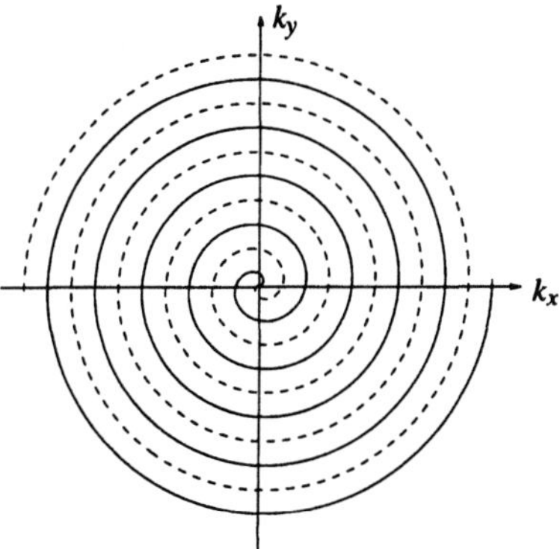

9.31 Justify that the following spiral trajectory has a constant angular velocity for $t \ll T$ and a constant linear velocity for $t \gg T$:

$$\mathbf{k}(t) = At\sqrt{1 + t/T}\, e^{i\omega_0 t \sqrt{1 + t/T}}$$

9.32 A rosette k-space trajectory is given by

$$\mathbf{k}(t) = k_{\max} \sin \omega_1 t\, e^{i\omega_2 t}$$

Derive the necessary gradient function and sketch the trajectory for $\omega_1/2\pi = 150$ Hz and $\omega_2 = 17$ Hz for $0 < t < 17$ ms.

9.33 Discuss the difference of T_2^*-weighting on k-space data between a zigzag trajectory and a spiral trajectory.

9.34 Assume that the spiral trajectory given in Eq. (9.55) reaches the maximum point $|\mathbf{k}(T_{\mathrm{acq}})| = k_{\max}$ at $t = T_{\mathrm{acq}}$. Determine A and the smallest ω_0 allowable by the Nyquist criterion for an object of radius R.

9.35 Modify the burst imaging sequence given in Fig. 9.16 so that the echoes are mapped to rectilinear lines in k-space.

9.36 For the burst imaging sequence given below, (a) discuss how slice selection is accomplished, (b) use the extended phase graph to predict the occurrence of the echo signals, and (c) sketch the k-space coverage.

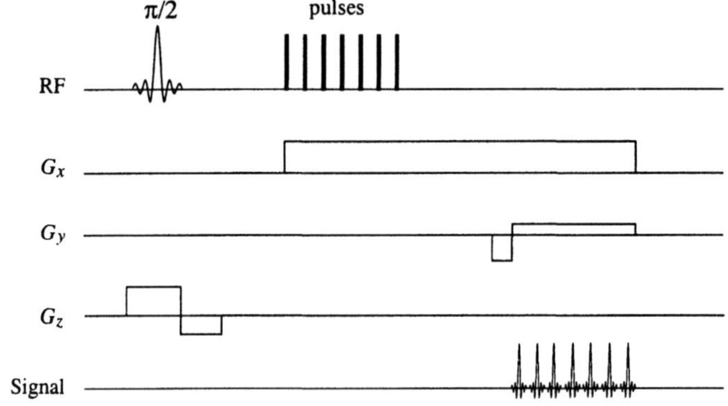

Chapter 10

Constrained Reconstruction

Everything should be made as simple as possible, but not simpler.

Albert Einstein

While the fast-scan methods discussed in Chapter 9 are widely used for high-speed imaging, reduced-scan approaches can further enhance imaging speed because imaging time is directly proportional to the number of encodings measured. In fact, reduced-scan is a popular way to shorten data acquisition time in conventional spin-echo imaging experiments. There are two main problems with reduced-scan imaging: (a) loss of spatial resolution and (b) image artifacts (most notably, spurious Gibbs ringing). To alleviate these problems, various methods have been proposed to utilize a priori information to compensate for the lack of sufficient measured data. In principle, the "best" reconstruction should result from incorporating the maximum amount of prior knowledge into the reconstruction process. However, if not used properly, a priori constraints may produce biased or even artifacted reconstructions. Therefore, an important goal of constrained reconstruction is to use the maximum amount of a priori information in an unbiased fashion. Although constrained reconstruction is still a relatively new area in MRI, a comprehensive review of the existing methods is beyond the scope of this chapter. The interested reader is referred to [80] for an in-depth review of methods developed before 1991. Some of the more recent methods are discussed in [109, 110, 111, 112, 113, 114, 181, 171, 265, 279, 287].

10.1   Half-Fourier Reconstruction

Recall that for a real-valued function $I(x)$, its frequency representation $S(k)$ is redundant. Specifically, if $S(k)$ is known for $k \geq 0$, then $S(-k)$ can be generated based on the Hermitian symmetry

$$S(-k) = S^*(k) \tag{10.1}$$

This simple fact has motivated the development of imaging methods that collect data from only half of k-space, thus the popular name *half-Fourier imaging*. In practice, however, the realness constraint is often violated because object motion and magnetic field inhomogeneities introduce a nonzero phase $\varphi(x)$ to the image function. Consequently, image artifacts arise when the phase term is not properly treated. The usual approach to cope with this problem is to collect a few additional encodings across the center of k-space, as illustrated in Fig. 10.1. In this way, the image phase $\varphi(x)$ can be estimated from the central symmetric k-space data.

According to the data acquisition scheme shown in Fig. 10.1, the half-Fourier reconstruction problem can be formally stated as follows:

$$\text{Given} \qquad S[n] = \int_{-\infty}^{\infty} I(x)e^{-i2\pi n\Delta k x}\,dx, \qquad -n_0 \leq n < N \tag{10.2}$$

$$\text{determine} \qquad I(x)$$

where it is assumed that n_0 is much smaller than N, typically, $n_0 = 16$ or 32. Most existing half-Fourier reconstruction methods follow a characteristic two-step procedure. The first estimates a phase function, and the second combines the

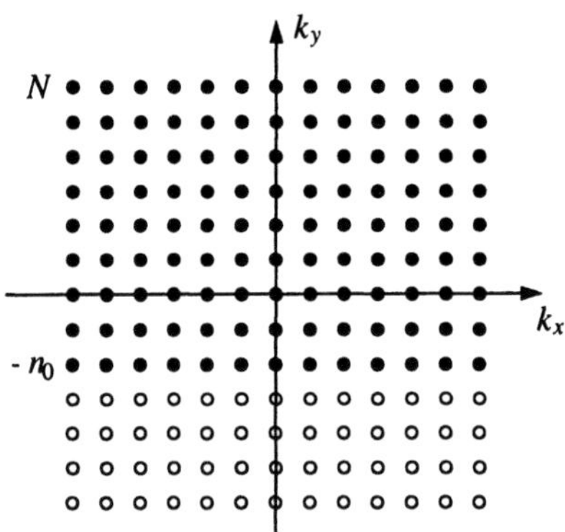

Figure 10.1 Asymmetric k-space sampling: $\bullet$ marks the locations of measured data and $\circ$ marks the locations of missing data in the conventional symmetric k-space coverage.

phase function and the measured data to get the final reconstruction. These two steps are discussed next.

10.1.1 Phase Estimation

A common approach to phase estimation is to first reconstruct a low-resolution image based on the central symmetric data and then extract the phase image from it. More specifically, let

$$\hat{I}(x) = \sum_{n=-n_0}^{n_0-1} \hat{S}[n]e^{-i2\pi n\Delta kx} \tag{10.3}$$

where $\hat{S}[n]$ represents the Hamming-filtered data, given by

$$\hat{S}[n] = S[n]\left[0.54 + 0.46\cos\left(\frac{n\pi}{n_0}\right)\right], \qquad -n_0 \le n < n_0 \tag{10.4}$$

Then, the phase estimate can be expressed as

$$\hat{\varphi}(x) = \angle\hat{I}(x) \tag{10.5}$$

10.1.2 Phase-Constrained Reconstruction

After $\hat{\varphi}(x)$ is available, the next step is to find an image function $\hat{I}(x)$ that satisfies both the measured data $S[n]$ and the phase constraint $\hat{\varphi}(x)$. Two types of methods have been used to solve this phase-constrained reconstruction problem. The first type, due mainly to Margosian, Schmitt, and Purdy [198] and Noll and Macovski [211], solves the problem using a one-step phase-compensation algorithm; the other type, originated from Cuppen and Van Est [128], solves the problem by iteratively regenerating the missing data. This section focuses on these basic two methods, although various variants of them also exist.

10.1.2.1 The Margosian Method

Consider a half echo $S_h(k) = S(k)u(k)$. In the continuous case, the Fourier reconstruction from $S_h(k)$ is related to the true image function $I(x)$ by the following formula:

$$I_h(x) = \mathcal{F}^{-1}\{S_h(k)\}$$

$$= I(x) * \left[\frac{1}{2}\delta(x) + i\frac{1}{2\pi x}\right]$$

$$= \frac{1}{2}|I(x)|e^{i\varphi(x)} + \left[|I(x)|e^{i\varphi(x)}\right] * \frac{i}{2\pi x} \tag{10.6}$$

If $\varphi(x)$ is a slowly varying function, the phase term $e^{i\varphi(x)}$ can be pulled outside the convolution in the second term of the above equation. That is,

$$\left[|I(x)|e^{i\varphi(x)}\right] * \frac{i}{2\pi x} \approx \left[|I(x)| * \frac{i}{2\pi x}\right] e^{i\varphi(x)} \tag{10.7}$$

With the above approximation, Eq. (10.6) reduces to

$$I_h(x) = \left[\frac{1}{2}|I(x)| + i|I(x)| * \frac{1}{2\pi x}\right] e^{i\varphi(x)} \tag{10.8}$$

Multiplying $I_h(x)$ with $e^{-i\hat{\varphi}(x)}$, which is known as the phase-compensation step, yields

$$I_h(x)e^{-i\hat{\varphi}(x)} = \left[\frac{1}{2}|I(x)| + i|I(x)| * \frac{1}{2\pi x}\right] e^{i[\varphi(x)-\hat{\varphi}(x)]} \tag{10.9}$$

If we further assume

$$\hat{\varphi}(x) \approx \varphi(x) \tag{10.10}$$

the following formula immediately results from Eq. (10.9):

$$I_h(x)e^{-i\hat{\varphi}(x)} \approx \frac{1}{2}|I(x)| + i\left[|I(x)| * \frac{1}{2\pi x}\right] \tag{10.11}$$

Inspection of Eq. (10.11) shows that the first term is the real part of the phase-compensated half-echo reconstruction, while the second term is its imaginary part. Therefore, $|I(x)|$ can be easily extracted from the phase-compensated half-echo reconstruction as follows:

$$|I(x)| \approx 2\Re\left[I_h(x)e^{-i\hat{\varphi}(x)}\right] \tag{10.12}$$

where $\Re$ denotes taking the real part of a complex number. The full complex image function can be expressed as

$$\hat{I}(x) = 2\Re\left[I_h(x)e^{-i\hat{\varphi}(x)}\right] e^{i\hat{\varphi}(x)} \tag{10.13}$$

If the magnitude image is desired as the final reconstruction, it can be obtained directly from Eq. (10.12). Alternatively, the complex image can be obtained from Eq. (10.13), from which the real part can be readily extracted as the final reconstruction if so desired.

Equations (10.12) and (10.13), though derived from continuous data, form the theoretical basis of the half-Fourier reconstruction method proposed by Margosian et al. [198] and Noll and Macovski [211]. With practical discrete data, the half-echo reconstruction $I_h(x)$ is obtained using the FFT. Instead of applying the FFT to the half echo, however, it is suggested [198, 211] that the entire asymmetric data set is used so that precise knowledge of the k-space center for the measured data is not necessary. Specifically, the asymmetric data set is first zero-filled to $-N$, and the central $2n_0$ data points are weighted with a ramp or asymmetric Hamming function as shown in Fig. 10.2. Then, the FFT is applied to this zero-padded, filtered data set to get $I_h(x)$. The purpose of the weighting function is twofold: (a) to roll off the sharp transition between the padded zeros and the measured data, and (b) to counter the imbalance between the low- and high-frequency data because of the lack of negative high-frequency data. A more detailed discussion of this topic can be found at [211].

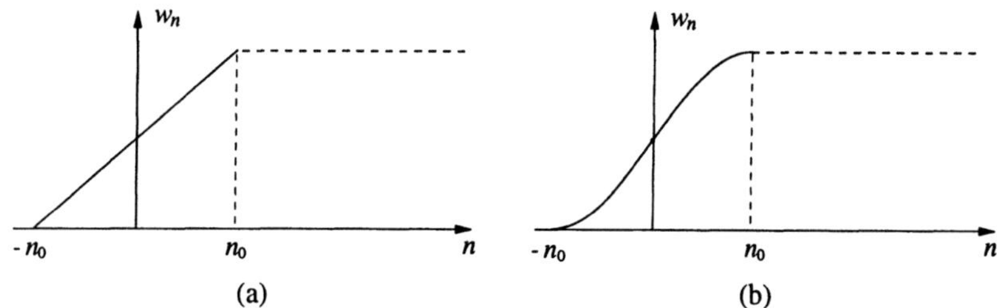

Figure 10.2   Weighting functions for half-Fourier reconstruction with the Margosian method: (a) a ramp function and (b) an asymmetric Hamming function defined as $w_n = 0.5 + 0.5 \cos[\pi(n - n_0)/(2n_0)]$, $-n_0 \leq n < n_0$.

10.1.2.2   The POCS Method

Projection onto convex sets (POCS) is a popular mathematical algorithm for solving a class of optimization problems, in which each constraint can be formulated as a convex set. Before describing how this algorithm is useful for half-Fourier reconstruction, let us first define what a convex set is.

Definition 10.1 *A set Ω is said to be convex if $x_1 \in \Omega$ and $x_2 \in \Omega$ implies that $\lambda x_1 + (1 - \lambda)x_2 \in \Omega$ for all x_1, x_2, and λ, $0 \leq \lambda \leq 1$.*

Based on the above definition, it is easy to show that the two constraints in half-Fourier reconstruction can be formulated as two convex sets:

(a) The phase-constraint:

$$\Omega_1 = \left\{ I(x) | \angle I(x) = \hat{\varphi}(x) \right\} \tag{10.14}$$

(b) The data-consistency constraint:

$$\Omega_2 = \left\{ I(x) | \mathcal{F}\{I(x)\} = S[n], -n_0 \leq n \leq N - 1 \right\} \tag{10.15}$$

Clearly, Ω_1 contains all the images satisfying the predetermined phase constraint, while Ω_2 contains all the images consistent with the measured data. The phase-constrained reconstruction problem can then be posed as finding an image function $I(x)$ in the intersection of Ω_1 and Ω_2. That is,

$$I(x) \in \Omega = \Omega_1 \cap \Omega_2 \tag{10.16}$$

When Ω is not empty (i.e., the phase constraints are not poorly chosen), $I(x)$ exists and can be found by alternating projections of an initial estimate onto these two sets.

Consider the following two operators

$$\wp_1\{I(x)\} = |I(x)|e^{i\hat{\varphi}(x)} \tag{10.17}$$

and

$$\wp_2\{I(x)\} = \mathcal{F}^{-1}\mathcal{R}\mathcal{F}\{I(x)\} \tag{10.18}$$

where $\mathcal{R}$ is a data replacement operator defined as

$$\mathcal{R}\{\hat{S}[n]\} = \begin{cases} S[n] & -n_0 \le n \le N-1 \\ \hat{S}[n] & \text{otherwise} \end{cases} \tag{10.19}$$

It is apparent that $\wp_1$ projects any image function $I(x)$ onto Ω_1, whereas $\wp_1$ projects it onto Ω_2. With $\wp_1$ and $\wp_2$, we can now succinctly express the POCS half-Fourier reconstruction algorithm as

$$I_{m+1}(x) = \wp_1\wp_2\{I_m(x)\} \tag{10.20}$$

or in a relaxed form

$$I_{m+1}(x) = (1-\lambda)I_m(x) + \lambda\wp_1\wp_2\{I_m(x)\} \tag{10.21}$$

where $0 < \lambda < 1$. The initial condition $I_0(x)$ for the above iterative equations is usually chosen to be the zero-filled Fourier reconstruction.

Note that $\wp_1$ and $\wp_2$ defined in Eqs. (10.17) and (10.17) are nonexpansive operators. Namely,

$$\|\wp_1\{I_1(x)\} - \wp_1\{I_2(x)\}\|_2 \le \|I_1(x)\} - I_2(x)\|_2 \tag{10.22}$$

and

$$\|\wp_2\{I_1(x)\} - \wp_2\{I_2(x)\}\|_2 \le \|I_1(x)\} - I_2(x)\|_2 \tag{10.23}$$

Consequently, the composite operator $\wp_1\wp_2$ is also nonexpansive. Convergence properties of iterative equations involving nonexpansive operators have been well analyzed in the literature; the interested reader may consult [255] for an in-depth discussion. Experimental studies of this algorithm have also been conducted [80], which indicate that Eq. (10.20) converges quickly, and four iterations appear to be sufficient in many practical situations.

10.1.3   Discussion

Asymmetric sampling of k-space is often used along the phase-encoding direction to reduce imaging time. It also occurs naturally in the frequency-encoding direction in gradient-echo imaging when a short echo time is used to avoid spin dephasing due to short T_2^* caused by local susceptibility changes or uncompensated motion effects. The source of data sampling asymmetry in sequences of this type can be due to gradient design or it can occur when field inhomogeneities shift the echo away from the expected echo time [149].

A noticeable limitation of half-Fourier imaging is the loss of image SNR. Specifically, as compared to symmetrical k-space sampling with the same number of encodings, a factor of 2 loss in SNR is expected,[1] but this loss is usually well compensated for by an improved contrast-to-noise in many applications, such as angiographic imaging [55].

In general, the quality of half-Fourier reconstruction is dependent on the phase constraint $\hat{\varphi}(x)$. If $\hat{\varphi}(x) = \varphi(x)$, the half-Fourier image can be as good as would be obtained from a symmetric data set. However, when the phase estimate is poor, image artifacts may result. This is particularly the case with the Margosian method because it is sensitive to both phase errors and large phase variations. Specifically, from Eq. (10.9), we have

$$2\Re\left[I_h(x)e^{-i\hat{\varphi}(x)}\right] \approx \cos[\varphi(x) - \hat{\varphi}(x)]|I(x)| \qquad (10.24)$$

The cosine modulation can be significant in regions where large phase errors exist. Additionally, when the true image has large phase variations, as is often the case with gradient-echo imaging, the Margosian method cannot guarantee the correct reconstruction even if $\hat{\varphi}(x) = \varphi(x)$. This is because the real part of the second term in Eq. (10.9) is significant when $\varphi(x)$ is not small. This term can contribute image artifacts in the form of geometric distortions [80]. The POCS method is less sensitive to phase errors and can produce "perfect" reconstruction if the phase constraint is accurate.

Figure 10.3 shows the magnitude and phase images from a phantom data set acquired using a gradient-echo sequence. The imaging parameters were $T_R = 45$ ms and $T_E = 12$ ms and the matrix size of the k-space data set was 256×256. By truncating this data set to 128 asymmetric points along the vertical direction, four half-Fourier reconstructions were obtained using the Margosian and POCS methods, respectively, as shown in Fig. 10.4. As can be seen, the images in Figs. 10.4a and 10.4b contain noticeable artifacts. These artifacts arose because the phase function $\hat{\varphi}(x)$, estimated from 16 data points in the central part of k-space, was a poor constraint for both the Margosian and POCS methods.

---

[1] Half-Fourier imaging with N encodings suffers a factor of $\sqrt{2}$ loss in SNR as compared to symmetrical k-space sampling with $2N$ encodings but a factor of 2 loss as compared to symmetrical k-space sampling with N encodings.

When the phase constraint was estimated from 64 central k-space data points, the half-Fourier images shown in Fig. 10.4c and 10.4d improved considerably, as expected. In practice, a simple way to improve the phase estimate is to use a large n_0. This, however, will reduce the number of high-frequency encodings available if the total number of encodings is fixed, thus sacrificing the spatial resolution of the final image. It should also be noted that image artifacts in half-Fourier reconstructions manifest themselves differently for different reconstruction methods. As can be seen from Fig. 10.4, phase errors result in geometric distortions and a "shadowing artifact" in the Margosian reconstruction, but they are in the form of spurious ringing in the POCS images.

Figure 10.5 shows the results from another experimental data set obtained from a sagittal head slice using a gradient-echo sequence with $T_E = 10$ ms and $T_R = 200$ ms. This data set has rapid phase changes and is a good test of the practical utility of half-Fourier imaging methods. For comparison, Figs. 10.5a and 10.5b show the reconstruction results from symmetric k-space data of 256 and 128 points, respectively. The images in Figs. 10.5c and 10.5d were reconstructed from 128 asymmetric data points ($-32 \leq n < 96$) using the Margosian and POCS methods, respectively. As can be seen, both half-Fourier images have better resolution than the Fourier image with an equal number of encodings in Fig. 10.5b. Although the Margosian reconstruction suffers from serious phase errors in the form of signal cancellation (signal voids) in regions near the pituitary gland, mouth cavity, and spinal cord, where large phase variations exist, the POCS method overcomes this problem effectively.

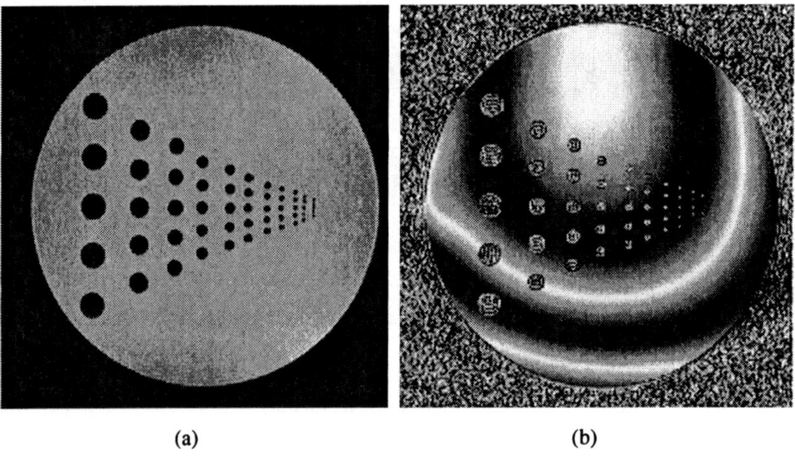

(a)   (b)

Figure 10.3 Magnitude and phase images of a phantom acquired using a gradient-echo sequence. The imaging parameters were $T_R = 45$ ms and $T_E = 12$ ms.

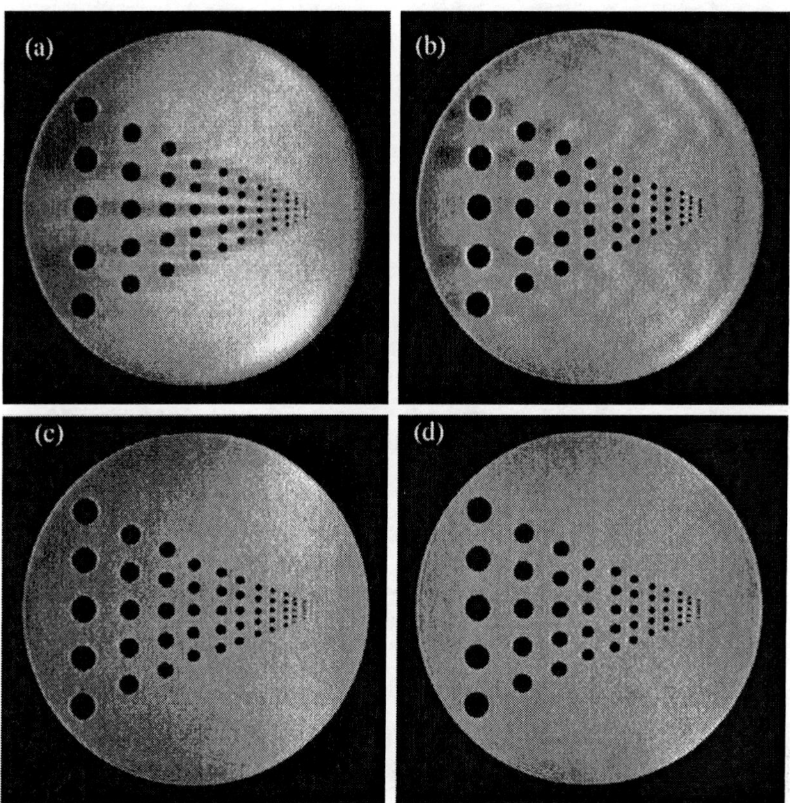

Figure 10.4 Half-Fourier images reconstructed from the phantom data set in Fig. 10.3. The horizontal direction was reconstructed from 256 symmetric echo data points, while the vertical direction was reconstructed using 128 asymmetric points. Specifically, $-8 \leq n < 112$ for (a) and (b), and $-32 \leq n < 96$ for (c) and (d). Images in (c) and (e) were reconstructed using the Margosian method, and images in (d) and (f) were reconstructed by the POCS method.

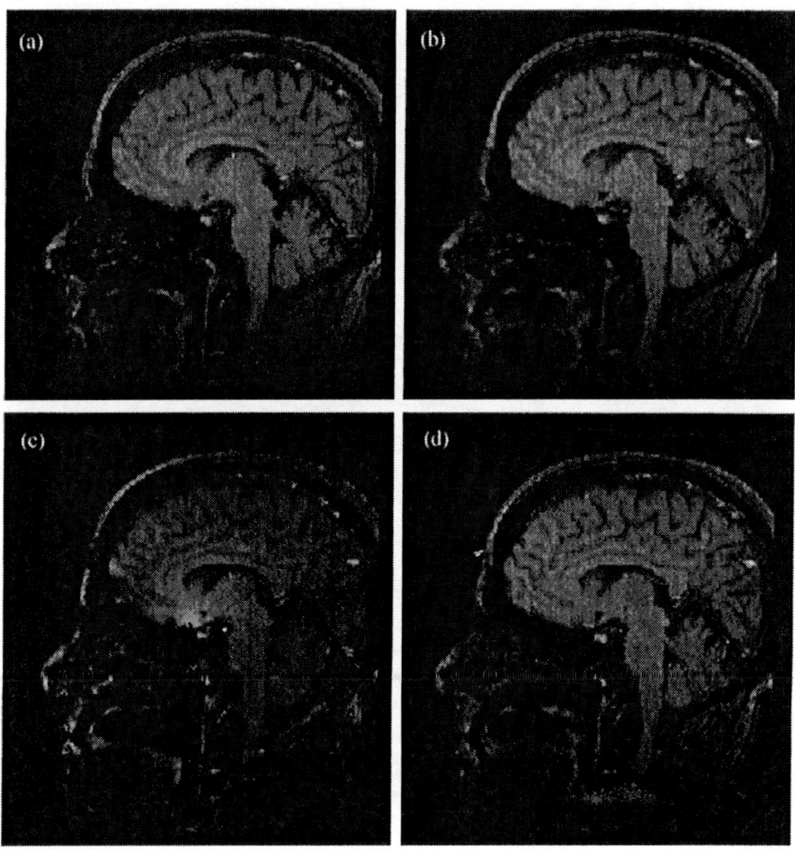

Figure 10.5 Reconstructions of a sagittal head slice. The vertical direction of all images was reconstructed using the Fourier method from full echoes of 256 data points. The horizontal direction was reconstructed using different methods. Images (a) and (b) were reconstructed from 256 and 128 symmetric data points, respectively, while images (c) and (d) were reconstructed from 128 asymmetric data points ($-32 \leq n < 96$) using the Margosian and POCS methods. Notice the phase artifacts in (c) and the resolution improvement of image (d) over image (b).

10.2   **Extrapolation-Based Reconstruction**

This section discusses two extrapolation-based methods for the classical problem of image reconstruction from a limited number of Fourier transform samples. For convenience, we limit our discussion to the one-dimensional case, in which the problem can be formally stated as follows:

$$\text{Given} \quad S[n] = \int_{-\infty}^{\infty} I(x)e^{-i2\pi n\Delta kx}dx, \quad -N/2 \leq n < N/2 \quad (10.25)$$

$$\text{determine} \quad I(x)$$

where N is assumed to be small (say, 64). Because N is small, direct application of the conventional Fourier reconstruction method is not desirable due to the reasons discussed in Chapter 8. An important goal of data extrapolation is to use a priori constraints to recover (explicitly or implicitly) some of the unmeasured high-frequency components so that $S[n]$ is defined for a bigger frequency range, as illustrated in Fig. 10.6. In this chapter, we denote the extrapolated frequency index range by $-\hat{N}/2 \leq n < \hat{N}/2$ where $\hat{N} > N$. With an extrapolated data set, an image function is often reconstructed using the conventional Fourier method as follows:

$$I(x) = \Delta k \sum_{n=-\hat{N}/2}^{\hat{N}/2-1} S[n]e^{-i2\pi n\Delta kx} \tag{10.26}$$

In the ensuing discussion of this section, we will examine the use of two popular constraints: the finite spatial support constraint and the maximum entropy constraint.

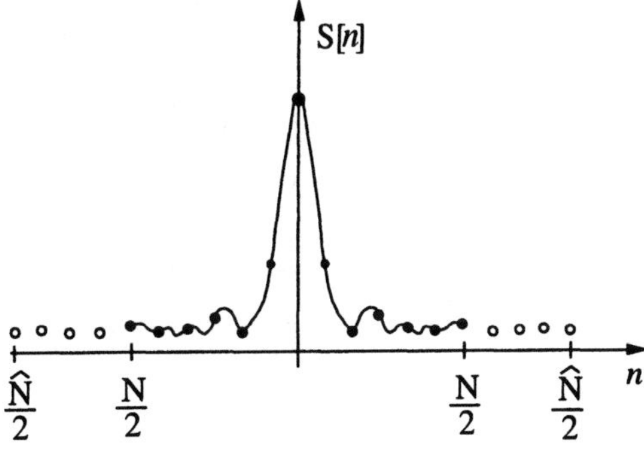

Figure 10.6   Extrapolation of a data set from N to $\hat{N}$ points.

10.2.1   Bandlimited Extrapolation

Recall that $I(x)$ is called a (spatially) bandlimited function if $I(x) = 0$ for $|x| > W_x/2$, where W_x is a finite number. This constraint can be explicitly used for data extrapolation, thus the name *bandlimited extrapolation*. The effectiveness of the bandlimitedness constraint is best understood by considering the continuous case (often known as analytical continuation). Let $S(k)$ be the Fourier transform of $I(x)$. Then, $S(k)$ is analytic over the entire real axis (see Section 2.5) and can be represented by, for example, the Taylor series. Specifically, assume that $S(k)$ is known for a finite interval $[k_0 - \delta, k_0 + \delta]$. Then

$$S(k) = S(k_0) + \sum_{n=0}^{\infty} \frac{S^{(n)}(k_0)}{n!}(k - k_0)^n \tag{10.27}$$

can be defined based on the known data. This expression is valid for all values of k because $S(k)$ is an analytic function. In other words, we have recovered the entire $S(k)$ from only a finite segment of it! Based on this property, several celebrated continuous extrapolation algorithms have been developed, most notably the method using the prolate spheroidal wave functions by Slepian and Pollack [244] and the iterative algorithm by Gerchberg [140] and Papoulis and Bertran [217]. In the case of discrete data, the analytic property of $S(k)$ becomes meaningless. Nonetheless, the bandlimitedness constraint is still useful for regenerating part of the missing data [169, 236, 237, 238]. We briefly describe the discrete extrapolation algorithm here because it is relevant to MRI.

Assuming that $I(x)$ is a bandlimited function, we can express it as

$$I(x) = \Pi\left(\frac{x}{W_x}\right) \sum_{m=-\infty}^{\infty} c_m e^{i2\pi m \Delta k x} \tag{10.28}$$

where $(-W_x/2, W_x/2)$ is called the spatial support region of $I(x)$. The series coefficients c_m in Eq. (10.28) are related to the measured data $S[n]$ by

$$S[n] = \sum_{m=-\infty}^{\infty} c_m \frac{\sin[\pi W_x (n - m)\Delta k]}{\pi(n - m)\Delta k} \tag{10.29}$$

Since $S[n]$ is known only for $-N/2 \le n < N/2$, it is evident that the solution for c_m is not unique. Therefore, unlike the continuous case, discrete extrapolation is inherently underdetermined. In practice, the minimum-norm solution is sought, namely,

$$c = \arg\min_{\{c_m\}} \sum_{m} |c_m|^2 \tag{10.30}$$

It has been shown [169] that the solution satisfies the following conditions:

$$\begin{cases} S[n] = \displaystyle\sum_{m=-N/2}^{N/2-1} c_m \frac{\sin[\pi W_x(m-n)\Delta k]}{\pi(m-n)\Delta k} & \frac{N}{2} \leq n < \frac{N}{2} \\[2ex] c_m = 0 & \text{otherwise} \end{cases} \tag{10.31}$$

which is the governing equation for discrete bandlimited extrapolation. Equation (10.31) can be solved directly for c. In matrix form, it can be written as

$$\mathbf{E}c = S \tag{10.32}$$

where $\mathbf{E}$ is an $N \times N$ matrix, and c and S are N-element column vectors defined respectively by

$$c = \left[c_{-N/2}, c_{-N/2+1}, \ldots, c_{N/2-1}\right]^T$$

$$S = [S[-N/2], S[-N/2+1], \ldots, S[N/2-1]]^T$$

$$E_{mn} = \frac{\sin[\pi W_x(m-n)\Delta k]}{\pi(m-n)\Delta k} \qquad m, n = 1, 2, \ldots, N$$

It has been shown [169] that the extrapolation matrix $\mathbf{E}$ has N positive eigenvalues such that $1 > \lambda_1 > \lambda_2 > \cdots > \lambda_N > 0$. The first $NW_x\Delta k$ eigenvalues are very close to 1, and the others gradually decay to zero. Since $\mathbf{E}$ is positive-definite, c is uniquely determined from Eq. (10.32). A major problem with this direct solution lies in its sensitivity to noise because the extrapolation matrix $\mathbf{E}$ is usually ill-conditioned. Paradoxically, the smaller the sampling interval Δk, the more information the support bound contains, but the more ill-conditioned the extrapolation matrix $\mathbf{E}$ becomes. The usual way to cope with this ill-conditioned problem is to regularize Eq. (10.32) by perturbing $\mathbf{E}$ with a diagonal matrix $\lambda\mathbf{I}$. In this case, Eq. (10.32) becomes

$$(\mathbf{E} + \lambda\mathbf{I})c = S \tag{10.33}$$

Other advanced regularization methods are available, which replace the diagonal matrix by a general regularization matrix incorporating additional constraints about the image function [131]. After c is known, one can extrapolate the measured data set to the desired frequency range using the following formula:

$$S[n] = \sum_{m=-N/2}^{N/2-1} c_m \frac{\sin[\pi W_x(n-m)\Delta k]}{\pi(n-m)\Delta k} \qquad |n| \geq N/2 \tag{10.34}$$

The extrapolated data set can then be Fourier transformed to get the final reconstruction. Alternatively, one can use Eq. (10.28) to get the final reconstruction, which corresponds to extrapolating $S[n]$ to the infinite frequency range.

Bandlimited extrapolation reconstruction is often carried out iteratively. The popular algorithm developed by Papoulis and Gerchberg is summarized below. The interested reader is referred to [51] for more details.

(a) Zero-fill the measured data set to $\hat{N}$ points and apply the inverse FFT to get a first approximation $\hat{I}_0(x)$ of the required reconstruction $I(x)$.

(b) In the mth iteration, force the previously estimated image $\hat{I}_{m-1}(x)$ to have the required spatial support bound by multiplying it with $\Pi(x/W_x)$

$$\hat{I}_m(x) = \hat{I}_{m-1}(x)\Pi\left(\frac{x}{W_x}\right) \tag{10.35}$$

(c) Apply the FFT to $\hat{I}_m(x)$ to get a new pseudo-data set $\hat{S}_m[n]$ and then fill the unsampled data region of the measured data set $S[n]$ with $\hat{S}_m[n]$.

(d) Apply the FFT to the extrapolated data set to get a new reconstruction and go back to step (b) if the maximum number of iterations is not reached; otherwise, accept it as the final reconstruction. To avoid noise amplification, this iterative process is often terminated after a few iterations, depending on the data signal-to-noise ratio.

10.2.2   Maximum Entropy Reconstruction

The maximum entropy principle has been widely used in various areas of science and engineering [9, 37]. Its application to image reconstruction from noisy incomplete data has also been investigated by several research groups [106, 122, 129, 130, 133, 145, 205, 206, 267]. However, the usefulness of the maximum entropy constraint for MR image reconstruction is not yet well established [122, 206]; so, this section will present only a brief review of the fundamental concepts underlying maximum entropy image reconstruction.

The core of maximum entropy image reconstruction is the entropy measure that guides the selection of an optimal reconstruction from the infinitely many feasible ones consistent with the measured data. So, let us begin with a review of the Shannon entropy definition.

Definition 10.2 *The entropy $\mathcal{H}$ of a discrete random variable ξ with probability distribution $\{p_1, p_2, \ldots, p_N\}$ is a measure of its uncertainty (or information content), defined by Shannon as*

$$\mathcal{H} = -\sum_{n=1}^{N} p_n \log p_n \tag{10.36}$$

Note that the base of the log function in the above definition can be arbitrary. However, it is customary to use the base 2 logs, and the resulting unit of entropy (information) is called a *bit*.

Entropy in one form or another is a rather old concept. Its origin dates back to the first work on thermodynamics in the nineteenth century. Nonetheless, most of the credit for defining entropy and promoting its use in signal processing (particularly, in communications) is due to Shannon. To better appreciate the above entropy definition, let us go through a couple of examples.

■ **Example 10.1**

Let ξ be a binary random variable such that

$$\xi = \begin{cases} 1 & \text{with probability } p \\ 0 & \text{with probability } 1-p \end{cases} \tag{10.37}$$

The entropy of ξ is given by

$$\mathcal{H}(\xi) = -p\log_2 p - (1-p)\log_2(1-p) \tag{10.38}$$

It is instructive to evaluate $\mathcal{H}$ for different values of p. In particular, $\mathcal{H}(\xi) = 0$ for $p = 0$ or 1, which is understandable because in this case ξ is not random and there is no uncertainty. It is also easy to show that $\mathcal{H}(\xi)$ reaches the maximum value of 1 bit when $p = 1/2$; that is, the uncertainty about ξ is maximum when ξ has an equal chance of taking the value of 1 and 0.

■ **Example 10.2**

This example shows that the entropy given in Eq. (10.36) reaches the maximum value $\log_2 N$ when $p_1 = p_2 = \cdots = p_N = 1/N$.

Consider the function

$$f(p_1, p_2, \ldots, p_N) = -\sum_{n=1}^{N} p_n \log_2 p_n + \lambda\left(\sum_{n=1}^{N} p_n - 1\right)$$

$$= -\frac{1}{\ln 2}\sum_{n=1}^{N} p_n \ln p_n + \lambda\left(\sum_{n=1}^{N} p_n - 1\right) \tag{10.39}$$

where λ is a Lagrangian multiplier. Taking the first-order derivative on both sides yields

$$\frac{\partial f}{\partial p_n} = -\frac{1}{\ln 2}(\ln p_n + 1) + \lambda, \qquad n = 1, 2, \ldots, N \tag{10.40}$$

Setting $\frac{\partial f}{\partial p_n}$ to zero yields the desired value of p_n for $\mathcal{H}(\xi)$ to reach the maximum. Inspection of Eq. (10.40) reveals that the p_n must be all equal. Noting that $\sum_{n=1}^{N} p_n = 1$, it is then apparent that

$$p_n = \frac{1}{N} \tag{10.41}$$

and, consequently,

$$\mathcal{H}(\xi) = \log_2 N \tag{10.42}$$

We now describe some entropy measures that are in use for an image function. First, for an image with positive pixel values $I[n]$, the normalized pixel intensity value is treated as the probability [106, 122, 129, 130, 133, 145, 206, 267]. That is, the probability to observe $I[n]$ is

$$p_n = \frac{I[n]}{\sum_m I[m]} \tag{10.43}$$

Then, the entropy of the entire image (treated as a random variable) is

$$\mathcal{H} = -\sum_n \left(\frac{I[n]}{\sum_m I[m]} \right) \log \left(\frac{I[n]}{\sum_m I[m]} \right) \tag{10.44}$$

In the case that $\sum_m I[m]$ is a constant, Eq. (10.44) can be written equivalently (apart from a constant term) as

$$\mathcal{H} = -\sum_n I[n] \log I[n] \tag{10.45}$$

The above entropy definitions can be extended to complex-valued image functions. Specifically, if one is primarily concerned with the magnitude image,[2] the probability distribution is calculated as

$$p_n = \frac{|I[n]|}{\sum_m |I[m]|} \tag{10.46}$$

and correspondingly,

$$\mathcal{H} = -\sum_n \left(\frac{|I[n]|}{\sum_m |I[m]|} \right) \log \left(\frac{|I[n]|}{\sum_m |I[m]|} \right) \tag{10.47}$$

or

$$\mathcal{H} = -\sum_n |I[n]| \log |I[n]| \tag{10.48}$$

---

[2]One can also treat the real and imaginary parts of a complex image function as independent quantities; see [205] for some discussion of this topic.

when $\sum_m |I[m]|$ is a constant.

Note that while the entropy measures in Eqs. (10.44) and (10.47) are commonly used for image reconstruction, they may not be useful for other image processing tasks. For example, in image registration the entropy of an image is defined as [196, 266]

$$\mathcal{H} = - \sum_{I=I_{\min}}^{I_{\max}} \left(\frac{n(I)}{N} \right) \log \left(\frac{n(I)}{N} \right) \tag{10.49}$$

where

$$
\begin{array}{ll}
I_{\min} : & \text{minimum image intensity value} \\
I_{\max} : & \text{maximum image intensity value} \\
n(I) : & \text{number of pixels with intensity value } I \\
N : & \text{total number of pixels}
\end{array}
$$

After $\mathcal{H}$ is defined, the next step in maximum entropy reconstruction is to maximize $\mathcal{H}$ under the data-consistency constraint, which is often expressed in terms of the following so-called χ^2 statistical test

$$\chi^2 = \sum_{n=-N/2}^{N/2-1} \frac{1}{\sigma_d} \left| S[n] - \sum_{m=-\hat{N}/2}^{\hat{N}/2-1} I[m] e^{-i2\pi mn/\hat{N}} \right|^2 \tag{10.50}$$

where σ_d is the standard deviation of the data noise. Note that in Eq. (10.50) the Fourier summation is used to calculate the k-space data values corresponding to a guess reconstruction $I[m]$; also, $\hat{N}$ is the total number of pixels in the resulting image, which equals to the number of data points in the extrapolated data set.

Maximization of $\mathcal{H}$ under the constraint of Eq. (10.50) is often transformed to an unconstrained problem through the introduction of a Lagrangian multiplier λ to form the following objective function:

$$Q = \mathcal{H} - \lambda \chi^2 \tag{10.51}$$

The desired solution corresponds to a critical point of Q where $\chi^2 \approx N$. However, there is no known closed-form solution to this problem in general, and iterative optimization algorithms are often employed to find an asymptotic solution. Detailed discussion of this topic can be found in [30, 106, 145].

10.2.3 Discussion

This section has discussed two constrained reconstruction methods using the bandlimited constraint and the maximum entropy constraint, respectively. The quality of bandlimited extrapolation reconstructions depends on the amount of information contained in the superimposed spatial support bound. If the measured data happen to be oversampled (i.e., the FOV is larger than the support bound), this constraint can help recover some of the unmeasured high-frequency data. Another advantage of this method is its computational efficiency. The iterative solution can be obtained with a few iterations; the noniterative solution can be obtained efficiently using the Levinson algorithm [177]. One drawback of band-limited extrapolation is its high sensitivity to noise. Moreover, if the measured data are taken at the Nyquist rate (i.e., $\Delta k = 1/W_x$, as is often the case in MRI applications), the support-bound constraint becomes trivial because $E = W_x I$ and $c = \Delta k S$. As a result, no meaningful data extrapolation will be gained. Therefore, the bandlimited extrapolation method may not be very effective for overcoming the truncation artifacts in general, although it has found useful applications in other MRI problems [167, 275, 277].

The effectiveness of the maximum entropy method depends, to a large extent, on how entropy is defined for a particular problem [206]. In the absence of any data constraints, maximization of the Shannon entropy measure $\mathcal{H}$ results in all the p_n being equal. This property seems to suggest that the maximum entropy principle selects the smoothest image consistent with the data. In other words, the maximum entropy reconstruction adds no new information beyond that contained in the measured data. This point has been demonstrated by examples from application of the maximum entropy principle to NMR spectroscopic data analysis and radio astronomy image reconstructions. However, some studies also indicate that this property is not generally true [122]. In fact, it is shown [133] that in some particular cases, the maximum entropy reconstruction is no more than a scaled version of the conventional Fourier reconstruction. Therefore, the maximum entropy method should be used with care.

A useful extension of the maximum entropy method is the incorporation of additional prior knowledge into the entropy expression. Specifically, if an initial estimate p_n^0 is available for p_n, it can be incorporated into the entropy expression as

$$\mathcal{H} = \sum_{n=-\hat{N}/2}^{\hat{N}/2-1} p_n \log \left(\frac{p_n}{p_n^0} \right) \tag{10.52}$$

This measure is often known as the cross-entropy [243], or the Kullback-Leibler distance between two probability distributions [15]. Note that the cross-entropy is always nonnegative and is zero if and only if $p_n = p_n^0$ [15]. Therefore, the final reconstruction should be obtained by minimizing the cross-entropy under the data-consistency constraint. Equivalently, one can maximize

$$\tilde{\mathcal{H}} = - \sum_{n=-\hat{N}/2}^{\hat{N}/2-1} p_n \log \left(\frac{p_n}{p_n^0} \right) \tag{10.53}$$

which is the minus cross-entropy.

Before concluding this section, it is worthwhile to point out that data extrapolation for superresolution reconstruction is often difficult to achieve; however, suppression of the Gibbs ringing artifact alone is much less challenging. A data extrapolation scheme based on sigma filtering [184] has proven rather effective for this purpose. The interested reader is referred to [86, 87, 124] for detailed discussion.

10.3   Parametric Reconstruction Methods

This section describes two parametric methods for image reconstruction. A distinct feature of these methods is the introduction of a parametric (or non-Fourier series) image model, and as a result, parameter estimation becomes a key step in the image reconstruction process. There are a couple of desirable properties with the parametric approach to image reconstruction. First, a non-Fourier series model, if optimally chosen, can represent the class of desired image functions with a finite number of unknowns, and consequently, only a finite number of data points are necessary. In other words, a parametric model can implicitly extrapolate the measured data set to the infinite frequency range, thereby completely removing the data truncation artifacts. Second, many of the parametric methods have a built-in filtering capability for noise removal. Specifically, if the number of model parameters is less than the number of data points, a least-squares parameter estimation procedure can effectively "smooth" out some of the measurement noise.

There are a variety of ways to set up a parametric image model. The general principles governing the selection of an (optimal) image model are the following:

- *Sufficiency*: The model can accurately represent the class of image functions of interest.

- *Efficiency/Parsimony*: The model can characterize the image functions with a small number of parameters.

- *Robustness*: The model should be stable with respect to perturbations, including random noise and systematic modeling offsets, of reasonable levels.

- *Computability*: The model parameters can be found efficiently when the model is fitted to the measured data.

Model sufficiency is usually not a problem if an unlimited number of parameters are used, such as is the case with the Fourier series. However, in practice, we are given only a finite number of degrees of freedom in setting up a model because only a finite number of data points are available for determining the model parameters. Therefore, only asymptotic sufficiency is obtained in practice, and as a result, model efficiency is important because it determines the level of modeling error with finite number of parameters. Hence, the challenge of parametric modeling lies in achieving an optimal compromise between model sufficiency and efficiency.

The robustness of a parametric model is important because we always have to deal with measurement random noise and systematic modeling errors. Ideally, the model should be stable so that the model parameters are insensitive to perturbations in the assumed working environments. Computational complexity of a model is also important for practical applications, since a priori constraints often require highly nonlinear models. In fact, suboptimal procedures are often used for parameter estimation to gain computational efficiency.

In the remainder of this section, we discuss two parametric models: the autoregressive moving average model and the generalized series model.

10.3.1   The Autoregressive Moving Average Model

The autoregressive moving average (ARMA) model is an important tool in modern spectral estimation [46, 68, 79, 82]. Application of this model to MR image reconstruction was first proposed by Smith et al. [246]. This section first reviews the definition of an ARMA model and then describes the corresponding image reconstruction algorithm.

10.3.1.1   Definition

In general, a (p, q)-order ARMA model is described by the following rational function

$$I(x) - \frac{\sum_{n=0}^{q} b_n e^{i2\pi n \Delta k x}}{1 + \sum_{n=1}^{p} a_n e^{i2\pi n \Delta k x}} - \frac{B_q(z)|_{z=e^{i2\pi \Delta k x}}}{A_p(z)|_{z=e^{i2\pi \Delta k x}}} \tag{10.54}$$

where

$$A_p(z) = 1 + a_1 z + \cdots + a_p z^p \tag{10.55a}$$
$$B_q(z) = b_0 + b_1 z + \cdots + b_q z^q \tag{10.55b}$$

It is useful to view $1/A_p(z)$, $B_q(z)$, and $B_q(z)/A_p(z)$ as the transfer functions of a digital filter. Then, the time-domain input-output relationships of these filters can be expressed, respectively, as

$$\frac{1}{A_p(z)} : \qquad d_n = -\sum_{m=1}^{p} a_m d_{n-m} + \epsilon_n \tag{10.56a}$$

$$B_q(z) : \qquad d_n = -\sum_{m=0}^{q} b_m \epsilon_{n-m} \tag{10.56b}$$

$$\frac{A_p(z)}{B_q(z)} : \qquad d_n = -\sum_{m=1}^{p} a_m d_{n-m} + \sum_{m=0}^{q} b_m \epsilon_{n-m} \tag{10.56c}$$

where ϵ_n is the input excitation sequence and d_n is the resulting output data sequence of each filter. It is clear from the above expressions that $1/A_p(z)$ is a pth-order AR (autoregressive) filter while $B_q(z)$ is a qth-order MA (moving average) filter. Since the transfer function of an AR filter has only poles in the z-plane, it is also known as an all-pole filter; likewise, an MA filter is an all-zero filter.

The ARMA model can be justified on the basis that any continuous function can be approximated arbitrarily closely by a rational function with sufficiently large values of p and q [68]. One can see from Eq. (10.54) that the ARMA model reduces to the conventional Fourier series model when $p = 0$ and to a strict AR model when $q = 0$. Recall that the Fourier series model is rather effective for representing smooth functions but becomes very inefficient for representing spiky image features. On the other hand, an AR model $1/A_p(z)$ lends itself well to representing spiky features because $1/A_p(z)$ will produce sharp peaks by poles located on or near the unit circle in the z-plane. A combination of these two features endows the ARMA model with the capability to represent a variety of image features efficiently. The widespread use of this model in various areas of data analysis is, to some extent, motivated by this property.

In the MRI application, the measured data $S[n] = S(n\Delta k)$ correspond to the Fourier transform of $I(x)$. That is,

$$S[n] = \int_{-\frac{1}{2\Delta k}}^{\frac{1}{2\Delta k}} \left[\frac{\sum_{m=0}^{q} b_m e^{i2\pi m \Delta k x}}{1 + \sum_{m=1}^{p} a_m e^{i2\pi m \Delta k x}} \right] e^{-i2\pi n \Delta k x} dx \qquad (10.57)$$

where it is assumed that $I(x)$ is bandlimited to $|x| \leq \frac{1}{2\Delta k}$. It is easy to show that

$$S[n] = -\sum_{m=1}^{p} a_m S[n-m] + \frac{1}{\Delta k} \sum_{m=0}^{q} b_m \delta_{n-m} \qquad (10.58)$$

where δ_n is the Kronecker delta function. For notational simplicity, the scaling factor $1/\Delta k$ is sometimes absorbed into the MA coefficients, resulting in the following recursion:

$$S[n] = -\sum_{m=1}^{p} a_m S[n-m] + \sum_{m=0}^{q} \hat{b}_m \delta_{n-m} \qquad (10.59)$$

where $b_m = \Delta k \hat{b}_m$. Comparing Eq. (10.58) with Eq. (10.56c), one can see that $S[n]$ is the output of an ARMA filter excited by a single pulse $\epsilon_n = \delta_n/\Delta k$, as illustrated in Fig. 10.7. Note that in the modified form given in Eq. (10.59), the filter is excited simply by δ_n.

A concept closely related to ARMA modeling is linear predictability of a data sequence. Formally, a data sequence d_n is called pth-order linearly predictable if any element in it can be expressed as a *linear combination* of its preceding (or ensuing) p elements with a fixed set of weightings. In the forward

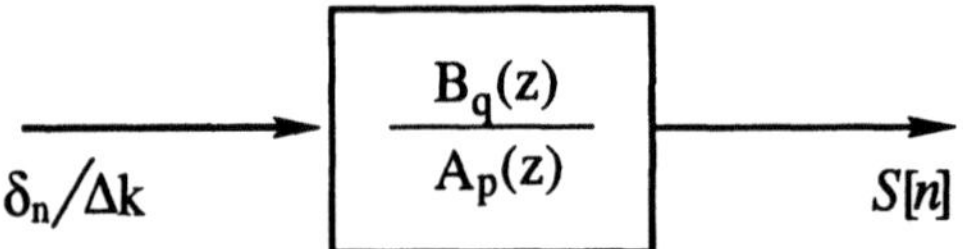

Figure 10.7 MR data modeled as the output of an ARMA filter activated by a single impulse.

prediction form,

$$d_n = -\sum_{m=1}^{p} h_m d_{n-m} \qquad (10.60)$$

where the weightings $\{h_m, m = 1, \ldots, p\}$ are called the linear predictor coefficients and p is the predictor order. Corresponding to Eq. (10.60), the following polynomial can be formed

$$P(z) = 1 + h_1 z^{-1} + \cdots + h_M z^{-M} \qquad (10.61)$$

which is called the *characteristic polynomial*. It is clear from Eq. (10.56a) that the impulse response of a pth-order AR filter can be expressed as

$$d_n = -\sum_{m=1}^{p} a_m d_{n-m}, \qquad n \geq p \qquad (10.62)$$

which is p-order linearly predictable.

■ **Example 10.3**

Let $d(t)$ be a transient signal consisting of M damped complex sinusoids. We show that the data sequence $d_n = d(n\Delta t)$ is Mth-order linearly predictable.

We first express $d(t)$ as

$$d(t) = \sum_{m=1}^{M} c_m e^{-(\beta_m + i\omega_m)t} \qquad (10.63)$$

for some values of c_m, β_m, and ω_m. (It is necessary that $\beta_m > 0$ for damped sinusoids.) Then,

$$d_n = \sum_{m=1}^{M} c_m z_m^n \qquad (10.64)$$

where

$$z_m = e^{-(\beta_m + i\omega_m)\Delta t}, \qquad m = 1, 2, \ldots, M \qquad (10.65)$$

Based on Eq. (10.64), we have

$$\begin{cases} d_n = \sum_{m=1}^{M} c_m z_m^n \\ d_{n-1} = \sum_{m=1}^{M} c_m z_m^{-1} z_m^n \\ \quad\vdots \\ d_{n-M} = \sum_{m=1}^{M} c_m z_m^{-M} z_m^n \end{cases} \qquad (10.66)$$

A linear combination of the above equations yields

$$d_n + h_1 d_{n-1} + \cdots + h_M d_{n-M} = \sum_{m=1}^{M} c_m \left(1 + h_1 z_m^{-1} + \cdots + h_M z_m^{-M}\right) z_m^n$$

$$(10.67)$$

We further assume that the weighting coefficients $h_m, m = 1, 2, \ldots, M$ are selected to satisfy the following equation:

$$1 + h_1 z^{-1} + \cdots + h_M z^{-M} = \prod_{m=1}^{M} \left(1 - z_m z^{-1}\right) \qquad (10.68)$$

Then,

$$1 + h_1 z_m^{-1} + \cdots + h_M z_m^{-M} = 0, \qquad m = 1, 2, \ldots, M \qquad (10.69)$$

Substituting Eq. (10.69) into Eq. (10.67) immediately yields

$$d_n = -h_1 d_{n-1} - h_2 d_{n-2} - \cdots - h_M d_{n-M} \qquad (10.70)$$

for $n \geq M$. Therefore, d_n is an Mth-order linearly predictable sequence according to Eq. (10.56).

10.3.1.2 Parameter Estimation

A key step in image reconstruction using an ARMA model is to determine all the model parameters, including the order parameters p and q, the AR coefficients a_m, and the MA coefficients b_m. Let d_n, for $n = 0, 1, \ldots, N - 1$, represent an FID signal or one wing of an echo signal, or these signals after some preprocessing. Fitting an ARMA model to d_n to determine all the parameters jointly is a challenging computational problem and is often avoided in practice. Therefore, most parameter estimation algorithms in practical use today find suboptimal solutions to these parameters in multiple steps. Specifically, the model order parameters p and q are first determined based on some statistical testing or ad hoc rules; then, the AR coefficients are determined by solving a linear least-squares problem, which is followed by calculation of the MA coefficients. One of these techniques called TERA (transient error reconstruction algorithm), developed by Smith et al. [246], has found useful applications in MRI applications and is summarized below. Note that a large number of algorithms have been proposed for ARMA model parameter estimation in connection with spectral estimation of a time series. The interested reader is referred to [46, 68, 79, 82] for excellent reviews of these algorithms.

Determination of the Model Order Parameters p and q. Finding the correct or the "best" value for p is difficult. Too low an order will lead to a loss of resolution and too high an order may cause model instability. The maximum value for p under the condition that the AR coefficients are not underdetermined is $N/2$; it is suggested [80] that p is chosen on the order of $N/3$. Rigorous treatments of model order selection can be found in [263, 283, 284].

Determination of the model order q for the MA part is more straightforward. In general, we select the largest possible value for q, which is N. By doing so, we can select the MA coefficients properly so that the resulting ARMA model is data-consistent [246].

Determination of the AR Parameters a_m. Temporarily ignoring the MA component of the ARMA model, the AR coefficients are related to the measured data sequence d_n by

$$d_n = -\sum_{m=0}^{p} a_m d_{n-m} + \epsilon_n, \qquad n = p+1, ..., N/2 - 1 \qquad (10.71)$$

where ϵ_n is the forward prediction error. Determination of the a_m from this set of linear equations is the classical linear prediction problem. After p is known, the a_m are usually determined by minimizing the total forward prediction error.[3] That is,

$$\min_{\{a_m\}} \sum_{n=p+1}^{N-1} |\epsilon_n|^2 = \min_{\{a_m\}} \sum_{n=p+1}^{N-1} \left| d_n + \sum_{m=0}^{p} a_m d_{n-m} \right|^2 \qquad (10.72)$$

In matrix form, Eq. (10.71) can be written as

$$\begin{bmatrix} d_0 & d_1 & \cdots & d_{p-1} \\ d_1 & d_2 & \cdots & d_p \\ \vdots & \cdots & \cdots & \vdots \\ d_{N-p-1} & d_{N-p} & \cdots & d_{N-2} \end{bmatrix} \begin{bmatrix} a_p \\ a_{p-1} \\ \vdots \\ a_1 \end{bmatrix} \approx - \begin{bmatrix} d_p \\ d_{p+1} \\ \vdots \\ d_{N-1} \end{bmatrix} \qquad (10.73)$$

---

[3]The resulting AR model is optimal in the least-squares sense, but it is not necessarily the correct one.

or simply,

$$\mathbf{D}\boldsymbol{a} \approx -\boldsymbol{d} \tag{10.74}$$

The solution for a_m given in Eq. (10.72) corresponds to the least-squares solution of Eq. (10.74) and is given by

$$\boldsymbol{a} = -\left(\mathbf{D}^H\mathbf{D}\right)^{-1}\mathbf{D}^H\boldsymbol{d} \tag{10.75}$$

Determination of the MA Coefficients b_n. Determination of the MA coefficients b_n for the current problem is rather simple. First, noting that

$$\sum_{m=0}^{q} b_m \delta_{n-m} = b_n \qquad n \leq N \tag{10.76}$$

we can rewrite Eq. (10.58) as

$$S[n] = -\sum_{m=1}^{p} a_m S[n-m] + \frac{1}{\Delta k} b_n \tag{10.77}$$

Second, comparing Eq. (10.77) to Eq. (10.71) yields the following simple relationship between the MA coefficients b_n and the prediction error sequence ϵ_n:

$$b_n = \Delta k \epsilon_n \tag{10.78}$$

Note that ϵ_n is defined only for $p < n < N$ in Eq. (10.71). However, after the AR coefficients a_n are known, we can use Eq. (10.71) to calculate the prediction error sequence for $0 \leq n \leq p$ as well. Specifically, since the measured data d_n for $n = 0, 1, \ldots, N-1$, is taken to be the impulse response of the ARMA model,[4] we can treat d_n as zero for $n < 0$.[5] Therefore,

$$\epsilon_n = d_n + \sum_{m=1}^{n} a_m d_{n-m} \tag{10.79}$$

for $0 \leq n \leq p$. Combining Eq. (10.79) with Eq. (10.71) yields

$$\epsilon_n = \begin{cases} d_n + \sum_{m=1}^{p} a_m d_{n-m} & n \geq p \\ d_n + \sum_{m=1}^{n} a_m d_{n-m} & n < p \end{cases} \tag{10.80}$$

Finally, according to Eq. (10.78), we have the following simple formula for calculating the MA coefficients b_n:

$$b_n = \Delta k \begin{cases} d_n + \sum_{m=1}^{p} a_m d_{n-m} & n \geq p \\ d_n + \sum_{m=1}^{n} a_m d_{n-m} & n < p \end{cases} \tag{10.81}$$

---

[4] Strictly speaking, d_n is modeled as the impulse response of the ARMA filter divided by Δk.

[5] It is assumed that the ARMA filter is a causal system.

Note that in [246], the $\hat{b}_n$ are calculated, which are given by

$$\hat{b}_n = \begin{cases} d_n + \sum_{m=1}^{p} a_m d_{n-m} & n \geq p \\ d_n + \sum_{m=1}^{n} a_m d_{n-m} & n < p \end{cases} \tag{10.82}$$

10.3.1.3 Discussion

There are a few subtle points in applying the ARMA model to MR data. First, it is useful to remove the zeroth- and first-order phase distortions of the data, which can be done using the techniques described in [202]. Removal of these phase terms has been found to substantially reduce the required AR model order, thus improving model stability. Second, it is necessary to split the measured echo data into Hermitian and anti-Hermitian sequences. This preprocessing step is necessary because fitting both wings of the data simultaneously would force the roots of the $A_p(z)$ filter onto the unit circle, thus leading to instability.

Assuming that the data $S[n]$ are available for $-N/2 \leq n < N/2$, the Hermitian ($S_+[n]$) and anti-Hermitian ($S_-[n]$) components can be calculated as

$$\begin{cases} S_+[n] = (S[n] + S^*[-n])/2 \\ S_-[n] = (S[n] - S^*[-n])/2 \end{cases} \qquad 0 \leq n < N/2 \tag{10.83}$$

The corresponding reconstructions I_+ and I_- from S_+ and S_-, respectively, can be combined to get the desired reconstruction I as follows:

$$I(x) = 2\Re\{I_+(x)\} + 2i\Im\{I_-(x)\} - S[0] \tag{10.84}$$

Note that in the ideal case, I_+ corresponds to the absorption mode and I_- corresponds to the dispersion mode, and one can simply use I_+ as the final reconstruction. In practice, both I_+ and I_- are needed, although I_- contributes only about 10% of the total energy to the final reconstruction [246].

The AR filter calculated from Eq. (10.75) is not guaranteed to be stable. To improve the stability of the resulting filter, Smith et al. [246] proposed to move its poles away from the unit circle (pole-pulling) by modifying the AR filter coefficients as follows:

$$\tilde{a}_m = a_m \alpha^m, \quad \alpha \leq 1.0 \tag{10.85}$$

A value of α around 0.99 or lower for very noisy signals is appropriate. Extreme pole-pulling is to be avoided as values of $\alpha \approx 0.95$ will give a TERA reconstruction with truncation artifacts similar to those in a standard Fourier reconstruction. Note that the use of $\tilde{a}_m$ would disturb the accuracy of the prediction, but not the final reconstruction since the MA coefficients are chosen based on the new AR coefficient values.

After the a_m and b_m have become available, an image can be directly obtained from the model given in Eq. (10.54). The numerator and the denominator can be evaluated using an FFT algorithm. Zero-padding is often used to get enough digital resolution to catch the high-resolution features embedded in such an image function. Based on Eq. (10.58), one can also extrapolate the data recursively to recover the missing high spatial frequency data. The normal Fourier method can then be applied to reconstruct the desired image from the extrapolated data.

To illustrate the performance of the ARMA modeling technique, a set of reconstruction results obtained from the phantom data set (Fig. 10.3) is shown in Fig. 10.8. As can be seen, the image in Fig. 10.8a has noticeable truncation artifacts (resolution loss and Gibbs ringing). The ringing artifact is considerably reduced in the ARMA reconstruction shown in Fig. 10.8b, and some improvement in resolution, particularly for the circles, can also be observed. More reconstruction examples comparing the ARMA model to other techniques can be found in [80].

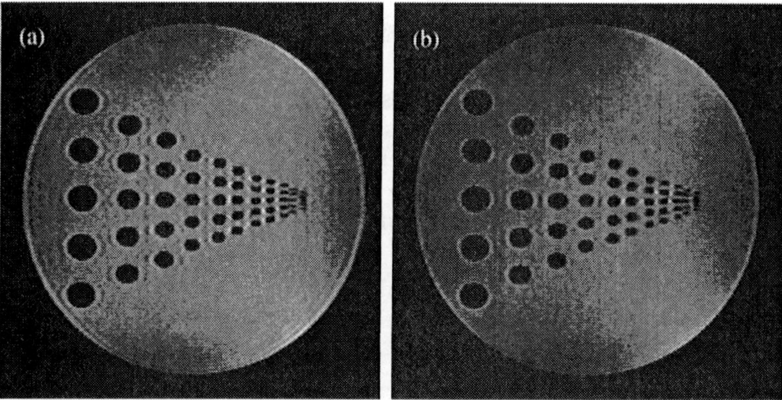

Figure 10.8 Reconstructions of a phantom image. The vertical direction of both images was reconstructed using the FFT reconstruction method from 256 symmetric Fourier transform samples, while the horizontal direction was reconstructed from 96 data points using (a) the conventional FFT method and (b) the ARMA modeling method.

10.3.2   The Generalized Series Model

The generalized series (GS) model was proposed as a general method for incorporating a priori constraints into the image reconstruction process [187, 189]. In this model, an image function is represented as

$$I(x) = \sum_{n} c_n \varphi_n(x) \tag{10.86}$$

where $\varphi_n(x)$ are the basis functions used to absorb any a priori information and c_n are the series coefficients chosen to match the measured data. This section describes the use of this model for constrained image reconstruction.

10.3.2.1 Selection of the Basis Functions

Selecting a set of "good" basis functions is essential for the GS model. A particular set of basis functions is given in the form of weighted complex sinusoids [187, 189]:

$$\varphi_n(x) = C(x)e^{i2\pi n\Delta kx} \tag{10.87}$$

where $C(x)$ is a nonnegative function incorporating a priori information. With this set of basis functions, the GS model becomes

$$I(x) = C(x)\sum_n c_n e^{i2\pi n\Delta kx} \tag{10.88}$$

This model has several useful properties. Specifically, when no nontrivial a priori information is available, namely, $C(x) = 1$, Eq. (10.88) automatically reduces to the conventional Fourier series model. This is desirable because the Fourier series model is indeed optimal in this case. On the other hand, if $C(x) = I(x)$, the multiplicative Fourier series factor will be forced to unity by the data-consistency constraint, and a perfect reconstruction will result. In general, if $C(x)$ is properly chosen, the new basis functions given in Eq. (10.87) enable the GS model to converge faster than the Fourier series model. Therefore, within a certain error bound, fewer terms can be used to represent an image function than are required by the Fourier series method, leading to a reduction of the truncation artifacts. The optimality of the GS model in Eq. (10.88) can also be justified from the minimum cross-entropy principle [243]. Specifically, treating the weighting function $C(x)$ as an initial estimate to a desired image function $I(x)$, the optimal reconstruction under this principle is the one that minimizes the cross-entropy measure. That is

$$I(x) = \arg\min_{\{I(x)\}} \int_{-\infty}^{\infty} I(x)\log\left[\frac{I(x)}{C(x)}\right] dx \tag{10.89}$$

subject to the data-consistency constraints

$$S[n] = \int_{-\infty}^{\infty} I(x)e^{-i2\pi n\Delta kx} dx \tag{10.90}$$

The solution to the above constrained problem is

$$I(x) = C(x)\exp\left(\sum_n \lambda_n e^{i2\pi n\Delta kx}\right) \tag{10.91}$$

where λ_n are appropriate Lagrangian multipliers. If $C(x)$ is a good estimate for $I(x)$, the exponential term can be reasonably approximated by the first two terms of its power series expansion [i.e., $\exp(x) \approx 1 + x$]. In this case, $I(x)$ becomes

$$I(x) \approx C(x) + \sum_n \lambda_n C(x) e^{i2\pi n \Delta k x}$$

$$= \sum_n (\delta_n + \lambda_n) C(x) e^{i2\pi n \Delta k x} \tag{10.92}$$

which is identical to the GS model function $I(x)$ defined in Eq. (10.88) with $c_n = \delta_n + \lambda_n$. Therefore, the GS model function can be viewed as an approximation to the optimal minimum cross-entropy solution. This approximate solution converts a highly nonlinear problem to a linear one so that fast reconstruction is possible.

We next consider the selection of the weighting function $C(x)$. For the limited data reconstruction problem, it was suggested [190] that $C(x)$ be chosen to be a summation of boxcar functions as

$$C(x) = \left| \sum_{m=1}^{M} a_m \Pi \left[\frac{x - \frac{1}{2}(\beta_m + \beta_{m+1})}{\beta_{m+1} - \beta_m} \right] \right| \tag{10.93}$$

where

M :	number of boxcar functions
β_m :	edge locations
a_m :	boxcar amplitudes

This function is particularly suitable for image functions containing sharp edges because they are explicitly built into the basis functions. Determination of the parameters in this model is described in the Appendix of this chapter.

The weighting function $C(x)$ can also be determined experimentally. A typical example is time-sequential imaging, which involves the acquisition of a time series of images, $I_1(x)$, $I_2(x)$, ..., $I_L(x)$, from the same anatomical site. For many of this type of imaging experiments, the underlying high-resolution morphology in the desired image sequence does not change from one image to another. As a result, it is not necessary to acquire each of these images independently. Specifically, with the GS model, we first acquire one high-resolution (reference) data set with N encodings followed by a sequence of reduced data set with M encodings, as shown in Fig. 10.9. In the image reconstruction step, the high-resolution reference image $I_{\text{ref}}(x)$ is used as the weighting function for the GS basis functions. That is, we set

$$C(x) = |I_{\text{ref}}(x)| \tag{10.94}$$

for the GS model when it is used for image reconstruction from the reduced data sets.

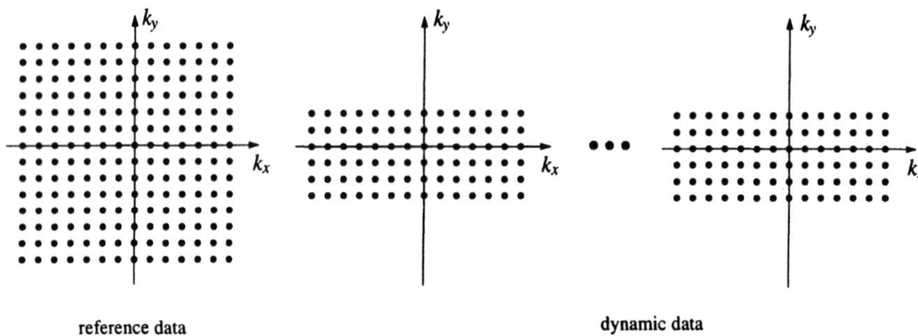

Figure 10.9 K-space coverage of time-sequential GS imaging.

Note that this GS imaging scheme, often called RIGR (reduced-encoding imaging by generalized-series reconstruction), offers a factor of N/M improvement in imaging efficiency (and temporal resolution) over the conventional Fourier imaging method. Similar imaging methods have also been proposed to achieve the same level of imaging efficiency [110, 171, 189, 225, 265]. Most notably, the "keyhole" imaging method [171] covers k-space in the same fashion, but uses a simpler method for image reconstruction. Specifically, it replaces the missing high-frequency data of the reduced data sets with the corresponding measurements from the high-resolution reference data set and then processes the merged data set with the conventional Fourier reconstruction method. An example comparing the GS reconstruction with the keyhole-Fourier reconstruction is shown later in this section.

10.3.2.2   Reconstruction Algorithm

After $\mathcal{C}(x)$ is known, the series coefficients c_n are determined under the data-consistency constraints. That is,

$$
S[n] = \int_{-\infty}^{\infty} \left\{ \mathcal{C}(x) \sum_{m=-N/2}^{N/2-1} c_m e^{i2\pi m \Delta k x} \right\} e^{-i2\pi n \Delta k x} \, dx
$$

$$
= \sum_{m=-N/2}^{N/2-1} c_m S_c[n-m] \tag{10.95}
$$

where

$$
S_c[n] = \int_{-\infty}^{\infty} \mathcal{C}(x) e^{i2\pi n \Delta k x} \, dx \tag{10.96}
$$

Rewriting Eq. (10.95) in matrix form, we have

$$\mathbf{H}c = S \tag{10.97}$$

where

$$c = [c_{-N/2}, \cdots, c_{N/2-1}]^T$$

$$S = [S[-N/2], \cdots, S[N/2 - 1]]^T$$

$$\mathbf{H} = \begin{bmatrix} S_c[0] & S_c[-1] & \cdots & S_c[-N+1] \\ S_c[1] & S_c[0] & \cdots & S_c[-N+2] \\ \vdots & \vdots & \ddots & \vdots \\ S_c[N-1] & S_c[N-2] & \cdots & S_c[0] \end{bmatrix}$$

which is a Toeplitz matrix. The GS model coefficients c can be found from Eq. (10.97) efficiently using the Levinson algorithm [4, 177]. The matrix $\mathbf{H}$ is sometimes ill-conditioned. In this case, Eq. (10.97) needs to be regularized. A simple method is to add a diagonal matrix $\lambda \mathbf{I}$ to $\mathbf{H}$ such that Eq. (10.97) becomes

$$(\mathbf{H} + \lambda \mathbf{I})c = S \tag{10.98}$$

The resulting regularized GS model can be expressed as

$$I(x) = \mathcal{C}(x) \sum_n c_n e^{i2\pi n \Delta k x} + \lambda \sum_n c_n e^{i2\pi n \Delta k x} \tag{10.99}$$

in which the second part can absorb broad-band noise. Therefore, this regularized GS model is to be preferred for numerical stability and noise insensitivity. The regularization parameter λ can be chosen on the basis of the data signal-to-noise ratio and the amount of regularization required to stablize $\mathbf{H}$, if that should be necessary. For example, λ can be chosen so that $S_c[0]/\lambda \sim \mathrm{SNR}$.

After $\mathcal{C}(x)$ and the c_n are available, evaluation of each pixel value directly from Eq. (10.88) will give the model reconstruction. Often a zero-filled FFT is applied to evaluate the Fourier series factor so that it has the same digital resolution as the $\mathcal{C}(x)$ does. Sometimes, the c_n may be filtered to remove any ringing artifacts resulting from inaccurate edge locations in $\mathcal{C}(x)$. Extrapolation reconstruction is also possible by using Eq. (10.95) to regenerate the missing high-frequency data. This step is desirable because filtering on the GS coefficients and model regularization could lead to data inconsistency beyond the noise level, and data extrapolation using the model can reinforce the data-consistency constraints in the final reconstruction.

10.3.2.3 Discussion

This section presents two examples to illustrate the performance of the GS modeling technique. The first example is parametric reconstruction using the GS model and the second is dynamic imaging.

Figure 10.10 shows the reconstruction results from actual MRI data of a transverse slice through a human leg. For comparison, the high-resolution image reconstructed using 256 Fourier data points along both the readout (horizontal) and phase-encoding (vertical) directions is shown in Fig. 10.10a. On reducing the number of phase encodings from 256 to 64, the Fourier series model produces the image in Fig. 10.10b, which shows significant Gibbs ringing artifact and a loss of spatial resolution, as expected. A simple way commonly used to reduce the ringing artifact is to multiply the measured data with a Hamming window function, but this causes a further loss of image resolution, as is evident in Fig. 10.10c. Using the generalized series method, the image in Fig. 10.10d was obtained. It shows a noticeable improvement both in resolution (compared to Fig. 10.10c) and in reduction of ringing (compared to Fig. 10.10b).

A practical limitation of this GS model-based reconstruction method is its significant computation requirement. Although fast algorithms are available for determining the GS coefficients $c(n)$, solving for the nonlinear parameters in the weighting function $C(x)$ of the basis functions is computationally expensive. Without a special array processor, this reconstruction algorithm is orders of magnitude slower than the FFT algorithm, which is a significant practical limitation.

Figure 10.11 shows a set of representative results from a dynamic imaging experiment with an injected contrast agent. In the experiment, a time series of data sets with 128 phase encodings was obtained before and after the injection of a contrast agent. The high-resolution preinjection image and one of the postinjection images are shown in the top row in this figure. The difference image between the preinjection image and the postinjection image is included in the third column to show how well the interimage variations are being reproduced. For the GS reconstruction, a subset of eight encodings from the postinjection data sets were used plus the preinjection image as the reference. For a comparison, results from the keyhole-Fourier reconstruction method [171] are also included. This method simply replaces the missing high-frequency encodings of the postinjection data sets with those from the reference preinjection data set, followed by conventional Fourier reconstruction.

As can be seen from Fig. 10.11, the keyhole-Fourier postinjection image appears to have the same resolution as the preinjection reference image, but the difference image suffers from the usual data truncation artifact. This means that the high-resolution images produced by the keyhole-Fourier method could be misleading, since they capture only low-resolution dynamic variations. This problem is significantly reduced in the GS image, since the dynamic image variations are produced at a much higher resolution. However, the GS model in the original form is not capable of reproducing the interimage variations at the resolution of the reference image either, as demonstrated in this example. This is because dynamic information in the GS model is contained exclusively in the series coefficients c_n. Since this model has only as many terms as the number of dynamic encodings, the dynamic information "registered" on the reference image may not have the same spatial resolution. This limitation can be alleviated by further improving the data acquisition and image reconstruction steps. For example, in some time-sequential imaging applications, it is possible to acquire two high-resolution images at different times of the dynamic imaging process such that their difference will reflect the dynamic signal changes. By building this difference image into the basis functions, one can reproduce the interimage variations at the resolution of the reference images [153].

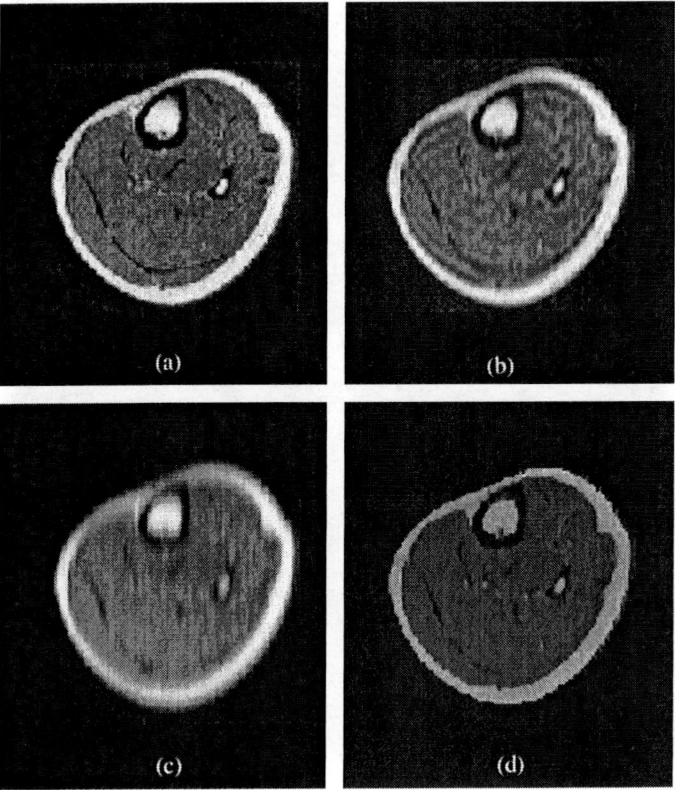

Figure 10.10   Cross-sectional images of a human leg. (a) The "gold standard" reconstructed from a data set with 256 encodings along both directions using the standard FFT method. The data set was truncated to 64 points along the vertical direction and then processed using three different reconstruction schemes: (b) the standard FFT, (c) the Hamming-windowed FFT, and (d) the GS model. Notice the ringing artifact in (b), the blurring artifact in (c), and the improvement of (d) over (b) and (c).

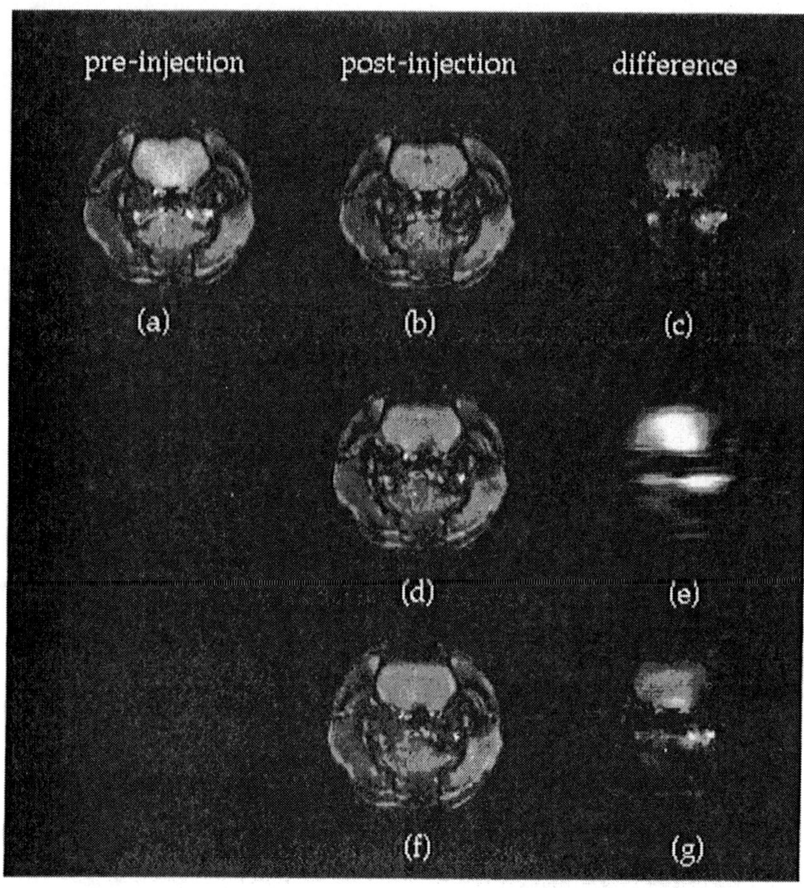

Figure 10.11 Cross-sectional images obtained from a rat during a dynamic study of an injected contrast agent: (a)-(c) high-resolution Fourier images reconstructed with 128 encodings along each direction; (d) and (f) postinjection images reconstructed with 8 postinjection encodings and the preinjection image as the reference using the keyhole-Fourier and GS modeling methods, respectively. The images in (c), (e) and (g) show the dynamic variations between the preinjection image and the corresponding postinjection image.

10.4 Appendix

This Appendix presents a brief review of several linear prediction (LP) estimation algorithms useful for determining the nonlinear parameters in a boxcar model introduced in Section 10.3.2.

Recall that a general boxcar model consisting of M boxcar functions can be expressed as[6]

$$C(x) = \sum_{m=1}^{M} a_m \Pi \left[\frac{x - \frac{1}{2}(\beta_m + \beta_{m+1})}{\beta_{m+1} - \beta_m} \right] \tag{10.100}$$

where it is assumed for convenience that $\beta_1 < \beta_2 < \cdots < \beta_{M+1}$. Fitting this model directly to a set of Fourier transform samples is a highly nonlinear problem. We describe here a linear prediction-based algorithm that can determine the nonlinear parameter β_m efficiently. After the β_m are known, the amplitude parameters a_m can be determined simply by solving a linear least-squares problem, which will not be discussed here.

First, noting that

$$\frac{dC(x)}{dx} = \sum_{m=1}^{p} \hat{a}_m \delta(x - \beta_m) \tag{10.101}$$

where $p = M + 1$ and

$$\begin{cases} \hat{a}_1 = a_1 \\ \hat{a}_m = a_m - a_{m-1} \quad \text{for } 2 \leq m < M \\ \hat{a}_{M+1} = -a_M \end{cases} \tag{10.102}$$

Let $S_c[n]$ be the sample values of the Fourier transform of $C(x)$

$$S_c[n] = \int_{-\infty}^{\infty} C(x) e^{-i2\pi n \Delta k x} \, dx \tag{10.103}$$

Then, based on the derivative property of the Fourier transform, we have

$$\hat{S}_c[n] = -i2\pi n \Delta k S_c[n] = \sum_{m=1}^{p} \hat{a}_m e^{-i2\pi n \Delta k \beta_m} \tag{10.104}$$

Finally, making use of the result in Example 10.3, we can state that the data sequence $\{\hat{S}_c[n]\}$ is $(M + 1)$th-order linearly predictable. Specifically, in the forward prediction form, we have

$$\hat{S}_c[n] = -\sum_{m=1}^{p} h_m \hat{S}_c[n - m] \tag{10.105}$$

---

[6]Note that only the magnitude part of this model should be used as the weighting function for the GS basis functions in Eq. (10.87).

for a proper set of coefficients h_m. An important consequence of Eq. (10.105) is that the corresponding characteristic polynomial given by

$$P(z) = 1 + h_1 z^{-1} + \cdots + h_p z^{-p} = 0 \qquad (10.106)$$

has roots on the unit circle of the z-plane, which are related to the edge locations β_m of the boxcar functions by

$$z_m = e^{-i2\pi \Delta k \beta_m}, \qquad m = 1, 2, \ldots, p \qquad (10.107)$$

This result suggests that the β_m can be determined efficiently by the way of finding the z_m.

Determining z_m from a given set of data is a classical LP estimation problem, for which a large number of algorithms have been proposed [46, 68, 79, 82]. In the ensuing discussion, we shall describe a few algorithms relevant to our problem. For notational simplicity, we use

$$d_n = \hat{S}_c[n - N/2] + e_n, \qquad n = 0, 1, \ldots, N - 1 \qquad (10.108)$$

to represent the available data that are corrupted by additive random noise e_n.

10.4.1   The Direct Least-Squares Method

According to Eqs. (10.105) and (10.108), we have

$$d_n \approx - \sum_{m=1}^{p} h_m d_{n-m} \qquad (10.109)$$

Let

$$\boldsymbol{h} = [h_p, h_{p-1}, \ldots, h_1]^T \qquad (10.110a)$$

$$\boldsymbol{d} = [d_p, d_{p+1}, \ldots, d_{N-1}]^T \qquad (10.110b)$$

$$\mathbf{D} = \begin{bmatrix} d_0 & d_1 & \cdots & d_{p-1} \\ d_1 & d_2 & \cdots & d_p \\ \vdots & \cdots & \cdots & \vdots \\ d_{N-p-1} & d_{N-p} & \cdots & d_{N-2} \end{bmatrix} \qquad (10.110c)$$

where it is usually true that $p < N - p$; therefore, there are more equations than unknowns in Eq. (10.109). Solving for $\boldsymbol{h}$ in the least-squares sense gives

$$\boldsymbol{h} = - \left(\mathbf{D}^H \mathbf{D} \right)^{-1} \mathbf{D}^H \boldsymbol{d} \qquad (10.111)$$

for which a number of numerical algorithms are available [31]. After the $\boldsymbol{h}$ is known, one can apply one of the polynomial rooting procedures to Eq. (10.106) to find the z_m [56].

10.4.2 SVD-Based Methods

Let us first review the basic concepts of singular value decomposition (SVD) of an arbitrary matrix $\mathbf{A}$. Assume that $\mathbf{A}$ is an M-by-N matrix. Its SVD is a product of three matrices

$$\mathbf{A} = \mathbf{U}\boldsymbol{\Sigma}\mathbf{V}^H \tag{10.112}$$

where $\mathbf{U}$ is an M-by-M unitary matrix, $\mathbf{V}$ is an N-by-N unitary matrix, and $\boldsymbol{\Sigma}$ is an M-by-N diagonal matrix. We may write these matrices as

$$\mathbf{U} = \begin{bmatrix} \boldsymbol{u}_1 & \boldsymbol{u}_2 & \cdots & \boldsymbol{u}_M \end{bmatrix} \tag{10.113a}$$

$$\mathbf{V} = \begin{bmatrix} \boldsymbol{v}_1 & \boldsymbol{v}_2 & \cdots & \boldsymbol{v}_N \end{bmatrix} \tag{10.113b}$$

$$\boldsymbol{\Sigma} = \mathrm{diag}\left[\lambda_1, \lambda_2, \ldots, \lambda_{\min\{M,N\}}\right] \tag{10.113c}$$

In this notation, the $\boldsymbol{u}_m$ and $\boldsymbol{v}_m$ are called the left and right singular vectors, respectively, and the λ_m (taking real and nonnegative values) are the singular values of $\mathbf{A}$. It is customary to order the λ_m such that $\lambda_1 \geq \lambda_2 \ldots \geq \lambda_{\min\{M,N\}}$. The SVD of $\mathbf{A}$ can also be expressed explicitly in terms of the $\boldsymbol{u}_m$, $\boldsymbol{v}_m$, and λ_m as

$$\mathbf{A} = \sum_{m=1}^{\min\{M,N\}} \lambda_m \boldsymbol{u}_m \boldsymbol{v}_m^H \tag{10.114}$$

where $\boldsymbol{u}_m \boldsymbol{v}_m^H$ represents the outer product of the two singular vectors. SVD has several desirable computational properties.

(a) The rank of $\mathbf{A}$ can be easily determined from its SVD. Specifically, rank($\mathbf{A}$) equals to the number of nonzero singular values of $\mathbf{A}$.

(b) The L_2-norm of $\mathbf{A}$ is given by

$$\|\mathbf{A}\|_2 = \sqrt{\sum_{m=1}^{\min\{M,N\}} \lambda_m^2} \tag{10.115}$$

(c) SVD is an effective computational tool for finding lower-rank approximations to a given matrix. Specifically, let $p < \mathrm{rank}(\mathbf{A})$. Then the rank p matrix $\mathbf{A}_p$ minimizing $\|\mathbf{A} - \mathbf{A}_p\|_2$ is given by

$$\mathbf{A}_p = \mathbf{U}\boldsymbol{\Sigma}_p\mathbf{V}^H = \sum_{m=1}^{p} \lambda_m \boldsymbol{u}_m \boldsymbol{v}_m^H \tag{10.116}$$

where $\boldsymbol{\Sigma}_p$ is obtained from matrix $\boldsymbol{\Sigma}$ after the singular values $\lambda_{p+1}, \lambda_{p+2}, \cdots$ are set to zero.

SVD was introduced to LP parameter estimation by Kumaresan and Tufts [179]. Their seminal work stimulated active research in this area in the 1980s, resulting in a large number of papers published on this topic. The following is a summary of these techniques; more detailed discussion can be found in the excellent review article by Kay and Marple [79].

10.4.2.1   The Original Kumaresan–Tufts Method

The Kumaresan–Tufts (KT) method (known as the LPSVD method in the MR literature) improves parameter estimation over the basic least-squares by the following two important steps.

First, we model the data with a higher-order linear predictor. Specifically, we assume that

$$d_n \approx - \sum_{m=1}^{\hat{p}} h_m d_{n-m} \tag{10.117}$$

where it is assumed that $\hat{p} \approx N/2 > p$. In matrix form, we have

$$\begin{bmatrix} d_0 & d_1 & \cdots & d_{\hat{p}-1} \\ d_1 & d_2 & \cdots & d_{\hat{p}} \\ \vdots & \cdots & \cdots & \vdots \\ d_{N-\hat{p}-1} & d_{N-\hat{p}} & \cdots & d_{N-2} \end{bmatrix} \begin{bmatrix} h_{\hat{p}} \\ h_{\hat{p}-1} \\ \vdots \\ h_1 \end{bmatrix} \approx - \begin{bmatrix} d_{\hat{p}} \\ d_{\hat{p}+1} \\ \vdots \\ d_{N-1} \end{bmatrix} \tag{10.118}$$

or

$$\mathbf{D}h \approx -d \tag{10.119}$$

Second, we find an optimal lower-rank approximation to $\mathbf{D}$. Note that in the noiseless case, $\mathrm{rank}(\mathbf{D}) = p$ (see Problem 10.18). With noisy data, $\mathbf{D}$ often becomes full rank. Restoring $\mathbf{D}$ to the closest rank p matrix will filter out some of the noise. Specifically, representing $\mathbf{D}$ in the SVD notation, we have

$$\mathbf{D} = \mathbf{U}\Sigma\mathbf{V}^H = \sum_{m=1}^{\min\{\hat{p}, N-\hat{p}\}} \lambda_m u_m v_m^H \tag{10.120}$$

The optimal rank p approximation to $\mathbf{D}$ is given by

$$\mathbf{D}_p = \sum_{m=1}^{p} \lambda_m u_m v_m^H \tag{10.121}$$

Replacing $\mathbf{D}$ with $\mathbf{D}_p$ in Eq. (10.119) gives

$$\mathbf{D}_p h \approx -d \tag{10.122}$$

Because h is now underdetermined by Eq. (10.122), the minimum-norm solution is often sought, which is given by

$$h = \sum_{m=1}^{p} \frac{1}{\lambda_m} (u_m^H d) v_m \tag{10.123}$$

After h is known, rooting the corresponding polynomial will give the desired values for z_m. Note that the KT method introduces $\hat{p} - p$ "extraneous" roots that need to be identified and removed. This is not necessary, however, for the boxcar model fitting because the additional edges associated with the extraneous roots can be absorbed into the model without creating a model instability problem if clustered edges are properly handled (see [186] for more details).

10.4.2.2   Total Least-Squares Method

In the original KT method, noise in d is not subject to numerical filtering by the truncated SVD and will perturb the accuracy of the estimated h. Moving d into the coefficient matrix results in the following homogeneous equation:

$$\begin{bmatrix} \mathbf{D} & \vdots & d \end{bmatrix} \begin{bmatrix} h \\ \cdots \\ 1 \end{bmatrix} \approx 0 \tag{10.124}$$

Noise in $\mathbf{D}$ as well as in d will be filtered by applying truncated-SVD to this new augmented coefficient matrix $\tilde{\mathbf{D}}$ and, thus the name *total-least-squares* (TLS) method [228]. Using the notation of Eq. (10.121), we can write the truncated coefficient matrix as

$$\tilde{\mathbf{D}}_p = \sum_{m=1}^{p} \lambda_m u_m v_m^H \tag{10.125}$$

Equation (10.124) then becomes

$$\mathbf{V}_p^H \begin{bmatrix} h \\ \cdots \\ 1 \end{bmatrix} \approx 0 \tag{10.126}$$

or

$$\mathbf{C}h \approx -c \tag{10.127}$$

where

$$\mathbf{C} = \begin{bmatrix} v_{11}^* & v_{21}^* & \cdots & v_{\hat{p}1}^* \\ v_{12}^* & v_{22}^* & \cdots & v_{\hat{p}2}^* \\ \vdots & \vdots & \cdots & \vdots \\ v_{1p}^* & v_{2p}^* & \cdots & v_{\hat{p}p}^* \end{bmatrix} \quad \text{and} \quad c = \begin{bmatrix} v_{(\hat{p}+1)1}^* \\ v_{(\hat{p}+1)2}^* \\ \vdots \\ v_{(\hat{p}+1)p}^* \end{bmatrix}$$

The minimum-norm solution for h is now given by

$$h = -\mathbf{C}^H (\mathbf{C}\mathbf{C}^H)^{-1} c \tag{10.128}$$

Making use of the identity

$$(\mathbf{C}\mathbf{C}^H)^{-1} = (\mathbf{I} - cc^H)^{-1} = \mathbf{I} + \frac{cc^H}{1 - \|c\|^2} \tag{10.129}$$

we get

$$h = -\mathbf{C}^H \left(\mathbf{I} + \frac{cc^H}{1 - \|c\|^2} \right) c \tag{10.130}$$

or

$$h = -\frac{\mathbf{C}^H c}{1 - \|c\|^2} \tag{10.131}$$

An equivalent expression can also be derived in terms of the noise singular vectors as

$$h = \frac{\tilde{\mathbf{C}}^H \tilde{c}}{\|\tilde{c}\|^2} \tag{10.132}$$

where

$$\tilde{\mathbf{C}} = \begin{bmatrix} v^*_{1(p+1)} & v^*_{2(p+1)} & \cdots & v^*_{p(p+1)} \\ v^*_{1(p+2)} & v^*_{2(p+2)} & \cdots & v^*_{p(p+2)} \\ \vdots & \vdots & \cdots & \vdots \\ v^*_{1(\hat{p}+1)} & v^*_{2(\hat{p}+1)} & \cdots & v^*_{p(\hat{p}+1)} \end{bmatrix} \quad \text{and} \quad \tilde{c} = \begin{bmatrix} v^*_{(\hat{p}+1)(p+1)} \\ v^*_{(\hat{p}+1)(p+2)} \\ \vdots \\ v^*_{(\hat{p}+1)(\hat{p}+1)} \end{bmatrix}$$

From expressions (10.131) or (10.132), one can see that the TLS method has a computational advantage over the KT method, since the former requires only the right singular vectors and thus eliminates the need for computing the full SVD.

10.4.2.3   The State-Space Method

The state-space formulation of the LP problem was initially developed by Kung, Arun, and Rao [180]. A more detailed and rigorous discussion of this method can be found in the review article [84]. This method has been used for NMR spectroscopic data processing, where it is called the HSVD method [92]. Following the derivation by Yan and Gore [276], one can treat the LP parameter estimation problem as finding a matrix $\mathbf{Z}$ satisfying

$$\mathbf{D}_b \mathbf{Z} = \mathbf{D}_t \tag{10.133}$$

where $\mathbf{D}_b$ and $\mathbf{D}_t$ are the matrices obtained by removing, respectively, the bottom and top rows of $\mathbf{D}$ constructed as follows,

$$\mathbf{D} = \begin{bmatrix} d_0 & d_1 & \cdots & d_{\hat{p}-1} \\ d_1 & d_2 & \cdots & d_{\hat{p}} \\ \vdots & \cdots & \cdots & \vdots \\ d_{N-\hat{p}} & d_{N-\hat{p}+1} & \cdots & d_{N-1} \end{bmatrix} \tag{10.134}$$

It can be shown that the solution to Eq. (10.133) is [276]

$$\mathbf{Z} = \begin{bmatrix} 0 & 0 & 0 & \cdots & 0 & -h_{\hat{p}} \\ 1 & 0 & 0 & \cdots & 0 & -h_{\hat{p}-1} \\ 0 & 1 & 0 & \cdots & 0 & -h_{\hat{p}-2} \\ \vdots & \vdots & \vdots & \cdots & \vdots & \vdots \\ 0 & 0 & 0 & \cdots & 1 & -h_1 \end{bmatrix} \tag{10.135}$$

where the h_m are defined through Eq. (10.118). Since the characteristic polynomial of $\mathbf{Z}$ is

$$\det(z\mathbf{I} - \mathbf{Z}) = \begin{vmatrix} z & 0 & 0 & \cdots & 0 & -h_{\hat{p}} \\ 1 & z & 0 & \cdots & 0 & -h_{\hat{p}-1} \\ 0 & 1 & z & \cdots & 0 & -h_{\hat{p}-2} \\ \vdots & \vdots & \vdots & \cdots & \vdots & \vdots \\ 0 & 0 & 0 & \cdots & 1 & -h_1 + z \end{vmatrix}$$

$$= z^{\hat{p}} + h_1 z^{\hat{p}-1} + \cdots + h_{\hat{p}} \tag{10.136}$$

the eigenvalues of $\mathbf{Z}$ provide exactly the desired roots of the LP characteristic polynomial but without explicitly solving for the polynomial coefficients h_m and the rooting step as is done in the KT or TLS methods. One further important result is that $\mathbf{D}_b$ and $\mathbf{D}_t$ in Eq. (10.133) can be replaced by the truncated left or right singular matrix of $\mathbf{D}$ without affecting the above property of $\mathbf{Z}$ [276]. For example, if the left truncated singular matrix $\mathbf{U}_p$ is used, the solution of $\mathbf{Z}$ from

$$\mathbf{U}_b \mathbf{Z} = \mathbf{U}_t \tag{10.137}$$

is given by [92]

$$\mathbf{Z} = \left(\mathbf{I} + \frac{\tilde{u}_{N-\hat{p}+1}^H \tilde{u}_{N-\hat{p}+1}}{1 - \|\tilde{u}_{N-\hat{p}+1}\|^2} \right) \mathbf{U}_b^H \mathbf{U}_t \tag{10.138}$$

where $\tilde{u}_{N-\hat{p}+1}$ is the $(N - \hat{p} + 1)$th row vector of $\mathbf{U}_p$ formed from the p principal left singular vectors of $\mathbf{D}$. A similar expression exists for the right singular vectors. The $\mathbf{Z}$ defined above has p eigenvalues, and they are exactly equal to the p signal roots of the KT linear predictor in the noiseless case. Therefore, one appealing feature of this state-space approach is that it directly gives the desired z_m values and thus no further measures are necessary to deal with the extraneous poles present in both the KT and TLS methods. Also, similar to the TLS method, this method requires only the left (or right) singular vectors and thus eliminates the need to compute the full SVD of $\mathbf{D}$.

Exercises

10.1 Describe the truncation effect of direct Fourier reconstruction from asymmetric k-space data.

10.2 Given that $\rho(x, y)$ is a real function, how many quadrants of k-space data are needed for its exact recovery?

10.3 Show that Ω_1 and Ω_2 defined in Eqs. (10.15) and (10.14), respectively, are convex sets.

10.4 Show that the points in any hyperplane form a convex set.

10.5 Show that $\wp_2$ defined in Eq. (10.18) is an orthogonal projection operator for Ω_2 but $\wp_1$ defined in Eq. (10.18) is not an orthogonal projection operator for Ω_1. *Note that if $\wp$ is an orthogonal projection operator of a convex set Ω, then $\|x - \wp x\| = \min_{y \in \Omega} \|x - y\|$.*

10.6 Show that the POCS method is identical to the conjugate symmetrization method when $\hat{\varphi}(x) = 0$.

10.7 Show that $\wp_1$ and $\wp_2$ defined by Eqs. (10.17) and (10.17) are nonexpansive operators.

10.8 In half-Fourier reconstruction, the phase constraint is estimated from the central symmetric portion of the measured k-space data. Assume that the phase constraint is calculated using the entire asymmetric data set as follows:

$$\hat{\varphi}(x) = \arg \left\{ \sum_{n=-n_0}^{N-1} \hat{S}[n] e^{-i 2\pi n \Delta k x} \right\}$$

Discuss what would happen to the Margosian and POCS half-Fourier reconstructions with this phase constraint.

10.9 Discuss why the support bandlimitedness constraint will have no extrapolation effect when $\Delta k = 1/W_x$, where Δk is the sampling interval of the k-space data from a one-dimensional object of width W_x.

10.10 Implement and test the bandlimited extrapolation algorithm.

10.11 The more random a variable is, the more entropy it will have. True or false?

10.12 Let $I[n] = \{0, 0, 3, 3, 3, 1, 1, 2\}$. Calculate the entropy of this image function according to the definitions in Eqs. (10.44) and (10.49), respectively.

10.13　Implement and test the maximum entropy reconstruction method.

10.14　What is parametric image reconstruction?

10.15　The transfer function of a digital filter is given by

$$H(z) = \frac{b_0 + b_1 z + \cdots + b_q z^q}{1 + a_1 z + \cdots + a_p z^p}$$

Let ϵ_n be the input excitation sequence to the filter and d_n be the resulting output data sequence. Show that

$$d_n = -\sum_{m=1}^{p} a_m d_{n-m} + \sum_{m=0}^{q} b_m \epsilon_{n-m}$$

10.16　Let

$$I(x) = \frac{\sum_{m=0}^{q} b_m e^{i2\pi m \Delta k x}}{1 + \sum_{m=1}^{p} a_m e^{i2\pi m \Delta k x}}$$

and

$$S(k) = \int_{-\frac{1}{2\Delta k}}^{\frac{1}{2\Delta k}} I(x) e^{-i2\pi k x} \, dx$$

Show that

$$S[n] = -\sum_{m=1}^{p} a_m S[n-m] + \frac{1}{\Delta k} \sum_{m=0}^{q} b_m \delta_{n-m}$$

where $S[n] = S(n\Delta k)$ and δ_n is the Kronecker delta function.

10.17　Let

$$d_n = a_1 e^{-i2\pi f_1 n} + a_2 e^{-i2\pi f_2 n}$$

(a)　Show that

$$d_n = -h_1 d_{n-1} - h_2 d_{n-2}$$

where

$$\begin{cases} h_1 = -e^{-i2\pi f_1} - e^{-i2\pi f_2} \\ h_2 = e^{-i2\pi (f_1 + f_2)} \end{cases}$$

(b)　Determine the two roots of $P(z) = 1 + h_1 z^{-1} + h_2 z^{-2}$.

10.18 Let

$$d_n = \sum_{m=1}^{p} c_m z_m^n$$

and

$$\mathbf{D} = \begin{bmatrix} d_0 & d_1 & \cdots & d_{\hat{p}} \\ d_1 & d_2 & \cdots & d_{\hat{p}+1} \\ \vdots & \cdots & \cdots & \vdots \\ d_{N-\hat{p}-1} & d_{N-\hat{p}} & \cdots & d_{N-1} \end{bmatrix}$$

where it is assumed that $\hat{p} > p$ and $N - \hat{p} < p$. Show that

$$\text{rank}(\mathbf{D}) = p$$

Appendix A

Mathematical Formulas

For easy reference, this appendix summarizes some commonly used mathematical formulas.

A.1 Sums

$$\sum_{n=0}^{N} r^n = \frac{r^{N+1} - 1}{r - 1} \qquad r \neq 1$$

$$\sum_{n=0}^{\infty} r^n = \frac{1}{1 - r} \qquad r < 1$$

A.2 Power Series

$$f(x) = f(x_0) + \frac{x - x_0}{1!} f'(x_0) + \frac{(x - x_0)^2}{2!} f^{(2)}(x_0) + \cdots$$

$$e^x = 1 + x + \frac{x^2}{2!} + \frac{x^3}{3!} + \cdots$$

$$\sin x = x - \frac{x^3}{3!} + \frac{x^5}{5!} - \frac{x^7}{7!} + \cdots$$

$$\cos x = 1 - \frac{x^2}{2!} + \frac{x^4}{4!} - \frac{x^6}{6!} + \cdots$$

$$\frac{1}{1 - x} = 1 + x + x^2 + x^3 + \cdots \qquad |x| < 1$$

A.3   Complex Numbers

$$e^{\pm\theta} = \cos\theta \pm i\sin\theta$$

$$a + ib = re^{i\theta}, \quad \text{where } r = \sqrt{a^2 + b^2} \text{ and } \theta = \tan^{-1}(b/a)$$

$$(re^{i\theta})^n = r^n e^{in\theta}$$

$$(r_1 e^{i\theta_1})(r_2 e^{i\theta_2}) = r_1 r_2 e^{i(\theta_1 + \theta_2)}$$

A.4   Trigonometric Identities

$$\cos x = \tfrac{1}{2}\left(e^{ix} + e^{-ix}\right)$$

$$\sin x = \tfrac{1}{2}\left(e^{ix} - e^{-ix}\right)$$

$$\cos(x \pm \tfrac{\pi}{2}) = \mp \sin x$$

$$\sin x \cos x = \tfrac{1}{2}\sin 2x$$

$$\sin^2 x + \cos^2 x = 1$$

$$\cos^2 x - \sin^2 x = \cos 2x$$

$$\cos^2 x = \tfrac{1}{2}(1 + \cos 2x)$$

$$\sin^2 x = \tfrac{1}{2}(1 - \cos 2x)$$

$$\sin(x \pm y) = \sin x \cos y \pm \cos x \sin y$$

$$\cos(x \pm y) = \cos x \cos y \mp \sin x \sin y$$

$$\tan(x \pm y) = \frac{\tan x \pm \tan y}{1 \mp \tan x \tan y}$$

$$\sin x \sin y = \tfrac{1}{2}[\cos(x - y) - \cos(x + y)]$$

$$\cos x \cos y = \tfrac{1}{2}[\cos(x - y) + \cos(x + y)]$$

$$\sin x \cos y = \tfrac{1}{2}[\sin(x - y) + \sin(x + y)]$$

$$a \cos x + b \sin b = r \cos(x + \theta)$$

$$\text{where } r = \sqrt{a^2 + b^2} \text{ and } \theta = \tan^{-1}(b/a)$$

A.5   Short Tables of Convolutions

Tables A.5a and A.5b list several pairs of functions (g and h) and their resulting convolution $g * h$.

Table A.5a   Continuous Convolution

$g(t)$	$h(t)$	$g(t) * h(t)$
$g(t)$	$\delta(t - t_0)$	$g(t - t_0)$
$e^{\alpha t} u(t)$	$u(t)$	$\dfrac{1}{\alpha}(e^{\alpha t} - 1)u(t)$
$u(t)$	$u(t)$	$tu(t)$
$e^{\alpha_1 t} u(t)$	$e^{\alpha_2 t} u(t)$	$\dfrac{1}{\alpha_1 - \alpha_2}(e^{\alpha_1 t} - e^{\alpha_2 t})u(t)$
$e^{\alpha t} u(t)$	$e^{\alpha t} u(t)$	$te^{\alpha t} u(t)$
$te^{\alpha t} u(t)$	$e^{\alpha t} u(t)$	$\frac{1}{2}t^2 e^{\alpha t} u(t)$

Table A.5b   Discrete Convolution

$g[n]$	$h[n]$	$g[n] * h[n]$
$g[n]$	$\delta(n - n_0)$	$g[n - n_0]$
$\alpha^n u[n]$	$u[n]$	$\dfrac{1}{1 - \alpha}(1 - \alpha^{n+1})u[n]$
$u[n]$	$u[n]$	$(n + 1)u[n]$
$\alpha_1^n u[n]$	$\alpha_2^n u[n]$	$\dfrac{1}{\alpha_1 - \alpha_2}(\alpha_1^{n+1} - \alpha_2^{n+1})u[n]$
$\alpha^n u[n]$	$\alpha^n u[n]$	$(n + 1)\alpha^n u[n]$

A.6   A Short Table of Fourier Transforms

$g(t)$	$\int_{-\infty}^{\infty} g(t) e^{-i2\pi ft}\, dt$
$\delta(t)$	1
1	$\delta(f)$
$u(t)$	$\frac{1}{2}\delta(f) + \dfrac{1}{i2\pi f}$
$\operatorname{sgn}(t)$	$\dfrac{1}{i\pi f}$
$e^{-at}u(t)$	$\dfrac{1}{a + i2\pi f} \quad a > 0$
$e^{-a|t|}u(t)$	$\dfrac{2a}{a^2 + 4\pi^2 f^2}$
$xe^{-at}u(t)$	$\dfrac{1}{(a + i2\pi f)^2} \quad a > 0$
$t^n e^{-at}u(t)$	$\dfrac{n!}{(a + i2\pi f)^{n+1}} \quad a > 0$
$e^{-i2\pi f_0 t}$	$\delta(t - t_0)$
$\cos(2\pi f_0 t)$	$\frac{1}{2}[\delta(f + f_0) + \delta(f - f_0)]$
$\cos(2\pi f_0 t)u(t)$	$\frac{1}{4}[\delta(f + f_0) + \delta(f - f_0)] + \dfrac{i2\pi f}{(2\pi f_0)^2 - (2\pi f)^2}$
$\sin(2\pi f_0 t)$	$\frac{i}{2}[\delta(f + f_0) - \delta(f - f_0)]$
$\sin(2\pi f_0 t)u(t)$	$\frac{i}{4}[\delta(f + f_0) - \delta(f - f_0)] + \dfrac{2\pi f_0}{(2\pi f_0)^2 - (2\pi f)^2}$
$e^{-at}\cos(2\pi f_0 t)u(t)$	$\dfrac{a + i2\pi f}{(2\pi f_0)^2 + (a + i2\pi f)^2} \quad a > 0$
$e^{-at}\sin(2\pi f_0 t)u(t)$	$\dfrac{2\pi f_0}{(2\pi f_0)^2 + (a + i2\pi f)^2} \quad a > 0$
$\Pi(t)$	$\operatorname{sinc}(\pi f)$
$\Lambda(t)$	$\operatorname{sinc}^2(\pi f)$
$\displaystyle\sum_{n=-\infty}^{\infty} \delta(t - n\Delta t)$	$\dfrac{1}{\Delta t}\displaystyle\sum_{n=-\infty}^{\infty} \delta\left(f - n\dfrac{1}{\Delta t}\right)$

Appendix B

Glossary

This appendix presents a glossary of technical terms used in this book. Note that some of the terms have broader meanings than are described here in the context of MRI applications. For a comprehensive glossary of MR terms, the reader is referred to a publication by the American College of Radiology: *Glossary of MR terms* (4th ed., ACR, Reston, VA, 1995).

Aliasing: Image error due to undersampling of k-space. In Fourier reconstruction, aliasing manifests itself as folding over (ghosting) of some parts of the object. In projection reconstruction, angular undersampling results in streaking artifacts.

Angiography: Application of MRI techniques to produce images of blood vessels.

Angular frequency: Frequency of oscillation or rotation commonly measured in radians/second.

Angular momentum: Inertial property of a rotating body that, in the absence of external forces (torques), tends to maintain the same axis of rotation. When an external torque is applied to a rotating body, the angular momentum changes, resulting in precession.

Angular velocity: Vector quantity specifying both the speed and direction of object rotation.

Artifacts: Spurious image features caused by imperfections in the imaging instrumentation and/or technique.

Asymmetric k-space sampling: Collection of more data points on one side of the k-space origin than on the other. This data acquisition scheme is often used in half-Fourier imaging experiments.

Bandlimited function: A function is called *frequency* bandlimited if its Fourier transform has nonzero values only inside a finite frequency band, whereas a function is said to be *space* bandlimited if it has nonzero values only over a finite spatial interval.

Bandwidth: Frequency interval over which the Fourier transform of a (frequency) bandlimited function has nonzero values.

Backprojection: Mathematical operation that maps a one-dimensional function (*projection profile*) to a higher-dimensional function by assigning (*backprojecting*) the value of each point in the projection to a line, or a plane, or a hyperplane.

Birdcage coil: RF volume coils with the appearance of a birdcage designed to produce homogeneous B_1 fields.

Bloch equations: Phenomenological equations of motion for the macroscopic magnetization vector in the presence of a magnetic field, including the effects of precession and relaxations.

Boltzmann distribution: If a system of particles that are able to exchange energy in collisions is in thermal equilibrium, then the relative number of particles, N_1 and N_2, in two particular energy states with corresponding energies, E_1 and E_2, is given by

$$\frac{N_1}{N_2} = e^{-(E_1 - E_2)/(KT)}$$

where K is the Boltzmann constant and T is absolute temperature.

Burst pulse: A sequence of uniform low flip-angle RF pulses used to excite a spin system for fast imaging.

Carr–Purcell sequence: RF pulse sequence consisting of a 90° pulse followed by a string of uniform 180° pulses to produce a train of spin echoes.

Carr–Purcell–Meiboom–Gill sequence: Modified Carr-Purcell sequence with a 90° phase shift in the rotating frame of reference between the 90° pulse and the subsequent 180° pulses to reduce accumulating effects of imperfections in the 180° pulses.

Chemical shift: Shifts in resonance frequency of a given nucleus when bound to different sites in a molecule, due to the magnetic shielding effects of the orbiting electrons. The amount of frequency shift is proportional to magnetic field strength and is usually specified in parts per million (ppm) of the resonance frequency relative to a reference.

Chemical shift artifact: Image artifact in the form of spatial shifts of regions along the frequency-encoding direction when the regions contain different chemical shifts.

Circular navigator: See *navigator echoes*.

Coil: Single or multiple loops of wire (or other electrical conductor, such as tubing, etc.) designed either to produce a magnetic field from current flowing through the wire or to detect a changing magnetic field by voltage induced in the wire.

Convolution: Mathematical operation between two functions, denoted by $*$ and defined, in the continuous case, by

$$f(t) * g(t) = \int_{-\infty}^{\infty} f(\tau)g(t - \tau)d\tau$$

or, in the discrete case, by

$$f_n * g_n = \sum_{m=-\infty}^{\infty} f_m g_{n-m}$$

Convolution kernel: In $f * g$, g is called the convolution kernel for f or f is the convolution kernel for g, depending on the context. For example, if $f * g$ is taken to be the output of a linear system with input f, then g is the kernel function, which is also called *point spread function* in imaging, because $f * g = g$ if $f = \delta$, a point source.

Data acquisition time: Time required to acquire an image, which equals to the product of the number of different encoded signals N_{enc}, the excitation repetition time T_R, and the number of signal averagings for each encoded signal N_{acq}.

DC artifact: A bright point in the center of an image caused by a constant offset in signal intensity of measured k-space data.

Demodulation: Conversion of the raw NMR signal to a lower frequency signal by removing the carrier signal.

Dephasing gradient: Magnetic field gradient pulse used to create spatial variations in the phase of transverse magnetization.

Diamagnetic: A substance that will slightly decrease a magnetic field when placed within it (its magnetization is oppositely directed to the magnetic field, that is, with a small negative magnetic susceptibility).

Diffusion: The process by which molecules or other particles intermingle and migrate as a result of their random thermal motion.

Echo: A form of NMR signal consisting of a recalled transient signal and a natural transient signal. Also see *gradient echo*, *spin echo*, and *stimulated echo*.

Echo-planar imaging: Ultra-fast imaging schemes that collects a complete set of two-dimensional k-space data from a single excitation.

Eddy currents: Electric currents induced in a conductor by a changing magnetic field or by motion of the conductor through a magnetic field.

Entropy: A measure of randomness of a random variable, or the uncertainty (or information content) of a random event.

Ergodic process: A stochastic process in which ensemble averages are equivalent to time sample averages.

Ernst angle: The RF excitation angle of a short-T_R spoiled steady-state sequence, at which the resulting signal is maximum.

Excitation: Putting energy into a nuclear spin system.

Expansive operator: An operator $\wp$ is called expansive if it amplifies the norm (magnitude), that is, $||\wp x|| > ||x||$.

Extended phase graph: Graph tool to show the phase evolution of the transverse and longitudinal magnetizations as a function of time.

Extrapolation: The mathematical process of extending the definition domain of a function.

Fast Fourier transform: An efficient algorithm to compute a discrete Fourier transform.

Feasible reconstruction: Any image function that is consistent with the measured data.

Ferromagnetic: A substance, such as iron, that has a large positive magnetic susceptibility.

Filtered backprojection: Mathematical technique used for image reconstruction from a set of projection profiles. It essentially involves filtering the projection profiles by suitable filter function and then backprojecting the filtered projections into image space.

Finite sampling: Acquisition of a finite number of samples or measurements from a continuous function or a physical process.

Flip angle: Amount of rotation of the bulk magnetization vector produced by an RF pulse, with respect to the direction of the static magnetic field.

Forced precession: Precession of the bulk magnetization about the excitation RF field.

Fourier transform: Integral transform whose kernel function is a complex sinusoidal function; a mathematical tool to separate out the frequency components of a signal from its temporal or spatial variations.

Fourier transform imaging: Imaging technique that collects raw data directly in the Fourier space. In MRI, the definition is narrower; it refers to techniques that sample the Fourier space in a rectilinear fashion so that the measured data can be processed directly by the discrete Fourier transform for image formation.

Free induction decay: Transient MR signal produced by the free precession of the transverse magnetization vector after an RF pulse has been switched off. The signal decays exponentially with a characteristic time constant T_2 (or T_2^*).

Free precession: Precession of the bulk magnetization vector about the static magnetic field after a pulse excitation. Free precession of the transverse magnetization at the Larmor frequency is responsible for the detectable NMR signal.

Frequency encoding: Technique to establish a *linear* correspondence between the spatial location and the oscillating frequency of an NMR signal.

Frequency-selective RF pulse: An RF pulse containing energy only within a specific frequency interval.

Gibbs artifact: Signal error associated with the approximation of a discontinuous function by a truncated Fourier series. This artifact is characterized by spurious ringings near the area of discontinuities.

Gradient coil: Current-carrying coil designed to produce a desired magnetic field gradient so that the magnetic field will be stronger in some location than others.

Gradient echo: Echo signal generated by first dephasing and then rephasing the transverse magnetization with a bipolar gradient pulse.

Gradient magnetic field: Magnetic field that changes in strength in a certain given direction. Magnetic field gradients are usually denoted by G_x, G_y, and G_z, where the subscripts represent the spatial direction along which the field strength changes.

Gradient pulse: Briefly applied gradient magnetic field.

Gyromagetic ratio: Physical constant measuring the ratio of the magnetic moment to the angular momentum of a particle.

Hahn echo: Echo signals created by multiple RF pulses.

Hard pulse: Short intense RF pulse; also see *nonselective pulse.*

Helmholtz coil: Pair of current-carrying coils used to create uniform magnetic field in the space between them.

Image contrast: The relative difference in image intensity of different tissues.

Inversion pulse: A 180° RF pulse that cause precessing nuclei to shift to the opposite state.

Inversion–recovery sequence: RF pulse sequence that applies a 180° inversion pulse before each 90° excitation pulse.

Inversion time: Time interval between the middle of a inversion pulse and that of the subsequent 90° excitation pulse in inversion-recovery pulse sequence.

Isochromat: A group of spins with the same resonance frequency.

K**-space:** Spatial-frequency domain; it is the mathematical space in which the Fourier transform of a spatial function is represented.

K**-space trajectory:** The path traced in k-space when a transient time signal is mapped to k-space by a magnetic field gradient function.

Laboratory frame: The Cartesian coordinates (x, y, z) that are stationary with respect to the observer.

Larmor equation: Equation relating the resonance frequency of a nuclear magnetic moment to the magnetic field it experiences via the gyromagnetic ratio, usually written as $\omega_0 = \gamma B_0$.

Larmor frequency: The frequency at which resonance can be induced from a nuclear spin system.

Line shape: Distribution of the relative strength of resonance as a function of frequency, which forms a particular spectral line.

Line width: Spread in frequency of a resonance line in an NMR spectrum. A common measure of line width is the full width at half-maximum of a resonance peak.

Linear navigator: See *navigator echoes*.

Longitudinal magnetization: Component of the macroscopic magnetization vector pointing along the direction of the static magnetic field.

Longitudinal relaxation: See *spin-lattice relaxation*.

Longitudinal relaxation time: See *spin-lattice relaxation time*.

Lorentzian line: Spectral line shape characterized by a narrow peak and long tails, with amplitude proportional to $1/[1/T_2^2 + (f - f_0)^2]$, where f is the frequency variable and f_0 is the frequency of the peak (i.e., central resonance frequency).

Magnetic field: The region surrounding a magnet (or current-carrying conductor) is endowed with certain properties. One is that a small magnet in such a region experiences a torque that tends to align it in a given direction. Magnetic field is a vector quantity whose direction is defined as the direction in which the north pole of the small magnet points when in equilibrium.

Magnetic moment: A measure of the net magnetic properties of an object or particle. A nucleus with an intrinsic spin will have an associated magnetic moment, so that it will interact with a magnetic field.

Magnetic resonance: See *nuclear magnetic resonance.*

Magnetic resonance imaging: Methods whereby NMR signals are spatially encoded using magnetic field gradients so that spatial distribution of a sample's NMR properties, such as spin density and relaxation times, can be reconstructed and presented in an image format.

Magnetic resonance spectroscopy: Method to obtain NMR spectra displaying chemically shifted resonance peaks that provide information on the chemical species present in the system and their relative concentrations.

MR spectroscopic imaging: MR imaging techniques to obtain spatially resolved NMR spectra.

Magnetic susceptibility: Measure of the ability of a substance to become magnetized.

Magnetization: Magnetic polarization of a material produced by a magnetic field (magnetic moment per unit volume).

Navigator echoes: Auxiliary echoes collected in the imaging process for detection of object motions or other purposes. Navigator echoes collected along a straight line in k-space are called *linear navigators*; similarly, navigator echoes collected along a circle centered at the k-space origin are called *circular* (or *orbital*) *navigators*.

NMR signal: Electrical (voltage) signal in the radio-frequency range produced by a precessing transverse magnetization.

Nonselective pulse: RF pulse with large frequency bandwidth that excites all nuclei of a particular type indiscriminately.

Nuclear magnetic resonance: The absorption or emission of electromagnetic energy by nuclei in a static magnetic field, after excitation by a suitable RF magnetic field.

Nuclear spin: An intrinsic property of certain nuclei that gives them an associated characteristic angular momentum and magnetic moment.

Nuclear spin quantum number: See *spin quantum number.*

Nyquist frequency: The critical sampling frequency of a signal beyond which aliasing will occur in the sampling process. The frequency is twice the maximum frequency of a bandlimited signal.

Nyquist interval: Inverse of Nyquist frequency. The critical sampling interval of a signal beyond which information loss will occur in the sampling process.

Off resonance: A state occurring when the Larmor frequency of a spin isochromat is different from that of an excitation RF field.

On resonance: A state occurring when the Larmor frequency of a spin isochromat matches that of an excitation RF field.

Paramagnetic: A substance with a small but positive magnetic susceptibility (magnetizability). The addition of a small amount of paramagnetic substance may greatly reduce the relaxation times of water. Typical paramagnetic substances usually possess an unpaired electron; examples are atoms or ions of transition elements, rare earth elements, some metals, and some molecules, including molecular oxygen and free radicals. Paramagnetic substances are considered promising for use as contrast agents in MR imaging.

Permanent magnet: Magnet whose magnetic field originates from permanently magnetized material.

Permeability: Tendency of a substance to concentrate magnetic field.

Partial saturation: Excitation technique applying repeated RF pulses in times on the order of or shorter than T_1.

Phase coherence: Maintenance of a constant phase relationship among all spin isochromats.

Phase encoding: Technique to establish a linear relationship between the spatial location and the phase of an NMR signal.

Phase sensitive detector: A detector whose output is the product of the input signal and a sinusoidal reference signal so that it depends on the amplitude of the input signal and its phase relative to the reference.

Pixel: Picture element.

Point spread function: See *convolution kernel.*

Precession: Comparatively slow gyration of the axis of a spinning body caused by the application of a torque. The magnetic moment of a nucleus with spin will experience such a torque when inclined at an angle to the magnetic field, resulting in precession at the Larmor frequency. Another example is the effect of gravity on the motion of a spinning top or gyroscope.

Precession frequency: See *Larmor frequency.*

Pulse length (width): The time duration of an RF pulse.

Pulse sequences: A timed diagram showing RF and/or gradient pulses used to manipulate a spin system.

Quadrature detection: Method to detect NMR signals that employs two phase-sensitive detectors, one measuring the x-component of the magnetization and the other measuring the y-component. The reference signals are 90° out of phase.

Radon transform: Mathematical operation to generate projection profiles from an object function by line, or planar, or hyperplanar integrals.

Receiver coil: RF coil converting a rotating magnetization to an electrical voltage signal.

Relaxation times: NMR time constants characterizing the longitudinal (spin-lattice) and transverse (spin-spin) relaxations. Most frequently mentioned are T_1, T_2, and T_2^*. T_1 (spin-lattice relaxation time) is a measure of the time required for a spin system to return to thermal equilibrium with its surroundings (lattice) following perturbations (e.g., by an RF pulse). T_2 (spin-spin relaxation time) is a measure of the decay time of the transverse magnetization due to spin-spin interactions; T_2^* accounts for the effect of both T_2 decay and magnetic field inhomogeneities.

Rephasing gradient: Magnetic field gradient pulse, of opposite polarity to the previously applied dephasing gradient, to rephase transverse magnetization. It is usually used for generation of a gradient-echo signal.

Resistive magnet: Magnet whose magnetic field originates from current flowing through an ordinary (nonsuperconducting) conductor.

Resonance frequency: Frequency at which the resonance phenomenon occurs; given by the Larmor equation for a nuclear spin system.

RF coil: Coil used to generate RF pulses and/or detect MR signals from a rotating magnetization. Commonly used are birdcage coils, saddle coils, and solenoid coils.

RF pulse: Burst of oscillating magnetic field rotating in the radio-frequency range about the direction of the static magnetic field.

Rotating frame of reference: Cartesian coordinate system (x', y', z') whose transverse plane is rotating about the z-axis with respect to the laboratory frame.

Rotating frame zeugmatography: Technique of MR imaging that uses a gradient of the RF excitation field (to give a corresponding variation of the flip angle along the gradient as a means of encoding the spatial location of spins in the direction of the RF field gradient) in conjunction with a static gradient magnetic field (to give spatial encoding in an orthogonal direction). It can be considered to be a form of Fourier transform imaging.

Saturation: A nonequilibrium state of a spin system, in which equal numbers of spins are aligned against and with the magnetic field, so that there is no net magnetization.

Saturation-recovery sequence: Particular type of pulse sequence in which the preceding pulses leave the spins in a state of saturation, so that recovery at the time of the next pulse has taken place from an initial condition of no magnetization.

Selective excitation: Frequency-selective RF pulses used to excite all but a desired region, such as a plane.

Shim coils: Coils carrying a relatively small current that are used to provide auxiliary magnetic fields to compensate for inhomogeneities in the main static magnetic field.

Shimming: Correction of inhomogeneities in the main static magnetic field.

Sinc pulse: RF pulse whose envelope is a sinc function.

Singular value decomposition: Generalized eigen decomposition of a rectangular matrix.

Slice selection: Excitation of spins in a predetermined plane using a selective RF pulse in the presence of a field gradient.

Soft pulse: RF pulses with a smooth envelope; also see *frequency-selective RF pulse* and *tailored pulse*.

Solenoid coil: A coil of wire wound in the form of a long cylinder. When a current is passed through the coil, it produces a relatively uniform magnetic field within the coil.

Spin: The intrinsic angular momentum of an elementary particle, or system of particles such as a nucleus. The spins of nuclei have characteristic fixed values. Pairs of neutrons and protons align to cancel out their spins (Pauli exclusion principle), so that nuclei with an odd number of neutrons and/or protons will have a net angular momentum, known as nuclear spin.

Spin echo: Echo signal generated by multiple RF pulses that refocus the dephased transverse magnetization.

Spin-echo imaging: MR imaging techniques in which spin-echo signals rather than the FID signals are used.

spin-lattice relaxation: The process by which the longitudinal magnetization returns to its equilibrium value after excitation; it involves exchange of energy between the nuclear spins and the lattice.

spin-lattice relaxation time: The characteristic time constant for nuclear spins to realign themselves with the external magnetic field. Starting from zero, the bulk magnetization will grow 63% of its final maximum value in a time T_1.

Spin quantum number: Property of all nuclei related to the largest measurable component of the nuclear angular momentum. Nonzero values of nuclear angular momentum are quantized (fixed) as integral or half-integral multiples of $(h/2)$, where h is Planck's constant. The number of possible energy states for a given nucleus in a fixed magnetic field is equal to $2I + 1$.

spin-spin relaxation: The process by which the transverse magnetization decays to zero due to spin-spin interactions resulting in a loss of phase coherence.

spin-spin relaxation time: The time constant characterizing spin-spin relaxation process. Starting from a nonzero value, the transverse magnetization will decay to 37% of its initial value in a time T_2.

Spin-warp imaging: Fourier transform imaging in which phase-encoding gradient pulses are applied for a constant duration but with varying amplitude, in contrast to the original FT imaging method in which phase encoding is performed by applying gradient pulses of constant amplitude but varying duration.

Spiral imaging: Ultra-fast imaging schemes that collect k-space data in spiral trajectories.

Spoiler gradient pulse: Magnetic field gradient pulse applied to effectively destroy a transverse magnetization by producing a rapid phase variation along the gradient direction.

Steady-state free precession: Method of MR excitation in which a sequence of uniform RF pulses are applied with interpulse intervals that are short compared to both T_1 and T_2.

Stimulated echo: A form of spin echo produced by a sequence of three RF pulses, appearing at a time delay after the third pulse, which is equal to the interval between the first two pulses.

Superconducting magnet: Magnet whose magnetic field originates from current flowing through a superconducting coil.

Surface coil: RF coil that is placed close to the surface of the object being imaged.

It increases signal-to-noise for regions close to the coil.

Tailored pulse: RF pulse whose envelope is varied with time in a predetermined manner, for example, a sinc function.

Thermal equilibrium: A state in which all parts of a system are at the same effective temperature. In thermal equilibrium, relative numbers of nuclear spins at different energy states is given by the Boltzmann distribution.

Tip angle: See *flip angle*.

Transceiver coil: RF coil used as both a transmitter and a receiver.

Transmitter coil: RF coil that produces an oscillating magnetic field.

Transverse magnetization: Component of the macroscopic magnetization vector at right angles to the static magnetic field.

Transverse relaxation: See *spin-spin relaxation*.

Transverse relaxation time: See *spin-spin relaxation time*.

Truncation artifact: Image artifact due to the loss of high spatial frequency data. With the Fourier reconstruction method, it manifests itself as image blurring and spurious ringing near sharp edges.

Vector: A quantity with both magnitude and direction.

Volume imaging: Imaging techniques in which NMR signals are gathered simultaneously from the whole object volume to be imaged.

Voxel: Volume element.

Zero-filled FFT: A data sequence is padded with zeros at one or both ends before the FFT algorithm is applied.

Zeugmatography: The original name given to MRI by Lauterbur.

Appendix C

Abbreviations

ARMA	Autoregressive moving average
ART	Algebraic reconstruction techniques
BP	Backprojection
CP	Carr–Purcell (sequence)
CPMG	Carr–Purcell–Meiboom–Gill (sequence)
CSI	Chemical shift imaging
CT	Computerized tomography
DANTE	Delays Alternating with Nutations for tailored excitation
DFT	Discrete Fourier transform
DIME	Dynamic imaging by model estimation
EPI	Echo-planar imaging
FBP	Filtered backprojection
fe	Frequency encoding
FFT	Fast Fourier transform (algorithm)
FID	Free induction decay
FISH	Fast Imaging with Steady-state Precession
FLASH	Fast Low-Angle SHot
FSE	Fast spin echo
FT	Fourier transform
FOV	Field of view
FWHM	Full width at half-maximum
G	Gauss
GE	Gradient echo
GPC	Ghost phase cancellation
GRASS	Gradient Recalled Acquisition in the Steady State
GS	Generalized series
Hz	Hertz (1 cycle/second)
IR	Inversion recovery
K	Kevin
kHz	Kilo Hertz
LP	Linear prediction

MEG	Magnetoencephalography
MHz	Mega Hertz
MR	Magnetic resonance
MRI	Magnetic resonance imaging
MRS	Magnetic resonance spectroscopy
NMR	Nuclear magnetic resonance
pe	Phase encoding
POCS	Projection onto convex set
ppm	Parts per million
PS	Partial saturation
PSD	Phase-sensitive detection
PSF	Point spread function
RARE	Rapid Acquisition with Relaxation Enhancement
RF	Radio frequency
RIGR	Reduced-encoding imaging by generalized-series reconstruction
s	Second
SAR	Synthetic aperture radar
SE	Spin echo
SNR (S/N)	Signal-to-noise ratio
SPECT	Single photon emission computed tomography
ss	Slice selection; steady state
SSFP	Steady-state free precession
STE	Stimulated echo
SVD	Singular value decomposition
T	Tesla

Appendix D

Mathematical Symbols

The following is a partial list of symbols used in the book. A few symbols are used for more than one purpose, and their meaning should be interpreted in the context.

$\vec{A}$, $\vec{a}$, and $\boldsymbol{a}$	Vector quantities
$\mathbf{A}$	Matrix
A_{E}	Maximum amplitude of an echo signal
A_{f}	Maximum amplitude of an FID signal
B	Magnetic field
B_0	Static magnetic field
B_1	Radio-frequency (RF) field
$B_{1,\mathrm{rot}}$	RF field in the rotating frame
B_1^e	Pulse envelope function
B_{eff}	Effective magnetic field in the rotating frame
B_G	Gradient field
B_r	Receiver sensitivity
$\mathrm{comb}(x)$	Comb function
$\mathrm{Dir}(N, x)$	$\sin(Nx)/\sin x$
E	Mathematical expectation operator
$E_\uparrow$	Spin energy in the pointing-up state
$E_\downarrow$	Spin energy in the pointing-down state
f_{max}	Frequency bandwidth of a time signal
f_{s}	Sampling frequency
$\mathcal{F}$, $\mathcal{F}^{-1}$	Forward/inverse Fourier transforms
$\mathcal{F}_m$, $\mathcal{F}_m^{-1}$	m-dimensional forward and inverse Fourier transforms
G_{fe}	Frequency-encoding gradient
G_{pe}	Phase-encoding gradient
G_{ss}	Slice-select gradient
G_x, G_y, G_z	Field gradients along the x-, y-, and z- directions
$G(\mu, \sigma, x)$	Gaussian window function

$h, \hbar = \frac{h}{2\pi}$	Planck's constant
$\mathcal{H}$	Shannon entropy
I	Spin quantum number
$\vec{i}, \vec{j}, \vec{k}$	Unit directional vectors of the x-, y-, and z-axes
$\vec{i}', \vec{j}', \vec{k}'$	Unit direction vectors of the x'-, y'-, and z'-axes
$\Im$	Taking the imaginary part of a complex number
$I(\cdot)$	Image function
$\mathbf{I}$	Identity matrix
$\vec{J}$	Angular momentum
$\mathbf{J}$	Jacobian matrix
$J_n(x)$	Bessel functions
k, k_x, k_y, k_z	Spatial frequency variables
K	Boltzmann's constant
$\vec{M}$	Bulk magnetization vector
$\vec{M}_{\mathrm{rot}}$	Bulk magnetization vector in the rotating frame
M_x, M_y, M_z	Components of $\vec{M}$
$\vec{M}_{xy} \triangleq M_x\vec{i} + M_y\vec{j}$	Transverse magnetization
$M_{xy} \triangleq M_x + iM_y$	Complex transverse magnetization
$M_{x'}, M_{y'}, M_{z'}$	Components of $\vec{M}_{\mathrm{rot}}$
$\vec{M}_{x'y'} \triangleq M_{x'}\vec{i}' + M_{y'}\vec{j}'$	Rotating frame transverse magnetization
$M_{x'y'} \triangleq M_{x'} + iM_{y'}$	Rotating frame complex transverse magnetization
M_z^0	Thermal equilibrium value of $\vec{M}$ established by B_0
$M_{x'}(0_-)$	Prepulse value of $M_{x'}$
$M_{y'}(0_-)$	Prepulse value of $M_{y'}$
$M_{z'}(0_-)$	Prepulse value of $M_{z'}$
$M_{x'y'}(0_-)$	Prepulse value of $M_{x'y'}$
$M_{x'}(0_+)$	Postpulse value of $M_{x'}$
$M_{y'}(0_+)$	Postpulse value of $M_{y'}$
$M_{z'}(0_+)$	Postpulse value of $M_{z'}$
$M_{x'y'}(0_+)$	Postpulse value of $M_{x'y'}$
m_I	Magnetic quantum number
$N_\uparrow, N_\downarrow$	Number of spins pointing up and down, respectively
N_s	Total number of spins in a sample
$p(f)$	Frequency selection profile of an RF pulse
$p_s(\cdot)$	Slice selection profile of an RF pulse
$P(p, \phi)$	Projections of an object
$\Re$	Taking the real part of a complex number
$\mathcal{R}, \mathcal{R}^{-1}$	Forward/inverse Radon transforms
$\mathcal{R}_m, \mathcal{R}_m^{-1}$	m-dimensional forward and inverse Radon transforms
$\mathbb{R}^n$	n-dimensional Euclidean space
$\mathbf{R}_{x'}(\alpha), \mathbf{R}_{y'}(\alpha), \mathbf{R}_{z'}(\alpha)$	Rotation matrix about the x'-, y'-, and z'-axes
$\mathrm{sgn}(x)$	Sign function

$\text{sinc}(x)$	$\sin x / x$
$S(k)$	k-space signal
$S(t)$	Measured time signal
T_1	Longitudinal relaxation time constant
T_2, T_2^*	Transverse relaxation time constants
T_{acq}	Data acquisition interval
T_{E}	Echo time
T_{I}	Inversion time in an inversion-recovery sequence
T_{pe}	Phase-encoding interval
T_{R}	Repetition time in an imaging sequence
T_{s}	Absolute temperature of a spin system
$V(t)$	Induced voltage signal
$V_{\text{psd}}(t)$	Voltage signal from a phase-sensitive detector
$u(\cdot)$	Unit step function
$w(\cdot)$	Window function
W_h	Effective width of $h(\cdot)$
W_x, W_y, W_z	Spatial support bounds of an object
x, y, z	Axes of the laboratory frame
x', y', z'	Axes of the rotating frame
α	Flip angle
δ	Shielding constant
$\delta(x)$	Dirac delta function
$\delta(n)$	Kronecker delta function
$\Delta k, \Delta k_x, \Delta k_y, \Delta k_z$	k-space sampling interval
Δt	Time sampling interval
$\Delta x, \Delta y, \Delta z$	Pixel size
$\Delta x_{\text{F}}, \Delta y_{\text{F}}, \Delta z_{\text{F}}$	Fourier pixel size
$\gamma, \curlyvee = \frac{\gamma}{2\pi}$	Gyromagnetic ratio
μ	Mean value of a Gaussian function
$\vec{\mu}$	Magnetic moment vector
μ_x, μ_y, μ_z	Components of $\vec{\mu}$
$\hat{\mu}$	Unit directional vector
$\vec{\mu}_{\text{G}}$	Gradient direction
$\vec{\mu}_{\text{s}}$	Slice direction
φ	Azimuthal angle; initial pulse angle
ϕ	Projection angle
$\Phi(t)$	Magnetic flux through a receiver coil
ω_0	Larmor frequency corresponding to the B_0 field
ω_1	Precessional frequency about the B_1 field
ω_{rf}	Excitation frequency of the RF field
ω_{eff}	Precessional frequency about the B_{eff} field
$\rho(\cdot)$	Spin density function
σ	Standard deviation

σ_d	Standard deviation of data noise
σ_I	Standard deviation of image noise
τ	Time interval between the 90°- and 180°-pulse
τ_p	Time duration of an RF pulse
∇	Gradient operator $\nabla \equiv \vec{i}\frac{\partial}{\partial x} + \vec{j}\frac{\partial}{\partial y} + \vec{k}\frac{\partial}{\partial z}$
$\Lambda(x)$	Triangular window function
$\Pi(x)$	Rectangular window function
$\cdot$	Dot product of vectors
$*$	Convolution operator (or Hermitian symmetry operator when used as a superscript)
$**$	Two-dimensional convolution
$***$	Three-dimensional convolution

Appendix E

Physical Constants

Boltzmann constant (K): Universal constant that relates macroscopic parameter to an absolute temperature; $K = 1.38 \times 10^{-23}$ J/K

Gyromagnetic ratio (γ): The ratio of the magnetic moment to the angular momentum of a particle. This constant is nucleus-specific; its values for some NMR-active nuclei are given in the following table.

$\gamma/2\pi$	^{1}H	^{13}C	^{19}F	^{31}P
MHz/T	42.58	10.71	40.05	11.26

Planck constant (h): Constant of proportionality (6.6×10^{-34} J-s) that relates the amount of energy emitted or absorbed by a photon to its oscillation frequency.

Bibliography

Books

1. A. Abragam, *Principles of Nuclear Magnetism*, Oxford University Press, New York, 1989.

2. G. Arfken, *Mathematical Methods for Physicists*, 3rd Ed., Academic Press, New York, 1985.

3. H. C. Andrew and B. R. Hunt, *Digital Image Restoration*, Prentice-Hall, Englewood Cliffs, NJ, 1977.

4. R. A. Blahut, *Fast Algorithms for Digital Signal Processing*, Addison-Wesley Publishing Company, Reading, MA, 1985.

5. M. Bertero and P. Boccacci, *Introduction to Inverse Problems in Imaging*, Institute of Physics Publishing, Bristol and Philadelphia, 1998.

6. R. N. Bracewell, *The Fourier Transform and Its Applications*, McGraw-Hill, New York, 1986.

7. E. O. Brigham, *The Fast Fourier Transform*, Prentice-Hall, Englewood Cliffs, NJ, 1974.

8. M. J. Bronskill and P. Sprawls, eds., *The Physics of MRI: 1992 AAPM Summer School Proceedings*, American Institute of Physics, Woodbury, NY, 1993.

9. B. Buck and V. A. Macaulay, eds. *Maximum Entropy in Action*, Oxford University Press, New York, 1991.

10. S. C. Bushong, *Magnetic Resonance Imaging: Physical and Biological Principles*, C. V. Mosby Company, St. Louis, 1988.

11. P. T. Callaghan, *Principles of Nuclear Magnetic Resonance Microscopy*, Oxford University Press, New York, 1991.

12. D. Canet, *Nuclear Magnetic Resonance: Concepts and Methods*, John Wiley & Sons, New York, 1996.

13. C.-N. Chen and D. I. Hoult, *Biomedical Magnetic Resonance Technology*, IOP Publishing Ltd., New York, 1989.

14. Z.-H. Cho, J. P. Jones, and M. Singh, *Foundations of Medical Imaging*, John Wiley & Sons, New York, 1993.

15. T. M. Cover and J. A. Thomas, *Elements of Information Theory*, John Wiley & Sons, New York, 1991.

16. S. R. Deans, *The Radon Transform and Some of Its Applications*, John Wiley & Sons, New York, 1983.

17. J. D. de Certaines, W. M. M. J. Bovée, and F. Podo, eds., *Magnetic Resonance Spectroscopy in Biology and Medicine: Functional and Pathological Tissue Characterization*, Pergamon Press, Oxford, 1992.

18. E. Feig, ed., *Advances in Magnetic Resonance Imaging*, Vol. I, Ablex Publishing Corporation, Norwood, NJ, 1989.

19. P. Diehl, E. Fluck, H. Günther, R. Kosfeld, and J. Seelig, eds., *In-Vivo Magnetic Resonance Spectroscopy I: Probeheads and Radiofrequency Pulses, Spectrum Analysis*, Springer-Verlag, New York, 1992.

20. P. Diehl, E. Fluck, H. Günther, R. Kosfeld, and J. Seelig, eds., *In-Vivo Magnetic Resonance Spectroscopy II: Localization and Spectral Editing*, Springer-Verlag, New York, 1992.

21. P. Diehl, E. Fluck, H. Günther, R. Kosfeld, and J. Seelig, eds., *In-Vivo Magnetic Resonance Spectroscopy III: Potential and Limitations*, Springer-Verlag, New York, 1992.

22. A. D. Elster, *Questions and Answers in Magnetic Resonance Imaging*, Mosby-Year Book, St. Louis, 1994.

23. R. R. Ernst, G. Bodenhausen, and A. Wokaun, *Principles of Nuclear Magnetic Resonance in One and Two Dimensions*, Oxford University Press, New York, 1991.

24. R. Fletcher, *Practical Methods of Optimization*, John Wiley & Sons, New York, 1987.

25. E. Fukushima and S. B. W. Roeder, *Experimental Pulse NMR: A Nuts and Bolts Approach*, Addison-Wesley Publishing Company, Reading, MA, 1981.

26. D. G. Gadian, *NMR and its Applications to Living Systems*, 2nd ed., Oxford University Press, Oxford, 1995.

27. D. M. Grant and R. K. Harris, eds., *Encyclopedia of Nuclear Magnetic Resonance, Vol. 1: Historical Perspective*, John Wiley & Sons, New York, 1996.

28. E. M. Haacke, R. W. Brown, M. R. Thompson, and R. Venkatesan, *Magnetic Resonance Imaging: Physical Principles and Sequence Design*, John Wiley & Sons, New York, 1999.

29. R. H. Hashemi and W. G. Bradley, Jr., *MRI: The Basics*, Williams & Williams, Baltimore, MD, 1997.

30. J. C. Hoch and A. S. Stern, *NMR Data Processing*, John Wiley & Sons, New York, 1996.

31. G. H. Golub and C. F. Van Loan, *Matrix Computations*, 2nd ed., Johns Hopkins University Press, Baltimore, MD, 1989.

32. G. T. Herman, *Image Reconstruction from Projection: The Fundamentals of Computerized Tomography*, Academic Press, New York, 1980.

33. S. W. Homans, *A Dictionary of Concepts in NMR*, Oxford University Press, New York, 1989.

34. J. Jin, *Electromagnetic Analysis and Design in Magnetic Resonance Imaging*, CRC Press, New York, 1998.

35. A. C. Kak and M. Slaney, *Principles of Computerized Tomographic Imaging*, IEEE Press, Piscataway, NJ, 1988.

36. P. A. Jansson, *Deconvolution with Applications in Spectroscopy*, Academic Press, New York, 1984.

37. J. H. Justice, ed., *Maximum Entropy and Bayesian Methods in Applied Statistics*, Cambridge University Press, New York, 1986.

38. C. L. Lawson and R. J. Hanson, *Solving Least Squares Problems*, Prentice-Hall, Englewood Cliffs, NJ, 1987.

39. D. Le Bihan, ed., *Diffusion and Perfusion Magnetic Resonance Imaging: Applications to Functional MRI*, Raven Press, New York, 1995.

40. A. Macovski, *Medical Imaging Systems*, Prentice-Hall, Englewood Cliffs, NJ, 1983.

41. S. Mallat, *A Wavelet Tour of Signal Processing*, Academic Press, New York, 1998.

42. P. Mansfield and P. G. Morris, *NMR Imaging in Biomedicine*, Academic Press, New York, 1982.

43. J. A. Markisz and J. P. Whalen, *Principles of MRI*, Appleton & Lange, Stamford, CT, 1998.

44. R. J. Marks II, *Introduction to Shannon Sampling and Interpolation Theory*, Springer-Verlag, New York, 1991.

45. R. J. Marks II, ed., *Advanced Topics in Shannon Sampling and Interpolation Theory*, Springer-Verlag, New York, 1993.

46. S. L. Marple Jr., *Digital Spectral Analysis with Applications*, Prentice-Hall, Englewood Cliffs, NJ, 1987.

47. J. Mattson and M. Simon, *The Pioneers of NMR and Magnetic Resonance in Medicine*, Bar-Ilan University Press, Israel (in the USA by Dean Books Co., Jericho, NY), 1996.

48. P. G. Morris, *Nuclear Magnetic Resonance Imaging in Medicine and Biology*, Oxford University Press, New York, 1986.

49. M. NessAiver, *All You Really Need to Know about MRI Physics*, Simply Physics, 5816 Narcissus Ave, Baltimore, MD, 1997.

50. T. H. Newton and D. G. Potts, eds., *Modern Neuroradiology, Volume II: Advanced Imaging Techniques*, Clavadel Press, San Anselmo, CA, 1993.

51. A. Papoulis, *Signal Analysis*, McGraw-Hill, New York, 1977.

52. A. Papoulis, *Probability, Random Variables, and Stochastic Processes*, 2nd ed., McGraw-Hill, New York, 1984.

53. A. M. Parikh, *Magnetic Resonance Imaging Techniques*, Science Publishing Company, New York, 1992.

54. J. A. Parker, *Image Reconstruction in Radiology*, CRC Press, Boca Raton, FLA, 1990.

55. E. J. Potchen, E. M. Haacke, J. E. Siebert, and A. Gottschalk, *Magnetic Resonance Angiography: Concepts and Applications*, Mosby-Year Book, St. Louis, 1993.

56. W. H. Press, B. P. Flannery, S. A. Teukolsky, and W. T. Vetterling, *Numerical Recipes in C: The Art of Scientific Computing*, 2nd ed., Cambridge University Press, New York 1992.

57. A. Rahman and M. I. Choudhary, *Solving Problems with NMR Spectroscopy*, Academic Press, New York, 1996.

58. W. J. Schempp, *Magnetic Resonance Imaging: Mathematical Foundations and Applications*, John Wiley & Sons, New York, 1998.

59. D. Shaw, *Fourier Transform NMR Spectroscopy*, 2nd ed., Elsevier Science Publishing Company, New York, 1984.

60. C. P. Slichter, *Principles of Magnetic Resonance*, 3rd ed., Springer-Verlag, New York, 1990.

61. R. C. Smith, R. C. Lange, eds., *Understanding Magnetic Resonance Imaging*, CRC Press LLC, 1998.

62. D. D. Stark and W. G. Bradley, Jr., *Magnetic Resonance Imaging*, vols. 1 and 2, 2nd ed., Mosby-Year Book, St. Louis, 1992.

63. H. Stark, *Image Recovery: Theory and Application*, Academic Press, New York, 1987.

64. S. R. Thomas and R. L. Dixon, eds., *NMR in Medicine: The Instrumentation and Clinical Applications*, American Association of Physicists in Medicine, 1986.

65. M. T. Vlaardingerbroek and J. A. Den Boer, *Magnetic Resonance Imaging: Theory and Practice*, Springer-Verlag, Berlin, 1996.

66. F. W. Wehrli, *Fast-Scan Magnetic Resonance: Principles and Applications*, Raven Press, New York, 1991.

67. S. W. Young, *Nuclear Magnetic Resonance Imaging: Basic Principles*, Raven Press, New York, 1984.

Major Review Articles

68. J. A. Cadzow, "Spectral estimation: An overdetermined rational model equation approach," *Proc. IEEE*, vol. 70, pp. 907–938, 1980.

69. Z. H. Cho, Y. M. Ro, and I. K. Hong, "FM DANTE fast imaging and variations: Emerging rf-based ultrafast imaging techniques," *Concepts Magn. Reson.*, vol. 10, pp. 33–54, 1998.

70. M. S. Cohen and R. M. Weisskoff, "Ultra-fast imaging," *Magn. Reson. Imag.*, vol. 9, pp. 1–37, 1991.

71. I. Daubechies, "Orthonormal bases of compactly supported wavelets," *Comm. Pure Appl. Math.*, vol. 41, pp. 909–996, 1988.

72. J. L. Duerk and O. P. Simonetti, "Review of MRI gradient waveform design methods with application in the study of motion," *Concepts Magn. Reson.*, vol. 5, No. 2, pp. 105–122, 1993.

73. E. M. Haacke, P. A. Wielopolski, and J. A. Tkach, "A comprehensive technical review of short T_R, fast, magnetic resonance imaging," *Rev. Magn. Reson. Imag.*, vol. 3, pp. 53–170, 1991.

74. E. L. Hahn, "Echo phenomena and nonlinearity," *Concepts Magn. Reson.*, vol. 6, pp. 193–199, 1994.

75. F. J. Harris, "On the use of windows for harmonic analysis with the discrete Fourier transform," *Proc. IEEE*, vol. 66, pp. 51–83, 1978.

76. R. M. Henkelman and M. J. Bronskill, "Artifacts in magnetic resonance imaging," *Rev. Magn. Reson. Med.*, vol. 2, pp. 1–126, 1987.

77. J. Hennig, "Echoes—How to generate, recognize, use or avoid them in MR imaging sequences, Part I: Fundamental and not so fundamental properties of spin echoes," *Concepts Magn. Reson.*, vol. 3, pp. 125–143, 1991.

78. J. Hennig, "Echoes—How to generate, recognize, use or avoid them in MR imaging sequences, Part I: Echoes in imaging sequences," *Concepts Magn. Reson.*, vol. 3, pp. 179–192, 1991.

79. S. M. Kay and S. L. Marple Jr., "Spectrum analysis—A modern perspective," *Proc. IEEE*, vol. 69, pp. 1380–1419, 1981.

80. Z.-P. Liang, F. Boada, T. Constable, E. M. Haacke, P. C. Lauterbur, and M. R. Smith, "Constrained reconstruction methods in MR imaging," *Rev. Magn. Reson. Med.*, vol. 4, pp. 67–185, 1992.

81. J. Listerud, S. Einstein, E. Outwater, and H. Y. Kressel, "First principles of fast spin echo," *Magn. Reson. Quarterly,* vol. 8, pp. 199–244, 1992.

82. J. Makhoul, "Linear prediction: A tutorial review," *Proc. IEEE*, vol. 63, pp. 561–580, 1975.

83. R. J. Nelson, Y. Maguire, D. F. Caputo, G. Leu, Y. Kang, M. Pravia, D. Tuch, Y. S. Winstein, D. G. Cory, "Counting echoes: Application of a complete reciprocal-space description of NMR spin dynamics," *Concepts Magn. Reson.*, vol. 10, pp. 331–341, 1998.

84. B. D. Rao and K. S. Arun, "Model based processing of signals: A state space approach," *Proc. IEEE*, vol. 80, pp. 283–309, 1992.

Articles

85. A. B. Ahn, J. H. Kim, and Z. H. Cho, "High-speed spiral-scan echo planar NMR imaging—I," *IEEE Trans. Med. Imag.*, vol. MI-5, pp. 1–6, 1986.

86. S. Amartur and E. M. Haacke, "Modified iterative model based on data extrapolation method to reduce Gibbs ringing," *J. Magn. Res. Imag.*, vol. 1, pp. 307–317, 1991.

87. S. Amartur, Z.-P. Liang, F. Boada, and E. M. Haacke, "A phase constrained data extrapolation method to reduce Gibbs ringing," *J. Magn. Reson. Imag.*, vol. 1, pp. 721–724, 1991.

88. D. Atkinson, D. L. G. Hill, P. N. Stoyle, P. E. Summers, and S. F. Keevil, "Automatic correction of motion artifacts in magnetic resonance images using an entropy focus criterion," *IEEE Trans. Med. Imag.*, vol. 16, pp. 903–910, 1997.

89. H. Barkhuijsen, R. D. Beer, W. M. M. J. Bovee, J. H. N. Creyghton, and D. Van Ormondt, "Application of linear prediction and singular value decomposition (LPSVD) to determine NMR frequencies and intensities from the FID," *J. Magn. Reson.*, vol. 62, pp. 86–89, 1985.

90. H. Barkhuijsen, R. D. Beer, and D. V. Ormondt, "Aspects of the computational efficiency of LPSVD," *J. Magn. Reson.*, vol. 64, pp. 343–346, 1985.

91. H. Barkhuijsen, R. D. Beer, and D. V. Ormondt, "Error theory for time-domain signal analysis with linear prediction and singular value decomposition," *J. Magn. Reson.*, vol. 67, pp. 371–375, 1986.

92. H. Barkhuijsen, R. D. Beer, and D. V. Ormondt, "Improved algorithm for noniterative time-domain model fitting to exponentially damped magnetic resonance signals," *J. Magn. Reson.*, vol. 73, pp. 553–557, 1987.

93. C. W. Barnes, "Object restoration in a diffraction-limited imaging system," *J. Opt. Soc. Am. A*, vol. 56, pp. 575–578, 1966.

94. I. Barrowdale and R. E. Erickson, "Algorithms for least squares prediction and maximum entropy spectral analysis—Part I: Theory," *Geophysics*, vol. 43, pp. 420–432, 1980.

95. I. Barrowdale and R. E. Erickson, "Algorithms for least squares prediction and maximum entropy spectral analysis—Part II: Fortran program," *Geophysics*, vol. 43, pp. 433–446, 1980.

96. E. M. Bellon, E. M. Haacke, P. E. Coleman, D. C. Sacco, D. A. Steiger, and R. E. Gangarosa, "MR artifacts: A review," *Am. J. Roentgenol.*, vol. 147, 1271-1281, 1986.

97. M. A. Dernstein, D. M. Thomasson, and W. H. Perman, "Improved detectability in low signal-to-noise ratio magnetic resonance images by means of a phase corrected real construction," *Med. Phys.*, vol. 16, pp. 813–817, 1989.

98. F. Bloch, "Nuclear induction," *Phys. Rev.*, vol. 70, pp. 460–474, 1946.

99. N. Bloembergen, E. M. Purcell, and R. V. Pound, "Relaxation effects in nuclear magnetic resonance absorption," *Phys. Rev.*, vol. 73, pp. 679–712, 1948.

100. L. Bolinger and J. Leigh, "Hadamard spectroscopic imaging (HSI) for multivolume localization," *J. Magn. Reson.*, vol. 80, pp. 162–167, 1988.

101. Y. Bresler and A. Macovski, "Three-dimensional reconstruction from projections with incomplete and noisy data by object estimation," *IEEE Trans. Acoust., Speech, Signal Process.*, vol. ASSP-35, pp. 1139–1152, 1986.

102. M. J. Bronskill, E. R. McVeigh, W. Kucharczyk, and R. M. Henkelman, "Syrinx-like artifacts on MR images of the spinal cord," *Radiology*, vol. 166, pp. 485–488, 1988.

103. H. R. Brooker, T. H. Mareci, and J. Mao, "Selective Fourier transform localization," *Magn. Reson. Med.*, vol. 5, pp. 417–433, 1987.

104. T. R. Brown, B. M. Kincaid, and K. Ugurbil, "NMR chemical shift imaging in three dimensions," *Proc. Natl. Acad. Sci. USA*, vol. 79, pp. 3523–3526, 1982.

105. J. R. Bunch, "Stability of methods for solving Toeplitz systems of equations," *SIAM J. Sci. Stat. Comput.*, vol. 6, pp. 349–364, 1985.

106. S. F. Burch, S. F. Gull, and J. Skilling, "Image restoration by a powerful maximum entropy method," *Computer Vision, Graphics, and Image Process.*, vol. 23, pp. 113–128, 1983.

107. J. A. Cadzow, "An extrapolation procedure for band-limited signals," *IEEE Trans. Acoust., Speech, Signal Process.*, vol. ASSP-27, pp. 4–12, 1979.

108. P. T. Callaghan and C. D. Eccles, "Sensitivity and resolution in NMR imaging," *J. Magn. Reson.*, vol. 71, pp. 426–445, 1987.

109. Y. Cao and D. N. Levin, "Imaging with spatially variable resolutions," *J. Magn. Reson. Imag.*, vol. 2, pp. 701–709, 1992.

110. Y. Cao and D. N. Levin, "Feature-recognizing MRI," *Magn. Reson. Med.*, vol. 30, pp. 305–317, 1993.

111. Y. Cao, D. N. Levin, and L. Yao, "Locally focused MRI," *Magn. Reson. Med.*, vol. 34, pp. 858–867, 1995.

112. Y. Cao and D. N. Levin, "On the relationship between feature-recognizing MRI and MRI encoded by singular value decomposition," *Magn. Reson. Med.*, vol. 33, pp. 140–142, 1995.

113. Y. Cao and D. N. Levin, "Using an image database to constrain the acquisition and reconstruction of MR images of the human brain," *IEEE Trans. Med. Imag.*, vol. 14, pp. 350–361, 1995.

114. Y. Cao and D. N. Levin, "Using prior knowledge of human anatomy to constrain MR image acquisition and reconstruction," *Magn. Reson. Imag.*, vol. 15, pp. 669–677, 1997.

115. H. Y. Carr and E. M. Purcell, "Effects of diffusion on free precession in nuclear magnetic resonance experiments," *Phys. Rev.*, vol. 94, pp. 630–638, 1954.

116. H. Y. Carr, "Steady-state free precession in nuclear magnetic resonance," *Phys. Review*, vol. 112, pp. 1693–1701, 1958.

117. S. Chavez and Q. S. Xiang, "Efficient ghost suppression by analytical gradient energy minimization," *Proc. 6th Ann. Conf. Int. Soc. Magn. Reson. Med.*, p. 132, 1998.

118. S. Chavez and Q. S. Xiang, "Fast ghost suppression using 1.5 or fewer excitations," *Proc. 7th Ann. Conf. Int. Soc. Magn. Reson. Med.*, p. 239, 1999.

119. S. Chavez and Q. S. Xiang, "Improved ghost suppression by two-parameter gradient energy minimization," *Proc. 7th Ann. Conf. Int. Soc. Magn. Reson. Med.*, p. 1999, 1999.

120. Z. H. Cho, H. S. Kim, H. B. Song, and J. Cumming, "Fourier transform nuclear magnetic resonance tomographic imaging," *Proc. IEEE*, vol. 70, pp. 1152–1173, 1982.

121. H. Choi and D. C. Munson Jr., "Direct-Fourier reconstruction in tomography and synthetic aperture radar," *Int. J. Imag. Syst. Techn.*, vol. 9, pp. 1–13, 1998.

122. R. T. Constable and R. M. Henkelman, "Why MEM does not work in MR image reconstruction," *Magn. Reson. Med.*, vol. 14, pp. 12–25, 1990.

123. R. T. Constable and R. M. Henkelman, "Contrast, resolution, and detectability," *J. Comp. Assist. Tomogr.*, vol. 15, pp. 297–303, 1991.

124. R. T. Constable and R. M. Henkelman, "Data extrapolation for truncation artifact removal," *Magn. Reson. Med.*, vol. 17, pp. 108–118, 1991.

125. R. T. Constable, A. W. Anderson, J. Zhong, and J. C. Gore, "Factors influencing contrast in fast spin-echo imaging," *Magn. Reson. Imag.*, vol. 10, pp. 497–511, 1992.

126. J. W. Cooley and J. W. Tukey, "An algorithm for the machine computation of complex Fourier series," *Mathematics of Computation*, vol. 19, pp. 297–301, 1965.

127. A. P. Crawley, M. L. Wood, and R. M. Henkelman, "Elimination of transverse coherence in FLASH MRI," *Magn. Reson. Med.*, vol. 8, pp. 248–260, 1988.

128. J. J. Cuppen and A. Van Est, "Reducing MR imaging time by one-sided reconstruction," *Topical Conference on Fast MRI Techniques*, Cleveland, 1987.

129. B. C. De Simone, F. De Luca, and B. Maraviglia, "Maximum entropy method in phase-encoding NMR imaging," *Magn. Reson. Med.*, vol. 4, 78-82, 1987.

130. B. C. De Simone, F. De Luca, and B. Maraviglia, "Maximum entropy and 2DFT NMR images,*Magn. Reson. Med.*, vol. 8, 332-339, 1988.

131. E. J. Diethorn and D. C. Munson, Jr., "A linear, time-varying system framework for noniterative discrete-time band-limited signal extrapolation," *IEEE Trans. Acoust., Speech, Signal Process.*, vol. ASSP-39, pp. 55–68, 1992.

132. G. T. di Francia, "Resolving power and information," *J. Opt. Soc. Am. A*, vol. 45, pp. 497–501, 1955.

133. D. L. Donoho, I. M. Johnstone, A. S. Stern, and J. C. Hoch, "Does the maximum entropy method improve sensitivity," *Proc. Natl. Acad. Sci. USA*, vol. 87, pp. 5066–5068, 1990.

134. W. A. Edelstein, G. H. Glover, C. J. Hardy, and K. W. Redington, "The intrinsic signal-to-noise ratio in NMR imaging," *Magn. Reson. Med.*, vol. 3, pp. 604–618, 1986.

135. R. L. Ehman and J. P. Felmlee, "Adaptive technique for high-resolution MR imaging of moving structures," *Radiology*, vol. 173, pp. 255–263, 1989.

136. R. R. Ernst and W. A. Anderson, "Application of Fourier transform spectroscopy to magnetic resonance," *Rev. Sci. Instrum.*, vol. 37, pp. 93–102, 1966.

137. F. Farzaneh, S. J. Riederer, and N. J. Pelc, "Analysis of T_2 limitations and off-resonance effects on spatial resolution and artifacts in echo-planar imaging," *Magn. Reson. Med.*, vol. 14, pp. 123–139, 1990.

138. D. A. Feinberg, J. D. Hale, J. C. Watts, L. Kaufman, and A. Mark, "Halving MR imaging time by conjugation: Demonstration at 3.5 kG," *Radiology*, vol. 161, pp. 527–531, 1986.

139. Z. W. Fu, Y. Wang, R. C. Grimm, P. J. Rossman, J. P. Felmlee, S. J. Riederer, and R. L. Ehman, "Orbital navigator echoes for motion measurements in magnetic resonance imaging," *Magn. Reson. Med.*, vol. 34, pp. 746–753, 1995.

140. R. W. Gerchberg, "Superresolution through error energy reduction," *Opt. Acta,* vol. 21, pp. 709–720, 1974.

141. G. H. Glover and J. M. Pauly, "Projection reconstruction techniques for reduction of motion artifacts," *Magn. Reson. Med.,* vol. 28, pp. 275–289, 1992.

142. G. H. Golub and V. Pereyra, "The differentiation of pseudo-inverses and non-linear least squares problems whose variables separate," *SIAM J. Numer. Anal.,* vol. 10, 413-432, 1973.

143. R. Gordon, "A tutorial on ART (Algebraic Reconstruction Techniques)," *IEEE Trans. Nucl. Sci.,* vol. NS-21, pp. 78–93, 1974.

144. S. Gull and J. Daniel, "Image reconstruction from incomplete and noisy data," *Nature,* vol. 272, 686-690, 1978.

145. S. F. Gull and J. Skilling, "Maximum entropy method in image processing," *Proc. IEE,* Pt. F, vol. 131, 646-659, 1984.

146. E. M. Haacke, "The effects of finite sampling in spin-echo or field-echo magnetic resonance imaging," *Magn. Reson. Med.,* vol. 4, 407-421, 1987.

147. E. M. Haacke, "Solving for nonideal conditions in two-dimensional Fourier transform magnetic resonance imaging using a generalized inverse transform," *Inverse Problems,* vol. 3, 421-435, 1987.

148. E. M. Haacke, Z.-P. Liang, and S. H. Izen, "Constrained reconstruction: A superresolution optimal signal-to-noise alternative to the Fourier transform," *Med. Phys.,* vol. 16, 388-397, 1989.

149. E. M. Haacke, J. A. Tkach, and T. B. Parrish, "Reduction of T_2^* dephasing in gradient field-echo imaging," *Radiology,* vol. 170, 457-462, 1989.

150. E. M. Haacke and J. Frahm, "A guide to understanding key aspects of fast gradient-echo imaging," *J. Magn. Reson. Imag.,* vol. 1, pp. 621–624, 1991.

151. E. L. Hahn, "Spin echoes," *Phys. Rev.,* vol. 80, pp. 580–594, 1950.

152. E. L. Hahn, "Free nuclear induction," *Physics Today,* vol. 6, November, pp. 4–9, 1953.

153. J. M. Hanson, Z.-P. Liang, E. C. Wiener, and P. C. Lauterbur, "Fast dynamic imaging using two reference images," *Magn. Reson. Med,* vol. 36, pp. 172–175, 1996.

154. A. Hasse, J. Frahm, D. Mattaei, et al., "FLASH imaging: Rapid NMR imaging using low flip angle pulses," *J. Magn. Reson.,* vol. 67, pp. 388–397, 1989.

155. D. M. Healy and J. B. Weaver, "Tow applications of wavelet transforms in magnetic resonance imaging," *IEEE Trans. Info. Theory,* vol. 38, pp. 840–860, 1992.

156. J. Hennig, A. Naureth, and H. Friedburg, "RARE imaging: A fast imaging method for clinical MR," *Magn. Reson. Imag.,* vol. 3, pp. 823–833, 1986.

157. J. Hennig and M. Hodapp, "Burst imaging," *MAGMA,* vol. 1, pp. 39–48, 1998.

158. G. T. Herman, A. Lent, and S. W. Rowland, "ART: Mathematics and applications— A report on the mathematical foundations and on the applicability to real data of the algebraic reconstruction techniques," *J. Theor. Biol.,* vol. 42, pp. 1–32, 1973.

159. C. P. Hess, Z.-P. Liang, and P. C. Lauterbur, "Maximum cross-entropy generalized series reconstruction," *Int. J. Imag. Syst. Techn.*, vol. 10, pp. 258–265, 1999.

160. W. S. Hinshaw and A. H. Lent, "An introduction to NMR imaging: From the Bloch equation to the imaging equation," *Proc. IEEE*, vol. 71, pp. 338–350, 1983.

161. D. I. Hoult and R. E. Richards. "The signal-to-noise ratio of the nuclear magnetic resonance experiment," *J. Magn. Reson.*, vol. 24, pp. 71–85, 1979.

162. X. Hu, "On the 'keyhole' technqiue," *J. Magn. Reson. Imag.*, vol. 4, p. 231, 1994.

163. X. Hu, "Simpler locally focused tomography in MR imaging," *J. Magn. Reson. Imag.*, vol. 4, pp. 103–104, 1994.

164. X. Hu, D. N. Levin, P. C. Lauterbur, and T. A. Spraggins, "SLIM: Spectral localization by imaging," *Magn. Reson. Med.*, vol. 8, pp. 314–322, 1988.

165. J. Hua and G. C. Hurst, "Noise and artifact comparison for Fourier and polynomial phase correction used with Fourier reconstruction of asymmetric data sets," *J. Magn. Reson. Imag.*, vol. 2, pp. 347–353, 1992.

166. T. S. Huang, J. L. C. Sanz, H. Fan, J. Shafii, and B.-M. Tsai, "Numerical comparison of several algorithms for band-limited signal extrapolation," *Appl. Opt.*, vol. 23, pp. 307–317, 1984.

167. J. Jackson, A. Macovski, and D. Nishimura, "Low frequency restoration," *Magn. Reson. Med.*, vol. 11, pp. 248–257, 1989.

168. J. Jackson, C. Meyer, D. Nishimura, and A. Macovski, "Selection of a convolution function for Fourier inversion using gridding," *IEEE Trans. Med. Imag.*, vol. MI-10, pp. 473–478, 1991.

169. A. K. Jain and S. Ranganath, "Extrapolation algorithms for discrete signals with application in spectral estimation," *IEEE Trans. Acoust., Speech, Signal Process.*, vol. ASSP-29, pp. 830–845, 1981.

170. E. T. Jaynes, "Prior probabilities," *IEEE Trans. Syst. Sci. Cybern.*, vol. SSC-4, pp. 227–241, 1968.

171. R. A. Jones, O. Haraldseth, T. B. Muller, P. A. Rinck, and A. N. Oksendal, "K-space substitution: A novel dynamic imaging technique," *Magn. Reson. Med.*, vol. 29, pp. 830–834, 1993.

172. S. Kaczmarz, "Angenaherte auflosung von systemen linearer gleichungen," *Bull. Acad. Pol. Sci. Lett. A*, vol. 6-8A, pp. 355–357, 1937.

173. N. Kalouptsidis, G. Carrayaannis, and D. Manolakis, "Fast algorithms for block Toeplitz matrices with Toeplitz entries," *Signal Process.*, vol. 6, pp. 77–81, 1984.

174. A. K. Katsaggelos and S. M. Estratiadis, "A class of iterative signal restoration algorithms," *IEEE Trans. Acoust., Speech, Signal Process.*, vol. ASSP-38, pp. 778–786, 1990.

175. L. Kaufman and V. Pereyra, "A method for separable nonlinear least squares problems with separable nonlinear equality constraints," *SIAM J. Numer. Anal.*, vol. 15, pp. 12–20, 1978.

176. E. L. Kosarev, "Shannon's superresolution limit for signal recovery," *Inverse Problems*, vol. 6, pp. 55–76, 1990.

177. H. Krishna and S. D. Morgera, "The Levinson recurrence and fast algorithms for solving Toeplitz systems of linear equations," *IEEE Trans. Acoust., Speech, Signal Process.*, vol. ASSP-35, pp. 839–848, 1984.

178. A. Kumar, D. Welti, and R. Ernst, "NMR Fourier zeugmatography," *J. Magn. Reson.*, vol. 18, pp. 69–83, 1975.

179. R. Kumaresan and D. W. Tufts, "Estimating the parameters of exponentially damped sinusoid and pole-zero modeling in noise," *IEEE Trans. Acoust., Speech, Signal Process.*, vol. ASSP-30, pp. 217–220, 1982.

180. S. Y. Kung, K. S. Arun, and B. D. Rao, "State-space singular value decomposition based methods for the harmonic retrieval problem," *J. Opt. Soc. Am. A*, vol. 73, pp. 1799–1811, 1983.

181. V. Y. Kuperman, S. K. Nagle, and D. N. Levin, "Locally focused MR imaging of interventions," *J. Magn. Reson. Imag.*, vol. 8, pp. 1288–1295, 1998.

182. P. C. Lauterbur, "Image formation by induced local interactions: Examples employing nuclear magnetic resonance," *Nature*, vol. 242, pp. 190–191, 1973.

183. P. C. Lauterbur, D. N. Levin, and R. B. Marr, "Theory and simulation of NMR spectroscopic imaging and field plotting by projection reconstruction involving an intrinsic frequency dimension," *J. Magn. Reson.*, vol. 59, pp. 536–541, 1984.

184. J.-S. Lee, "Image smoothing and the sigma filter," *Comput. Vision, Graphics and Image Process.*, vol. 24, pp. 255–269, 1983.

185. A. Lent, "An iterative method for the extrapolation of band-limited functions," *J. Math. Anal. Appl.*, vol. 83, pp. 554–565, 1981.

186. Z.-P. Liang, E. M. Haacke, and C. W. Thomas, "High resolution spectral estimation through a localized polynomial approximation," *Inverse Problems*, vol. 5, pp. 831–847, 1989.

187. Z.-P. Liang and P. C. Lauterbur, "A generalized series approach to MR spectroscopic imaging," *IEEE Trans. Med. Imag.*, vol. MI-10, pp. 132–137, 1991.

188. Z.-P. Liang and P. C. Lauterbur, "A theoretical analysis of the SLIM technique," *J. Magn. Reson., B.*, vol. 102, pp. 54–60, 1993.

189. Z.-P. Liang and P. C. Lauterbur, "Efficient magnetic resonance imaging using a generalized series model," *IEEE Trans. Med. Imag.*, vol. 13, pp. 677–686, 1994.

190. Z.-P. Liang and P. C. Lauterbur, "Constrained imaging: Overcoming the limitations of the Fourier series," *IEEE EMB Magazine*, vol. 15, pp. 126–132, 1996.

191. Z.-P. Liang, "A model-based method for phase unwrapping," *IEEE Trans. Med. Imag.*, vol. 15, pp. 893–897, 1996.

192. Z.-P. Liang, H. Jiang, C. P. Hess, and P. C. Lauterbur, "Dynamic imaging by model estimation," *Int. J. Imag. Syst. Techn.*, vol. 8, pp. 551–557, 1997.

193. I. J. Lowe and R. E. Wysong, "DANTE ultra fast imaging sequence (DUFIS)," *J. Magn. Reson. Ser. B.*, vol. 101, pp. 106–109, 1993.

194. R. B. Lufkin, E. Pusey, D. D. Stark, R. Brown, B. Leikind, and W. N. Hanafee, "Boundary artifact due to truncation errors in MR imaging," *Am. J. Roentgenocology*, vol. 147, pp. 1283–1287, 1986.

195. A. Macovski, "Noise in MRI," *Magn. Reson. Med.*, vol. 36, pp. 494–497, 1996.

196. F. Maes, A. Collignon, G. Marchal, and P. Suetens, "Multimodality image registration by maximization of mutual in formation," *IEEE Trans. Med. Imag.*, vol. 16, pp. 187–198, 1997.

197. P. Mansfield, "Multi-planar image formation using NMR spin echoes," *J. Phys. C: Solid State Phys.*, vol. 10, pp. L55–L58, 1977.

198. P. Margosian, F. Schmitt, and D. E. Purdy, "Faster MR imaging: Imaging with half the data," *Health Care Instrum.*, vol. 1, pp. 195–197, 1986.

199. J. F. Martin and C. F. Tirendi, "Modified linear prediction modeling in magnetic resonance imaging, *J. Magn. Reson.*, vol. 82, pp. 392–399, 1989.

200. S. Matej and I. Bajla, "A high-speed reconstruction from projections using direct Fourier method with optimized parameters—an experimental analysis," *IEEE Trans. Med. Imag.*, vol. 9, pp. 421–429, 1990.

201. A. A. Maudsley, G. B. Matson, J. W. Hugg, and M. W. Weiner, "Reduced phase encoding in spectroscopic imaging," *Magn. Reson. Med.*, vol. 31, pp. 645–651, 1994.

202. S. R. McFall, N. J. Pelc, and R. M. Vaurek, "Correction of spatially dependent phase shifts for partial Fourier Imaging," *Magn. Reson. Imag.*, vol. 6, pp. 143–155, 1988.

203. S. Meiboom and D. Gill, "Modified spin-echo method for measuring nuclear relaxation times," *Rev. Sci. Instrum.*, vol. 29, pp. 668–691, 1958.

204. C. H. Meyer, B. S. Hu, D. G. Nishimura, and A. Macovski, "Fast spiral coronary artery imaging," *Magn. Reson. Med*, vol. 28, pp. 202–213, 1992.

205. A. Mohammad-Djafari and G. Demoment, "Maximum entropy image reconstruction in X-ray and Diffraction tomography," *IEEE Trans. Med. Imag.*, vol. 7, pp. 345–354, 1988.

206. P. R. Moran, "Observations on maximum entropy processing of MR imaging," *Magn. Reson. Imag.*, vol. 9, pp. 213–222, 1991.

207. G. A. Morris and R. Freeman, "Selective excitation in Fourier transform nuclear magnetic resonance," *J. Magn. Reson.*, vol. 29, pp. 433–462, 1978.

208. J. P. Mugler III, "Potential degradation in image quality due to selective averaging of phase-encoding line in Fourier transform MRI," *Magn. Reson. Med.*, vol. 19, pp. 170–174, 1991.

209. J. P. Mugler III and J. R. Brookeman, "Evaluation of a simple method for reconstructing asymmetrically sampled echo data," *J. Magn. Res. Imag.*, vol. 1, pp. 487–491, 1991.

210. S. K. Nagle and D. N. Levin, "Multiple Region MRI," *Magn. Reson. Med.*, vol. 41, pp. 774–786, 1999.

211. D. C. Noll, D. G. Nishimura, and A. Macovski, "Homodyne detection in magnetic resonance imaging," *IEEE Trans. Med. Imag.*, vol. MI-10, pp. 154–163, 1991.

212. J. O'Sullivan, "A fast sinc function gridding algorithm for Fourier inversion in computer tomography," *IEEE Trans. Med. Imag.*, vol. MI-4, pp. 200–207, 1985.

213. L. P. Panych, P. D. Jakab, and F. A. Jolesz, "An implementation of wavelet encoded MRI," *J. Magn. Reson. Imag.*, vol. 3, pp. 649–655, 1993.

214. L. P. Panych and F. A. Jolesz, "A dynamically adaptive imaging algorithm for wavelet encoded MRI," *Magn. Reson. Med.*, vol. 32, pp. 738–748, 1994.

215. L. P. Panych, C. Oesterle, G. P. Zientara, and J. Hennig, "Implementation of fast gradient-echo SVD encoding technique for dynamic imaging," *Magn. Reson. Med.*, vol. 35, pp. 554–562, 1995.

216. L. P. Panych, "Theoretical comparison of Foruier and wavelet encoding in magnetic resonance imaging," *IEEE Trans. Med. Imag.*, vol. 15, pp. 141–153, 1996.

217. A. Papoulis and M. S. Bertran, "Digital filtering and prolate functions," *IEEE Trans. Circuit Theory*, vol. CT-19, pp. 674–681, 1972.

218. A. Papoulis, "A new algorithm in spectral analysis and band-limited extrapolation," *IEEE Trans. Circuits Syst.*, vol. CAS-22, pp. 735–742, 1975.

219. D. L. Parker, G. T. Gullberg, and P. R. Frederick, "Gibbs artifact removal in magnetic resonance imaging," *Med. Phys.*, vol. 14, pp. 640–645, 1987.

220. D. L. Parker and G. T. Gullberg, "Signal-to-noise efficiency in magnetic resonance imaging," *Med. Phys.*, vol. 17, pp. 250–257, 1990.

221. T. Parrish and X. Hu, "Continuous update with random encoding (CURE): A new strategy for dynamic imaging," *Magn. Reson. Med.*, vol. 33, pp. 326–336, 1995.

222. J. Pauly, D. Nishimura, and A. Macovski, "A k-space analysis of small-tip-angle excitation," *J. Magn. Reson.*, voil. 81, 43-56, 1989.

223. J. Pauly, P. Le Roux, D. Nishimura, and A. Macovski, "Parameter relations for the Shinnar-Le Roux selective excitation pulse design algorithm," *IEEE Trans. Med. Imag.*, Vol. 10, pp. 53–65, 1991.

224. R. D. Peters and M. L. Wood, "Multilevel wavelet-transform encoding in MRI," *J. Magn. Reson. Imag.*, vol. 6, pp. 529–540, 1996.

225. S. K. Plevritis and A. Macovski, "Spectral extrapolation of spatially bounded images," *IEEE Trans. Med. Imag.*, vol. MI-14, pp. 487–497, 1995.

226. D. B. Plewes, J. Bishop, I. Soutar, and E. Cohen, "Errors in quantitative dynamic three-dimensional Keyhole MR imaging of the breast," *J. Magn. Reson. Imag.*, vol. 5, pp. 361–364, 1995.

227. I. L. Pykett and R. R. Rzedzian, "Instant images of the body by magnetic resonance," *Magn. Reson. Med.*, vol. 5, pp. 563–571, 1987.

228. M. A. Rahman and K. B. Yu, "Total least squares approach for frequency estimation using linear prediction," *IEEE Trans. Acoust., Speech, Signal Process.*, vol. ASSP-35, pp. 1440–1454, 1987.

229. R. Rangayyan, A. P. Dhawan, and R. Gordon, "Algorithm for limited-view computed tomography: An annotated bibliography and a challenge," *Appl. Opt.*, vol. 24, pp. 4000–4012, 1985.

230. V. Rasche, R. Proksa, R. Sinkus, P. Börnert, and H. Eggers, "Resampling of data between arbitrary grids using convolution interpolation," *IEEE Trans. Med. Imag.*, vol. 18, pp. 385–392, 1999.

231. P. A. Rattey and A. G. Lindgren, "Sampling the 2-D Radon Transform," *IEEE Trans. Acoust. Speech, Signal Process.*, vol. ASSP-29, pp. 994–1002, 1994.

232. S. J. Riederer, "Recent advances in magnetic resonance imaging," *Proc. IEEE*, vol. 76, pp. 1095–1105, 1988.

233. D. J. Rossi and A. S. Willsky, "Reconstruction from projections based on detection and estimation of objects—Part I and II: Performance analysis and robustness analysis," *IEEE Trans. Acoust., Speech, Signal Process.*, vol. ASSP-32, pp. 886–906, 1984.

234. V. M. Runge and M. L. Wood, "Half-Fourier MR imaging of CNS disease," *Am. J. Neuroradiol.*, vol. 11, pp. 77–82, 1990.

235. C. K. Rushforth, "Restoration, resolution, and noise," *J. Opt. Soc. Am. A*, vol. 58, pp. 539–545, 1968.

236. J. L. C. Sanz and T. S. Huang, "Discrete and continuous band-limited signal extrapolation," *IEEE Trans. Acoust., Speech, Signal Process.*, vol. ASSP-31, pp. 1276–1285, 1983.

237. J. L. C. Sanz and T. S. Huang, "Unified Hilbert space approach to iterative least-squares linear signal restoration," *J. Opt. Soc. Am. A*, vol. 73, pp. 1455–1465, 1983.

238. J. L. C. Sanz and T. S. Huang, "Some aspects of band-limited signal extrapolation: Models, discrete approximations, and noise," *IEEE Trans. Acoust., Speech, Signal Process.*, vol. ASSP-31, pp. 1492–1501, 1983.

239. T. K. Sarkar, D. D. Weiner, and V. K. Jain, "Some mathematical considerations in dealing with the inverse problem," *IEEE Trans. Antennas Propag.*, vol. AP-29, pp. 373–379, 1981.

240. R. W. Schafer, R. M. Mersereau, and M. A. Richards, "Constrained iterative restoration algorithms," *Proc. IEEE*, vol. 69, pp. 432–450, 1981.

241. M. I. Sezan and H. Stark, "Image restoration by the method of convex projection: Part 2—Applications and numerical results," *IEEE Trans. Med. Imag.*, vol. MI-1, pp. 95–101, 1982.

242. M. I. Sezan and H. Stark, "Tomographic image reconstruction from incomplete view data by convex projections and direct Fourier inversion," *IEEE Trans. Med. Imag.*, vol. MI-3, pp. 91–98, 1984.

243. J. E. Shore and R. W. Johnson, "Axiomatic derivation of the principle of maximum entropy and the principle of minimum cross-entropy," *IEEE Trans. Inf. Theory*, vol. IT-26, pp. 26–37, 1980.

244. D. Slepian and H. O. Pollack, "Prolate spheroidal wavefunctions, Fourier analysis, and uncertainty," *Bell Syst. Tech. J.*, vol. 40, pp. 43–60, 1961.

245. D. Slepian, "On bandwidth," *Proc. IEEE*, vol. 64, pp. 292–300, 1976.

246. M. R. Smith, S. T. Nichols, R. M. Henkelman, and M. L. Wood, "Application of auto-regressive moving average parametric modeling in magnetic resonance image

reconstruction," *IEEE Trans. Med. Imag.*, vol. MI-5, pp. 132–139, 1986.

247. S. P. Souza, J. Szumowski, C. L. Dumoulin, D. P. Plewes, and G. Glover, "SIMA: Simultaneous multislice acquisition of MR images by Hadamard-encoded excitation," *J. Comp. Assist. Tomogr.*, vol. 12, pp. 1026–1030, 1988.

248. T. A. Spraggins, "Simulation of spatial and contrast distortions in keyhole imaging," *Magn. Reson. Med.*, vol. 31, pp. 320–322, 1994.

249. H. Stark, "Sampling theorems in polar coordinates," *J. Opt. Soc. Am.*, vol. 69, pp. 1519–1525, 1979.

250. H. Stark, J. W. Woods, I. Paul, and R. Hingorani, "Direct Fourier reconstruction in computer tomography," *IEEE Trans. Acoust., Speech, Signal Process.*, vol. ASSP-29, pp. 237–245, 1981.

251. H. Stark, J. W. Woods, I. Paul, and R. Hingorani, "An investigation of computerized tomography by direct Fourier inversion and optimum interpolation," *IEEE Trans. Biomed. Eng.*, vol. BME-29, pp. 496–505, 1981.

252. H. Stark and M. Wengrovitz, "Comments and corrections on the use of polar sampling theorems in CT," *IEEE Trans. Acoust., Speech, Signal Process.*, vol. ASSP-31, pp. 1329–1331, 1983.

253. A. E. Stillman, D. N. Levin, D. B. Yang, R. B. Marr, and P. C. Lauterbur, "Back projection reconstruction of spectroscopic NMR images from incomplete sets of projections," *J. Magn. Reson.*, vol. 69, pp. 168–175, 1986.

254. K. Tanabe, "Projection method for solving a singular system," *Numer. Math.*, vol. 17,, pp. 203–214, 1971.

255. V. T. Tom, T. F. Quatieri, M. H. Hayes, and J. H. McClellan, "Convergence of iterative nonexpansive signal reconstruction algorithms," *IEEE Trans. Acoust., Speech, Signal Process.*, vol. ASSP-29, pp. 1052–1058, 1981.

256. H. C. Torrey, "Bloch equations with diffusion terms," *Phys. Rev.*, vol. 140, pp. 563–565, 1956.

257. H. J. Trussell and M. R. Civanlar, "The feasible solution in signal restoration," *IEEE Trans. Acoust., Speech, Signal Process.*, vol. ASSP-32, pp. 201–212, 1984.

258. D. A. Turner, M. I. Rapoport, W. D. Erwin, M. McGould, and R. I. Silvers, "Truncation artifact: A potential pitfall in MR imaging of the menisci of the knee," *Radiology*, vol. 179, pp. 629–633, 1991.

259. D. B. Twieg, "The k-trajectory formulation of the NMR imaging process with applications in analysis and synthesis of imaging methods," *Med. Phys.* vol. 10, pp. 610–621, 1983.

260. J. J. van Vaals, M. E. Brummer, W. T. Dixon, H. H. Tuithof, H. Engels, R. C. Nelson, B. M. Gerety, J. L. Chezmar, and J. A. den Boer, "'Keyhole' method for accelerating imaging of contrast agent uptake," *J. Magn. Reson. Imag.*, vol. 3, pp. 671–675, 1993.

261. M. von Kienlin and R. Mejia, "Spectral localization with optimal point spread function," *J. Magn. Reson.*, vol. 94, pp. 268–287, 1991.

262. M. Wax and T. Kailath, "Efficient inversion of Toeplitz-block Toeplitz matrix," *IEEE Trans. Acoust., Speech, Signal Process.*, vol. ASSP-31, pp. 1218–1221, 1983.

263. M. Wax and T. Kailath, "Detection of Signals by Information Theoretic Criteria," *IEEE Trans. Acoust., Speech, Signal Process.*, vol. ASSP-33, pp. 387–392, 1985.

264. J. B. Weaver, Y. Xu, D. M. Healy, and L. D. Cromwell, "Filtering noise images with the wavelet transform," *Magn. Reson. Med.*, vol. 21, pp. 288–295, 1991.

265. J. B. Weaver, Y. Xu, D. M. Healy, and J. R. Driscoll, "Wavelet-encoded MR imaging," *Magn. Reson. Med.*, vol. 24, pp. 275–287, 1992.

266. W. M. Wells III, P. Viola, H. Atsumi, S. Nakajima, and R. Kikinis, "Multi-modal volume registration by maximization of mutual information," *Med. Image Analysis*, vol. 1, pp. 35–51, 1996.

267. S. J. Wernecke and L. R. D'Addario, "Maximum entropy image reconstruction," *IEEE Trans. Comput.*, vol. C26, pp. 351–364, 1977.

268. D. E. Woessner, "Effects of diffusion in nuclear magnetic resonance spin-echo experiments," *J. Chem. Phys.*, vol. 34, pp. 2057–2061, 1961.

269. M. L. Wood and R. M. Henkelman, "MR image artifacts from periodic motion," *Med. Phys.*, vol. 12, pp. 143–151, 1985.

270. M. L. Wood and R. M. Henkelman, "Truncation artifacts in magnetic resonance imaging," *Magn. Reson. Med.*, vol. 2, pp. 517–526, 1985.

271. Q.-S. Xiang and R. M. Henkelman, "Motion artifact reduction with three-point ghost phase cancellation," *J. Magn. Reson.*, vol. 1, pp. 633–642, 1991.

272. Q.-S. Xiang and R. M. Henkelman, "Dynamic image reconstruction: MR movies from motion ghosts," *J. Magn. Reson. Imag.*, vol. 2, pp. 679–685, 1992.

273. Q.-S. Xiang and R. M. Henkelman, "K-space description for MR imaging of dynamic objects," *Magn. Reson. Med.*, vol. 29, pp. 422–428, 1993.

274. Q. S. Xiang, M.J. Bronskill, and R.M. Henkelman, "Two-point interference method for suppression of ghost artifact due to motion," *J. Magn. Reson. Imag.*, vol. 5, pp. 529–534, 1995.

275. H. Yan and J. C. Gore, "An efficient algorithm for MR image reconstruction without low spatial frequencies," *IEEE Trans. Med. Imag.*, vol. MI-9, pp. 184–189, 1990.

276. H. Yan and J. C. Gore, "The relation of HSVD to LPSVD for fitting time domain signals," *J. Magn. Reson.*, vol. 80, pp. 324–327, 1988.

277. H. Yan and J. Mao, "The relation of low frequency restoration methods to the Gerchberg-Papoulis algorithm," *Magn. Reson. Med.*, vol. 16, pp. 166–172, 1990.

278. H. Yan and M. Braun, "Image reconstruction from Fourier domain data sampled along a zig-zag trajectory," *Magn. Reson. Med.*, vol. 18, 405-410, 1991.

279. L. Yao, Y. Cao, and D. N. Levin, "2D locally focused MRI: Applications to dynamic and spectroscopic imaging," *Magn. Reson. Med.*, vol. 36, pp. 834–846, 1996.

280. D. C. Youla, "Generalized image restoration by the method of alternating orthogonal projections," *IEEE Trans. Circuits Syst.*, vol. CAS-25, pp. 694–702, 1978.

281. D. C. Youla and H. Webb, "Image restoration by the method of convex projections: Part I -Theory," *IEEE Trans. Med. Imag.*, vol. MI-1, pp. 81–94, 1982.

282. L. Zha and I. J. Lowe, "Optimized ultra-fast imaging sequence (OUFIS)," *Magn. Reson. Med.*, vol. 33, pp. 377–395, 1995.

283. L. C. Zhao, P. R. Krishnaiah, and Z. D. Bai, "On detection of the number of signals in presence of white noise," *J. Multivariate Anal.*, vol. 20, 1-25, 1986.

284. L. C. Zhao, P. R. Krishnaiah, and Z.-D. Bai, "Remarks on certain criteria for detection of number of signals," *IEEE Trans. Acoust., Speech, Signal Processing*, vol. ASSP-35, 129-132, 1987.

285. X. Zhou, Z.-P. Liang, G. P. Cofer, C. F. Beaulieu, S. A. Suddarth, and G. A. Johnson, "Reduction of ringing and blurring artifacts in fast spin-echo imaging," *J. Magn. Reson. Imag.*, vol. 3, pp. 803–807, 1993.

286. X. Zhuang, R. B. Harolick, and Y. Zhao, "Maximum entropy image reconstruction," *IEEE Trans. Acoust., Speech, Signal Process.*, vol. ASSP-39, 1478-1480, 1991.

287. G. P. Zientara, L. P. Panych, and F. A. Jolesz, "Dynamically adaptive MRI with encoding by singular value decomposition," *Magn. Reson. Med.*, vol. 32, pp. 268–274, 1994.

Index

About the Authors

Zhi-Pei Liang received the B.S. degree in electric engineering from South China University of Technology in 1982 and the Ph.D. degree in biomedical engineering from Case Western Reserve University in 1989. From 1989 to 1991, he was a postdoctoral fellow in the National Center for Supercomputing Applications at the University of Illinois at Urbana-Champaign (UIUC). He subsequently worked as a research assistant professor in the UIUC Biomedical Magnetic Resonance Laboratory from 1991 to 1993. Dr. Liang joined the faculty of the UIUC Department of Electrical and Computer Engineering (ECE) in 1993, and is currently an associate professor in the ECE Department, the Beckman Institute for Advanced Science and Technology, the Coordinated Science Laboratory, the Biophysics Program, and the Bioengineering Program at UIUC.

Dr. Liang's research interests include magnetic resonance imaging, superresolution image reconstruction using a priori constraints, statistical and scale-space approaches to image segmentation and analysis, bioinformatics, and computational intelligence. He is a member of the International Society of Magnetic Resonance in Medicine and a senior member of the IEEE. He organized and chaired a special session on magnetic resonance imaging for the IEEE First International Conference on Image Processing in 1994, and organized the First Workshop on MR Signal Processing in 1996. He was a member of the Program Committee of the 1996 IEEE Workshop on Mathematical Methods in Biomedical Image Analysis, a member of the Organizing Committee of the 1998 IEEE International Conference on Image Processing, and a charter member of the MR Engineering Group of the International Society of Magnetic Resonance in Medicine. He has been serving as an associate editor of the *IEEE Transactions on Medical Imaging* since 1995, and was the guest editor of a special issue on MR Signal Processing for the *International Journal of Imaging Systems and Technology* in 1997.

Dr. Liang is a recipient of the Sylvia Sorkin Greenfield Best Paper Award of the *Medical Physics Journal* (1990) and the National Science Foundation Career Award (1995). He was named a Beckman Fellow of the UIUC Center for Advanced Study in 1997 and was appointed as a Henry Magnuski Scholar for Outstanding Young Faculty Member in the ECE Department in 1999.

Paul C. Lauterbur, a native of Sidney, Ohio, received the B.S. degree in chemistry (1951) from Case Institute of Technology, Cleveland, Ohio, and the Ph.D. degree in chemistry (1962) from the University of Pittsburgh, Pennsylvania. From 1951 to 1963, with the exception of a two-year period of military service, he was affiliated with the Mellon Institute, Pittsburgh. In 1954 during his service in the army, Dr. Lauterbur helped to set up a nuclear magnetic resonance (NMR) laboratory and began research on NMR spectroscopy and the development of its analytical applications, work that resulted in several publications. When he returned to the Mellon Institute in 1955, he collaborated on the first investigation of ^{29}Si NMR spectra, and set up his own NMR laboratory. The initial publication from that laboratory was the first description of ^{13}C NMR spectroscopy. A series of papers followed that established the foundations of ^{13}C NMR spectroscopy. In 1963 he moved to the State University of New York at Stony Brook. There he again set up a new laboratory and measured the first hydrogen and lead shielding tensors in single crystals, intramolecular and solvent isotope effects on chemical shifts, and the first ^{13}C NMR spectra of proteins in 1970.

In 1971 Dr. Lauterbur realized that NMR signals could be used to make a new kind of image. After independently devising an image reconstruction technique, he published the first NMR images in 1973. That work was followed by a series of papers establishing the foundations of many techniques and applications now in use. He collaborated on a fundamental analysis of the sensitivity of MR imaging, developed a number of new techniques and mathematical algorithms for NMR imaging, and carried out the first in-depth study and implementation of NMR microscopy.

In 1985 Dr. Lauterbur joined the faculty of the University of Illinois and established the Biomedical Magnetic Resonance Laboratory (BMRL) on the Urbana-Champaign campus. He holds appointments in the College of Medicine, the Department of Chemistry, the Center for Biophysics and Computational Biology, the Neuroscience and Bioengineering Programs, and the Beckman Institute. He is a professor in the Center for Advanced Study, and Head of the Department of Medical Information Sciences, College of Medicine at Urbana-Champaign.

Dr. Lauterbur continues to work on the development of new imaging methods and image processing techniques. A project begun by his group during 1995 has made it possible to control MRI systems over the World Wide Web from any computer with widespread potential applications in education and scientific collaborations. Dr. Lauterbur's work in these and other MRI-related areas continues, with the aid of graduate and undergraduate students from programs in chemistry, physics, biophysics, physiology, bioengineering, and electrical and computer engineering. Among his numerous awards are the 1987 National Medal of Science, 1990 Bower Award and Prize for Achievement in Science, and 1994 Kyoto Prize for Advanced Technology. Dr. Lauterbur is a member of the National Academy of Sciences.